AF779617

VISUAL ANALYSIS

LEO MANAS, M.A., O.D.

Editors
Robert A. Hohendorf, OD
Joseph Sullivan, OD
Wayne Yorkgitis, OD
Paul Harris, OD

Fourth Edition

OPTOMETRIC EXTENSION PROGRAM FOUNDATION

Copyright © 2009 OEP Foundation, Inc.
The OEP Foundation, founded in 1928, is an international non-profit organization dedicated to continuing education and research for the advancement of human progress through education in behavioral vision care.

OEP Foundation, Inc.
1921 E. Carnegie Ave., Suite 3-L
Santa Ana, CA 92705
www.oep.org

Managing editor: Sally Marshall Corngold
Cover design: Kathleen Patterson

Library of Congress Cataloging-in-Publication Data
Manas, Leo, 1910-1989.
Visual analysis / Leo Manas. -- 4th ed. / editors, Robert A. Hohendorf ... [et al.].
p. ; cm.
Includes bibliographical references and index.
ISBN 978-0-929780-19-1 (alk. paper)
1. Optometry. 2. Eye--Accommodation and refraction. I. Hohendorf, Robert A. II. Optometric Extension Program Foundation. III. Title.
[DNLM: 1. Vision Disorders--diagnosis. 2. Vision Tests--methods. 3. Vision, Ocular. 4. Visual Perception. WW 141 M241v 2009]
RE925.M275 2009
617.7'5--dc22

2009021225

****

Optometry is the health care profession specifically licensed by state law to prescribe lenses, optical devices and procedures to improve human vision. Optometry has advanced vision therapy as a unique treatment modality for the development and remediation of the visual process. Effective vision therapy requires extensive understanding of:

- the effects of lenses (including prisms, filters and occluders)
- the variety of responses to the changes produced by lenses
- the various physiological aspects of the visual process
- the pervasive nature of the visual process in human behavior

As a consequence, effective vision therapy requires the supervision, direction and active involvement of the optometrist.

****

TABLE OF CONTENTS

Dedication

These efforts of mine in clarifying and extending the basic concepts of functional optometry would have been impossible without the constant inspiration received from one man. This gentleman and scholar devoted his life to bringing post-graduate education to our profession. It is with humility, that I dedicate these efforts to that man--Dr. A.M. Skeffington.

Leo Manas, O.D.

FOREWORD

When a book so long out of print and largely out of sight is to be republished, it is fitting that we look at the reasons for doing so and to acknowledge the efforts of our editors who spent many hours making certain the material and principles in the book remained accessible to the modern reader.

First let us acknowledge the hours of effort that our principle editors put in. When editing a book, it must be read multiple times, shared, and discussed before it can be brought to print. What may be only a few hours reading is the product of days of work. Our editors not only read the book, but consulted class notes and shared personal experiences with Dr. Manas to assure that this new fourth edition remains true to the teaching of Dr. Manas and reasonably reflects his philosophy and intent.

Thank you to Wayne Yorkgitis, Joe Sullivan, Bob Hohendorf, and Paul Harris for their exhaustive efforts to bring this edition to us. A special thank you to Sally Corngold and Koe Johnson who took what the editors gave them and produced this fourth edition in an attractive and easily useable form.

Last we should remember that it was the life's work of Leo Manas that made this work possible.

Dr. Leo Manas received his OD degree from the Illinois College of Optometry in 1946 after earning BS and MA degrees from the University of Cincinnati. He was in private practice in Chicago, IL and served on the Illinois College of Optometry faculty for many years. He taught binocular vision and vision therapy before retiring in 1975. He was an OEP Associate for more than 50 years. He donated the copyright of Visual Analysis to the OEP Foundation prior to his death.

In chapter one, Dr. Manas provides a rationale, supported by science, for a more sophisticated form of case analysis than was in common use at that time. He explains that "Optometrists originally supplied glasses as a means of restoring acuity, depending merely on the distance subjective to tell when to supply glasses." Dr. Manas makes a carefully reasoned case for the understanding that the visual process is pervasive in human life and that appropriate visual care for the human being involves more than care for the eye and closely associated structures.

In the second chapter, Dr. Manas explains that "...vision is not an isolated function of the human organism, but it is a complex function of many action systems of the body." He proceeds in that context to explain the roles and interaction of accommodation and convergence that produce and preserve the ability of the person to successfully direct his behavior to a constructive conclusion.

Following, in Chapter 3, he describes the developing visual problem in terms of the person's response to stress within the environment, "...the organism tends to retreat or narrow the visual environment that it can function effectively." He expands from there to explain the optometrist's role in assessing human visual behavior and to introduce the analytical examination that is central to optometric visual evaluation.

The fourth chapter contains an exhaustive description of the case history and explains its importance to the ultimate success of optometric health care including the visual process. Dr. Manas explains the importance of an interactive case history set in the context of the patient's life. He explains the importance of understanding a child in the context of visual development. This leads to the optometrist providing visual solutions that fit comfortably and efficiently into the patient's life.

In chapter five Dr. Manas provides a logical, straightforward and well reasoned approach to evaluating what he calls visual skills. Others have called this chair testing. These are aspects of the visual assessment performed without a phoropter, or the equivalent. In addition to an extremely thorough methodology, Dr. Manas points out the principles underlying the assessment of overall visual skill. "It is extremely difficult to isolate a single simple visual skill out of a complex visual act." "A visual skills profile informs us what the patient has done about his visual problem, [it] tells us what adaptations have been made... in order to maintain survival in his visual environment."

Chapter six is a how-to guide for what has often been called the 21 point visual examination. This examination battery has long been the standard for full scope optometric care. The first two points are an assessment of the health and structure of the eye as it was done at that time. About 10% of the examination is dedicated to physical health and structure. Now, with improved instrumentation and more in depth health education, we, as optometrists, can do more in the same or even less time than it took when this work was first published. The remaining parts of the analytical are devoted a dynamic assessment of visual function. About 40% of the evaluation is dedicated to the assessment of visual function at distance. Fully half of the evaluation is dedicated to assessing dynamic visual function at the near test distance.

Chapter seven explains the significance of the 21 point analytical sequence. I can do no better than to quote Dr. Manas who said, "In the beginning, when our concept of a visual problem was merely acuity, it was sufficient to consider only the magnitude of a visual test. As our concept of... a visual problem broadened to include visual performance and visual achievement, it became evident that the magnitude of a test value was not sufficient identification for a visual problem." Dr. Manas provides a reasoned explanation for not only the use of each particular component of the analytical examination, but also explains the significance of the interrelationships between various findings in preparation for an introduction of the mechanics of case analysis covered in chapters eight and nine.

Chapters eight and nine include a traditional form of case analysis often called check, chaining and typing. Originally this form of analysis was designed to provide a reliable mechanism for applying the information gained in the analytical evaluation. It does not require an in depth knowledge of the visual process beyond the ability to perform the steps of the analytical evaluation, but Dr. Manas provides the reason behind the ritual and helps us understand how such an approach provides reliable access for those who do not yet have an understanding of the importance of visual function at near.

In chapter ten, Dr. Manas describes the behavioral factors and measures observed in the development of myopia including evidence on the incidence and development of myopia by age and environment. His conclusions are in accord with current physiological evidence in primate studies and are in good accord with more recent study of the physiological means by which the changes take place.

Chapter Eleven is titled Esophoria. Dr. Manas explains the appearance of esophoria as a personal response to stress. The causes range from a systemic response to environmental toxicity to a protective response that enables the person to continue to perform in the face of increasing demand. Dr. Manas closes the chapter with case based illustrations of the factors influencing successful nearpoint prescribing.

Chapter 12 includes a glossary of terms relevant to the behavioral philosophy of optometry. Of special significance are answers to over 60 questions that are often asked about the "21 point" examination and behavioral analysis.

This volume is published in honor of Dr. Leo Manas in order to showcase his teachings on how to prescribe and provide behavioral vision care.

Robin Lewis, O.D.
OEP Foundation

EDITORS' NOTES

In several places in this manuscript the author makes brief mention of the use of a small amount of base in prism, particularly in cases of esophoria. In chapter 11 he states, "*The esophoric traces (memory traces in the central nervous system) do not erase this easily, and we may find if careful visual supervision is not followed that we will have a gradual return to the esophoric condition through the prescribed plus spheres. If the patient is not willing to perform the home visual training chores, it is advisable to include in your prescription at least one diopter of base-in prism.*"

The editors agree that if asked now, that the author would say that the small amount of base in prism is a training or treatment lens that would be used on a temporary basis and that the patient should be evaluated in a short period of time to see if the desired change had occurred. At that point, once the "memory traces" of the esophoria had been altered, then the patient would benefit from the removal of the prism. One of the editors who spent time in the clinic with Dr. Manas states that he frequently saw prescriptions written by Dr. Manas of +0.50 spheres in both eyes with an interpupillary (PD) distance of 50 mm, which for most adults would result in a very small amount of base in prism depending on their PD. It would have been nice to find more original text on this topic. Unfortunately, we do not have this benefit.

The following are class notes taken during lectures by Dr. Manas: Under the topic of lens application for esophores he gave a general rule for hyperopia: *Under prescribe in plus and decenter for a base in effect.* The notes continue: *The reason for this seems to lie in the fact that you train an esophore with base in and minus. These then act as initial training aids. Also it has been found, clinically, that by prescribing plus to an esophore, we set up a vicious cycle in which he becomes more hyperopic and esophoric. This is due to the difference between the initial effect of plus and the long term effect of plus. For example: when you prescribe plus to reduce the eso he will go into less eso initially (due to accommodation/convergence hookup) but since his visual pattern is still basically the same, the forgetting curve is very steep and he will drift back to his prior level or lower. When he comes back to you, you may give him more plus again, with the same thing occurring, thus setting up an unwanted cycle which embeds the esophoria.*

It should be noted that the references herein are taken exactly from the original text and are not in a format commonly used in today's optometric literature.

Robert A. Hohendorf, O.D.
Joseph Sullivan, O.D.
Wayne Yorkgitis, O.D.
Paul Harris, O.D.

CHAPTER I
Vision and the Eye

There are many different ways in which clinical data can be analyzed. At this time we are interested in the functional method or nearpoint method of analysis. The functional method of analysis was developed over 25 years ago by a group of practicing optometrists in the Midwest. Up to now, tradition stated that the lens or lenses which restored the patient to emmetropia was the correct prescription, presuming absence of presbyopia. The practicing optometrist found that many of his hyperopic patients were more comfortable if he "cut" the correction, rather than if he prescribed the full plus of the subjective test. The search for an explanation led eventually into the psychological and developmental literature.

The physiological and anatomical literature was barren. Exploration, however, of the psychological and developmental fields and their application to optometry has given optometry great impetus in the past 25 years.

There is no question that any method of analysis of visual data will arrive at the same answer for 40% of the cases seeking optometric services, i.e., prescribing the subjective refraction. In fact, this 40% could refract themselves at the bargain counter. They do not present the real problem. Even the ability to prescribe for the remaining 60% who seek optometric services, and who need modified subjective refraction prescriptions, is not the serious problem of today.

The optometric horizon of today is rapidly being expanded in two directions: first, toward the field of preventive optometry; and second, the field of visual enhancement. The advancement of optometry into the field of prevention means that optometrists are no longer satisfied in prescribing lenses as a prosthetic device, but consider them a means of maintaining the visual efficiency of the patient in spite of the impact of school or industry. Optometry can perform its greatest service in the field of visual enhancement. We optometrists possess the key to increased visual efficiency for these patients so that they can perform their jobs easily, quickly and accurately.

In the foreword of the handbook published by the Minnesota State Board of Optometry, it is stated:

> *Optometry is founded upon an old science that has been developed and expanded and later professionalized by law and education.*

Modern optometry stresses the fact that the profession is dealing with the visual act and not altogether with the eyeball: that it bears a relation to neurology, physiology and psychology, as well as optics, and that the recognition of these facts places optometry in the sciences and arts dealing with human efficiency and well-being.

Modern optometry is based on the realization that vision is a psycho-physiological correlation, and that such psycho-physiological interpretation is more important than mere mechanical optics. Optometry is concerned with the proper adaptation of a visual mechanism to the nearpoint task to which mankind, as yet, has not been able to properly adjust itself.

In 1941, Dr. E. B. Alexander wrote as follows regarding the functional philosophy:

This school accepts the eyeball as the receptor of visual stimuli but postulates an interpretative quality in the brain and bases its work not so much on the difficulty of interpreting faulty retinal images, but on the concept that most visual problems are at the nearpoint; and that this problem is further complicated by the fact that two nervous systems are involved in seeing; that these two nervous systems are forced in the accommodative-convergence act to work simultaneously and in harmony with each other. In reaching an unaided balance, these two nervous systems make compromises, concessions and other mutual inter-relations under the compulsion of the use to which the seeing sense is put.

These compromises and concessions may be (or may not be) satisfactory from the point of view of the internal organism, but they are usually totally unsatisfactory when the organism is required to adapt itself to the requirements and responsibilities of modern economic life. The old idea was a correction of refractive errors-the new is to provide an environment in which the individual can re-adapt himself to his life necessities. This is not a difference in words; it is a difference in attitudes . . . It is also the difference between an optometrist and a refractionist.

1. The Modern Approach to Science

In every branch of science revolutionary changes have occurred. These changes all reveal the same pattern, all repudiate the old mechanistic conceptions based upon absolutistic philosophies. In the physical sciences, these changes are based upon the principle of relativity. In the biological sciences, these changes are based upon the concept that the whole organism is more than the sum total of its isolated parts. In psychology, they are based upon the concept of Gestalt. In the field of optometry, they are based upon the concept that vision is a function that involves the whole organism. Eyes cannot be studied in isolation from the rest of the human body.

During the 44th Annual Congress of the American Optometric Association, Emmett A. Betts stated:

> *Recent studies on the psycho-physiology of seeing have contributed new ideas, if not new concepts of visual problems. More emphasis is placed on binocular vision and more attention is given to nearpoint seeing problems. The mere mechanical refraction approach to the visual problems of both children and adults has proved to be quite inadequate. At least, from the viewpoint of prevention, the sheer mechanical or anatomical approaches are characterized by unmistakable elements of futility. In short, it appears that the dynamics of seeing merit consideration in the prevention and correction of seeing difficulties.*[1]

He continues:

> *. . . Mechanistic psychology, which has dominated educational practice for generations, is slowly being uprooted and new growth in terms of Gestalt, configuration and/or organismic principles is being substituted. Structural, anatomical, or mechanistic concepts of certain vision problems gradually are being discarded in favor of psycho-physiological or functional concepts. In short, many areas of human endeavor (such as in physical and social sciences) are being transformed by changing the emphasis from the static considerations, in which the structural entities are stressed, to the study of dynamics. The trend in this direction is unmistakable.*

Wheeler and Perkins, in the preface of their textbook, *The Principles of Mental Development, Reference* state:

> *Since man first attempted to give a rational account of natural phenomena, mechanistic assumptions have prevailed. That they are now being abandoned independently in practically every branch of human thought is reason for the supposition that progress in science, including the conceptions of problems for experimental attack, is a product of evolution. That the progress should have been made independently by specialists in various fields gives added weight to its significance."*

In the transitional stage, confusion arises while proceeding from mechanist concepts to functional concepts. This is due to our inability to free our minds of the habits we have developed in trying to explain phenomena in terms of mechanisms. I refer to the usual student experience when he studies physical systems. He has very little difficulty in reconstructing and analyzing one component system. When he advances to the study of two component systems, here, again, he can draw these on two-dimensional paper. When he advances to three component systems, the period of model building begins. Hours are spent constructing three-dimensional models representing this system. Unfortunately, most of the ingredients of our civilization are made up of multi-component systems. Would you like to construct what such a system would look like in three-dimensional space? To further complicate this picture, we have assumed molecular reactions; whereas, actually these reactions are usually colloidal in nature. We, therefore, have difficulty in dealing with complex systems primarily because we strive to visualize them on a three-dimensional datum. We try to analyze the complex system in terms of its simple system prototype, and when we fail to see the comparison, confusion and doubt arise.

Goldstein,[2] in explaining his holistic approach to biology states:

> *Hitherto, the aim of biological research has been to divide the organism, like any physical object, into parts, and then to reconstruct it. But this procedure has yielded few satisfactory results either in respect to the physical or the psychic phenomena of an organism . . .The real crisis arises when, even in the face of new findings, the investigator cannot free himself from the former theory. Rather, he attempts to preserve it and, by constant emendations, to reconcile it with these new facts, instead of replacing it with a new theory fit to deal with both the new and old facts. This error has not been avoided in the evolution of the classical doctrine.*

2. The Modern Approach to Optometry

Vision is the dominant function in all the actions of the organism in relation to its space world. Vision includes the visual activity of the individual in his environment. It includes the way the individual organizes his space world so that he can function optimally. (See Figure 1. Space World Development.)

We have been so busy supposedly measuring the physical sizes of eyes that we may have forgotten that the eye is only one portion of the total chain of activity that ends in the experience we describe as seeing. We have been functioning under the theory of defective eyes, just as the dentist of the last decade dealt with defective teeth. The successful dentist of that era was the

1. SKELETAL - convergence - Seeks and holds a visual image

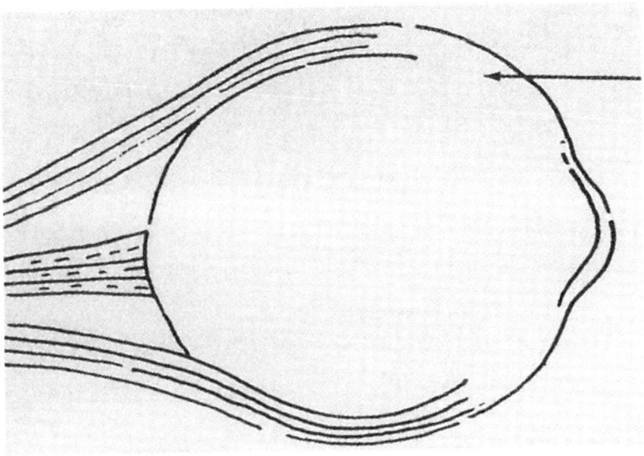

Extrinsic eye muscles
- striated muscles - quick acting.
Large in size for the job they do.

2. VISCERAL - accommodation image - Discriminates and defines the image

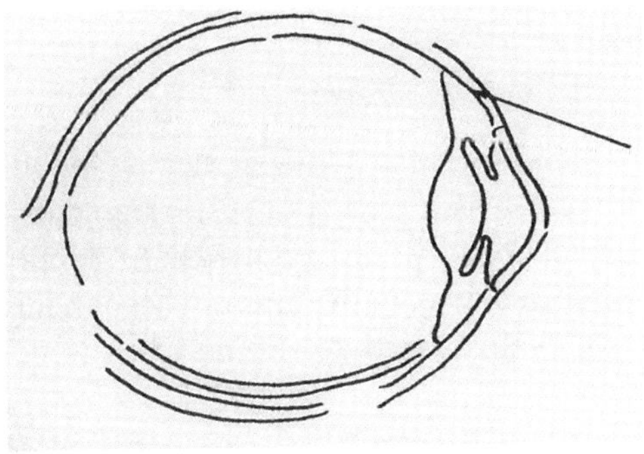

Intrinsic eye muscles
- smooth muscles - slow acting

3. CORTICAL - perceptual - "Unifies, elaborates and interprets the image."

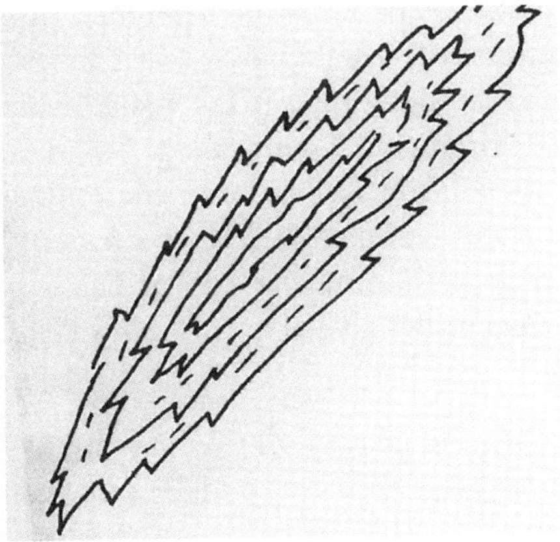

The only image existing in the brain is electrochemical fields which are ever in motion, fluctuating in amount and intensity.

Figure 1. Space World Development.

one who had in his window the greatest mound of extracted teeth, just as the successful optometrist was the one who had fitted the greatest number of glasses. The false teeth and the glasses supplied to the patient were prosthetic devices to restore capacity. Dentistry truly became a profession when it changed its concept from mechanical extraction to prevention and enhancement. Preventive dentistry demanded that the patient be examined at frequent intervals, not to extract teeth, but to maintain the oral state of the patient at a high level.

Arnold Gesell, director of the Child Development Clinic, Yale University, addressing the 1948 Great Lakes Optometric Congress commented, in part, regarding the future of optometry:

> *If optometry is to become a profession of highest standards, it will inevitably move into the fields of prevention. It will operate largely at the childhood level. It must build high standards of professional techniques and of mores. It must begin to provide systematic, periodical visual analysis, adequate in all ways to protect the visual health of our children."*

Optometry now is progressing through this same series of steps. Optometrists originally supplied glasses merely as a means of restoring acuity, depending merely upon the distant subjective to tell when to supply glasses. Functional case analysis points the way to the future. Through this method of analysis optometrists can evaluate and determine when remedial measures should be inaugurated.

Through the application of case analysis, the visual achievement level of the patient can be determined. If the visual achievement level is not sufficient for the environmental demands on the patient, remedial measures can be instituted. In this manner, optometry is operating on the highest professional plane. In utilizing the techniques of visual analysis, it is important to see the patient at regular intervals to determine if his visual achievement level is still adequate for his environmental demands. If a significant change has occurred either in his visual achievement or in environmental demands, remedial procedures can be instituted before the patient has suffered structural modification of the visual mechanism or has experienced discomfort. Optometry can thus be defined as the *art and science of visual care.*

The patient poses three questions for us to answer: (1) What is my visual problem? (2) What have I done to meet this problem? and (3) What can be done to eliminate this problem?

To answer these three questions, the optometrist must perform:

1. A case study to determine the cause of the problem:
2. A visual skills profile to determine what the patient did to meet this problem;
3. Corrective procedures to eliminate the problem;
4. A progress report to determine the amount of visual improvement obtained by the patient and to ascertain if the problem has been eliminated.

It is only after the practitioner has gone through all four of these steps that he can be sure that the patient had adequate professional aid.

3. The Value of Case Analysis

Case analysis gives a procedure for summing up optometric analytical data for purposes of classification.

Without this method of classification, it would be extremely difficult to come to any decision regarding the proper visual rehabilitation procedure to follow in any particular case. Binocular case analysis gives the wherewithal to take this large mass of data is about the various components of the visual pattern at both farpoint and nearpoint and from it determine the kind, type and extent of the visual problem. The solution of binocular dysfunction cases calls not only for good technical and manipulative skill, but also for the ability to determine the degree and extent of the visual adaptations and concessions made by the patient.

The purpose of case analysis is threefold: (a) to find the limitations of the prescriptible lens for distance and for near; (b) to determine whether the case can be handled by lens application alone, by vision training and lenses, or by vision training alone; (c) to follow the changes in relationship between accommodation and convergence brought about by the new Rx or the vision training program or both (progress report examination). Without the aid of binocular case analysis, the solution of visual problems becomes a hit-and-miss affair - a grave injustice to the patient.

4. Normal Eye

In optometry, "normal" is generally defined as "that which agrees with the regular and established type" or it is "conformance to the natural order of things." There are three different approaches to the problem of classifying objects or "things" as to whether they are normal or abnormal as follows:

1. The *normative* or *physical* viewpoint which requires that the system must possess certain ideal values in order to be considered normal. It establishes an arbitrary set of standards for the variables of the system

which it must possess in order to be considered normal. The standards selected are usually based upon logic.

2. The *pathological* viewpoint: a normal system is one which is free of pathology, a system which has no abnormal disturbances. We do not consider the degenerative processes associated with aging as being of a pathological nature.

3. The *statistical* viewpoint: a normal system is one which agrees with the statistics established for a group of similar systems.

The pathological viewpoint does not enter into our system of analysis, since it is screened for referral to the medical or dental specialist. The normative or physical viewpoint considers vision from the standpoint of the immobilized eyeball - the eye in which all functional structures have been paralyzed by a cycloplegic. The comparison is made to the camera. The normative or physical normal eye is one in which the optical system needs no auxiliary lenses to obtain a sharp focus at the retinal plane. It establishes an arbitrary value of emmetropia and orthophoria as the normal conditions for efficient vision.

These standards bear little recognition to the existing facts. First, optometric data is obtained from the measurement of the visual mechanism without a cycloplegic. Although the "fogging" method is used to inhibit accommodation to its fullest extent, optometrists all realize that this mechanism will change because some residual accommodation is active. We never examine the visual mechanism as if it were a fixed system. This is illustrated by the following data taken on students over a 10-week period, using the same standard test procedures and instrumentation:

(1)	(2)	(3)
1. plano	+.25	+.25-.25x155°
plano	+.50	+.50
2. -0.25	plano -.25x25°	plano
-0.25	+.25	+.50-.50x120°
3. plano	+.25	+.50-.25x110°
plano	+.50	+.50
4. plano	+.25 -.50x20°	+.25
plano	+.50	+.50-.25x135°
5. plano	+.50	+.25
plano	+.75	+.50-.25x145°
6. plano	+.25	plano
plano	+.25	plano
7. plano	+.25 -.50x15°	(did not complete
plano	+.50 -.25x160°	remainder of tests)
8. plano	+.50 -.25x20°	
plano	+.50	
9. +.25	+.25	
+.25	+.50	
10. plano	+.25	
plano	+.50	

All of the subjects listed stated that they have always had the same refractive error in the past three years of examinations. Almost invariably, the maximum change in refractive error was found when the student was confronted by school examinations.

Second, our existing data indicates that emmetropia and orthophoria, instead of being ideal conditions for the visual mechanism, are in reality abnormal conditions which are prevalent in those individuals classified as reading disabled. In fact, emmetropia and orthophoria, when found in an individual, seem to indicate the presence of a visual problem. The data of Tiffin, (*Industrial Psychology* 1944:144) on the relationship of the distant phoria test with the percentage of the individuals having serious accidents, revealed that those individuals who had exophoria had fewer accidents than those with orthophoria or esophoria.

Neither does emmetropia seem to be the desirable condition for the ideal, efficient visual mechanisms. A study made by Frank (graduate thesis at Chicago College of Optometry, 1949) reveals that the average refractive error of good readers in this study was nearly one diopter of myopia, while the average refractive error of poor readers was about emmetropia.

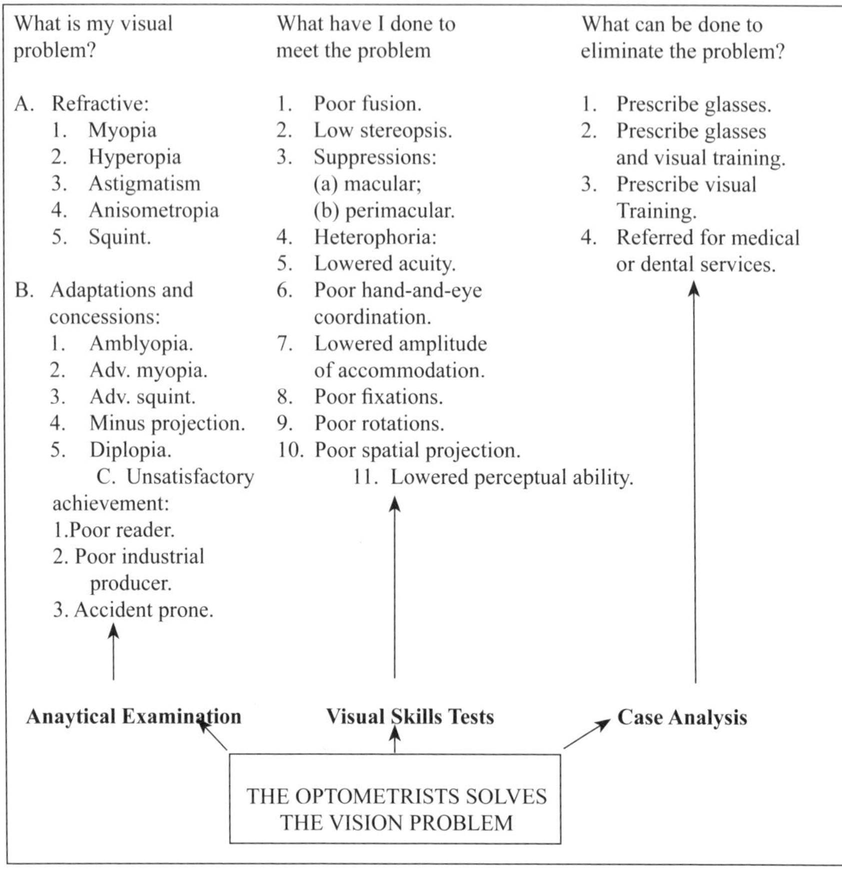

Figure 2.

If any biological variable (height, weight, phoria, stereopsis, etc.) is measured for a group of individuals, a range in value is found of this particular statistic. The normal value of this variable is determined by finding the arithmetic average for the group. *This average value is said to be the normal value for that particular biological variable.* The refractive status of a great number of people was measured and it was found that the normal value for this variable is 0.75D of hyperopia. From an optometric viewpoint, the *normal* eye is hyperopic and exophoric. In fact, since the emmetropic and orthophoric eye differs significantly from the normal eye, we can state that these conditions when found are *not normal.* The lowered performance rates of the emmetrope and orthophore support this contention.

The chief objection to the statistical viewpoint lies in the seeming contradiction that an eye may be statistically normal, but physiologically abnormal.

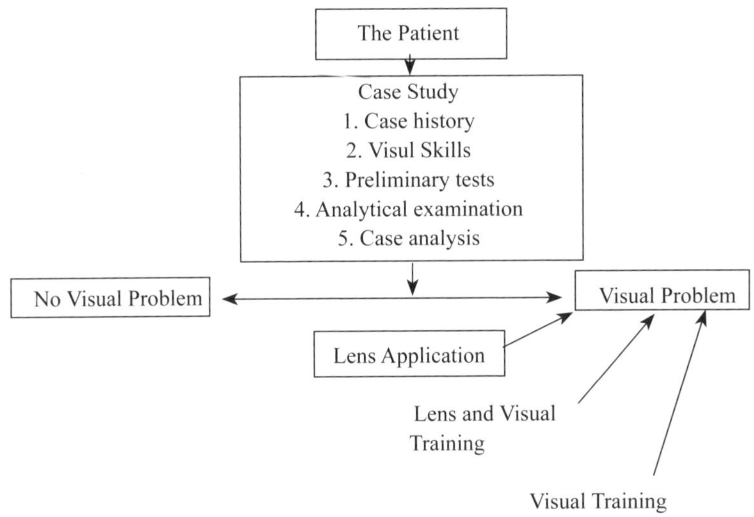

No Visual Problem: Adequate ability to perform visually, above environmental demands.
Visual Problem:

Lens application: Simple visual problem; visual efficiency can be restored by a lens.

Visual training: Complex visual problem; high deterioration problem has existed for a considerable period; basic visual skills must be restored before lenses can be used.

Visual training and lens application: A complex visual problem which has some plus acceptable or when visual problem is disorganized; lens application can be used simultaneously with visual training.

Figure 3. Case analysis

We may cite the presbyope and myope as examples. The presbyope may have only 2.00D of amplitude. This amplitude may be statistically normal for his age, but would be considered as physiologically abnormal on the basis that the patient needs a minimum of 5.00D for sustained nearpoint activity. This individual who possesses 2.00D of amplitude is actually physiologically normal if this amplitude agrees with the statistical average for his age. The abnormal individual would be the person of the same age who has only 1.00D of amplitude. This second individual deviates from the normal (for his age group) and he must receive special consideration in evaluating his visual problem in order to determine why he has an abnormally low amplitude.

In the case of the myope, we again have the seemingly paradoxical situation of an individual who is statistically normal, but is physiologically abnormal. Again we have a distortion of the related facts. If the refractive condition of nearpoint workers who are efficient at their jobs were determined, it might be found that the statistical normal would be the myope.

He is more efficient at nearpoint, but he has sacrificed distant acuity ability to reach this status. He, therefore, is physiologically abnormal at farpoint. Does this mean that we must create more myopes in order to obtain this nearpoint normality of an efficient producer? Obviously the answer is *no.* The one diopter myope, when looking at 16", must accommodate 1.50D and converge 15PD. How can we obtain this same situation without the individual becoming a myope?

Let us consider an individual who is an emmetrope. This individual, even though he is an emmetrope at far, can, through training, increase his plus acceptance at nearpoint. If a plus one diopter lens was placed before his eyes for all nearpoint work, what would be the effect at near? This emmetrope with the plus one lenses at near would now accommodate 1.50D and converge 15PDs at 16". We see that these figures are the same as for the myope, with this basic difference: the emmetrope now has the efficiency of the myope at near without the subsequent loss of distance acuity.

We are measuring a complex psycho-physiological system which has many components. To understand this system, we must determine by means of statistical methods the normal or expected values for our various tests. *Any arbitrary standards of perfection which are not based on statistical data have little optometric significance.*

5. Emmetropia

Emmetropia has been defined as:

> *An eye so constructed that parallel rays of light come to a focus in the retina without any effort of accommodation.* (James Thorington)
>
> *It is the condition of a normal eye in which the retina is situated at the posterior principal focus distance of the refracting system so that, with accommodation at rest, parallel light is brought to a focus at the retina.* (Laurance and Wood)
>
> *An eye in which point images are formed and in which (the eye being un-accommodated) these fall on the retina when the object is at infinity is called an emmetropic eye.* (H. H. Emsley)
>
> *An eye structure in which, with accommodation inactive, the secondary focal point of its optical system lies coincident with the fovea.* (F.L. Mason)

For the purpose of case analysis, none of these given definitions can be used. The phrase "normal eye" cannot be used in a definition of emmetropia because the normal eye is hyperopic. The expression "accommodation inactive" or "un-accommodated" cannot be used because in optometric testing procedures (non-cycloplegic) accommodation is always active. Since the eye is a living organ directly integrated into the visual behavior pattern of the individual, it is never inactive, regardless of the probe (lenses or prisms) being used, but is always under stress or strain, depending upon the external environment, internal environment, past experience, emotional level of the patient and many other variables. The use of the "fogging technique" does not force the patient to give up all accommodative effort, but merely to maintain it at a minimum level which is conducive to that individual. We must define emmetropia for our purposes on a functional basis. *Emmetropia can only refer to an individual who possesses standard acuity without the use of concave lenses and who refuses plus lenses (letters blur).* We can make no statement as to the accommodative status of the patient or where the focus might be located in his eyeball. We can only state that his acuity is at a maximum without the aid of any concave lenses and if we place plus lenses before his eyes, he will experience a blur. Such an individual is emmetropic.

Emmetropia means that there is no accommodation free of association with convergence at the fixation distance. It can be found at near as well as far. The one diopter hyperope, if he has single binocular vision, must be able to accommodate one diopter while looking at a distant object, without affecting convergence. If he cannot inhibit those impulses proceeding from accommodation towards convergence, he may experience diplopia. Similarly, an emmetrope, since he possesses no "refractive error" which can be corrected by a lens, must have no accommodation free from association with convergence for the test distance in question.

Since the emmetropic individual deviates considerably from the statistical norm of 0.75D of hyperopia, we consider him a visual defective. This is borne out by clinic and office experience which has shown that the emmetropic individual usually has a visual symptom. Emmetropia is a transition point between hyperopia and myopia. The patient who is moving toward an emmetropic condition is heading for trouble and is not attaining an ideal status.

This transition of the normally hyperopic organism toward emmetropia is a sign of coming danger, particularly in the young child, (nine years of age or younger). The organism, under the continued stress of the socially compulsive intensified nearpoint environment, can only move in the direction of myopia or retain his emmetropia and become a poor reader. Emmetropia is a biological mistake. It reduces one of the important psycho-physiological abilities; that of changing accommodation without causing a change in convergence, to a zero range. If the stress situation continues, the organism must make some type of emergency adaptation in order to preserve the functioning unity. This usually means the appearance of minus projection.

6. Orthophoria

Orthophoria is defined as:

> *The condition in which, the motor muscles being at rest, the visual axes are parallel to each other. This state of normal balance obtains not only when the eyes are in ordinary use, but also when they are subjected to a balance test.* (Laurance and Wood)
>
> *The ideal state of binocular balance; there exists no manifest deviation under dissociation.* (C. H. Giles)
>
> *When the passive position of functional rest is also the primary position, such a perfectly balanced condition of the ocular-motor system is described as orthophoria.* (H. H. Emsley)

The motor muscles are not at rest in the state of orthophoria. Stimuli are constantly proceeding to these muscles. It is not an ideal condition because the efficiency of those who are orthophoric is lower than those who are exophoric. Orthophoria is not a balance point, as far as equating muscle strength. The muscle bulk of esophores and exophores are all the same. What then is orthophoria? From a functional viewpoint, orthophoria is an equilibrium state in which the eyes under dissociation have the same posture as the eyes have when they are not dissociated.

The presence of orthophoria indicates that all of the latitude of protection in the convergence pattern has been used up due to a stress situation; and that any continuation of the stress situation will result in the presence of esophoria. The presence of orthophoria is undesirable, and remedial measures should be instituted to regain the buffer of exophoria as soon as possible.

7. Static or Dynamic Eye

If the eye were a static organ similar to a camera, the obvious solution to the presence of a visual problem would be to measure the power of the optical system under cycloplegia. Ophthalmologic experience, as well as optometric experience, has shown that the great majority of patients will not tolerate such a full correction, but that it must be modified. The modification used is usually less plus. The refractive power of the eye is subject to change because of the stimulatory effects of accommodation and convergence and because of the intimate linkage with the autonomic and skeletal nervous systems of the body. As a result of these influences, it is difficult to apply the term *static* to any aspect of vision short of death itself.

Normally, visual changes occur gradually due to growth, aging, vocational and social demands. Emotional factors arising from our environment are also a source of stimulation. We are all familiar with the patient who develops visual difficulty after the sudden loss of a loved one. This visual mechanism is capable of making dramatic changes in its refractive status. One need only refer to the literature on traumatic myopia to read of these sudden changes. Magitot *(Traumatic Myopia, Ann d'Ocul 1920;157:680)* reported on four cases of traumatic myopia. In three of these cases, foreign bodies had penetrated the orbit, but had not penetrated the eyeball. The observations showed that the myopia created was not affected by atropine, general anesthesia or by puncture of the anterior chamber. Bekes *(Klin Mf Augen 1925;75:535)* reports on a case of traumatic myopia following contusion due to a blow from a tennis ball. The first examination revealed a shallow anterior chamber, mydriasis, hypotomy, edema, and retinal hemorrhages with about six to seven diopters of myopia. On the fourth day after the injury, the fundus was normal, but the patient still exhibited 5.50D of myopia. On the 10th day after the injury, the vision was normal without any correction.

The sudden change exhibited by the visual mechanism of an individual after shock and trauma shows the extreme ability of the mechanism to react to this situation.

C. E. Ferree and G. Rand in their research on the *Refractive Condition for the Peripheral Field of Vision (Report of A Joint Discussion on Vision, 1932:244)* reported on the effect of prolonged fixation upon the refractive status of the eye that, "As fixation was prolonged, a tendency towards myopia was found; that is, if hyperopic, the eye tended to become less hyperopic; if emmetropic, the eye tended to become myopic; if myopic, it tended to become more myopic. This change was observed in all the eyes examined when an eccentric fixation was taken; also for some eyes when a far fixation was taken in the median plane. *Further, the change was found to take place whether the examination was made with or without a cycloplegic.*

The work of Spooner *(Br J Phys Optics 1954;11:158)* illustrates the effect of body posture upon vision. In his third experiment, he was interested in determining the effect of rotation of the head on the manifest refractive error, as measured by an objective optometer. The head of the subject was rotated a known number of degrees, and he was instructed to look into the optometer. Spooner then measured the manifest refractive error for various degrees of rotation. He sums up his results as follows:

> *It will be seen that most of the eyes used were stable up to 40°, though fluctuations up to 1.0 diopter are to be seen. However, a picture of increasing conflict, in the form of minor oscillations of accommodation, was common as the excursion was increased. . . Two subjects, the top myope and the bottom hyperope, have lost accommodative control altogether at 30°; the myope rocketing off into a spasm, and the hyperope diving into a defocused condition. . . . From our present point of view, these experiments are sufficient evidence of increasing instability of the visual apparatus, with postures involving extreme rotation of the eyes. Postural abnormalities, therefore, may adversely affect the visual apparatus.*

Schwartz and Sanberg, in a report on the effect of time in submarine service on vision *(Med Res Lab, USN Submarine base, NL 1954 ;13(14)* state:

> *The comparison of submariners' entrance scores and of candidates for submarine school with submariners, both show a loss of visual acuity with time in submarine service for distant vision: candidates 11.50; submariners 10.19. This change in acuity was significant at better than the 1% level. . . . These changes in visual characteristics may be brought about by the submarine environment in which most work is performed at distance of two feet or less. It is rare to be able to view an object at more than 10 feet. Thus, the eyes are always accommodating and always converging, a circumstance which may cause a relatively fixed posturing of the crystalline lens in an accommodative state and a neuromuscular tendency to over convergence. This is further abetted by the mutual reinforcement of the accommodative and convergence functions. The more time spent in this situation, the firmer the neuromuscular pattern becomes established. With the invention of the snorkel and now of the atomic submarine, this condition may become even more accentuated due to the decrease in opportunity for distance vision afforded by surface running.*

Duke-Elder *(Br J Ophthalmol 1930;14:609)* investigated the effect upon the eye of occupations involving close work. The subjects were obtained from the London School of Printing. The 244 subjects who were examined were in the age group of 14 to 20 years. This group was divided into two sections. The first section consisted of 80 subjects who almost always did near work. The second section consisted of 164 subjects who worked at various distances not involving great eye strain. Four successive examinations were tabulated each at a nine-month interval:

Initial Refraction	Near Workers	Others
1. Emmetropes	15%	2%
2. Myopes	42.5%	31%
3. Hypermetropes	40%	64%
4. Mixed	2.5%	3%

Change of Refraction	Near Workers	Others
1. Emmetropes		
A. Stationary	83.5%	100%
B. Became Myopic	16.7%	0%
2. Myopes		
A. Stationary	23%	55%
B. Progressed	77%	45%
3. Hypermetropes		
A. Stationary	69%	78%
B. Became Myopic	31%	20%
C. Became More Hypermetropic	0%	2%

Duke-Elder concludes:

> *It is obvious that the near workers do not compare well with those engaged in other occupations. Not only do their numbers contain initially a considerable higher percentage of myopes; but the number in which the refractive error increases towards myopia is also higher. . . . These figures suggest that the occupation which entails the greatest degree of eyestrain has the most deleterious effect upon vision, and that one of the results of such an occupation is to encourage the development of myopia.*

In all of the examples cited it is impossible for these changes to have occurred because of the growth of the eyeball. These changes or fluctuations in refractive errors can only occur because of a change in the relationship between accommodation and convergence. It is also significant that Ferree and Rand obtained their refractive changes even when they used a cycloplegic. These pattern changes between accommodation and convergence can occur even when the known existing accommodative mechanism has been paralyzed by drugs. We must realize that when we are examining the visual pattern of an individual by means of lenses and prisms, that we are investigating a dynamic mechanism capable of making dramatic changes in its refractive power. *We are investigating a relatively simple receptor combined with a complex integrating system.*

We have seen that changes in the visual environment will create changes in the refractive condition of the organism. The first reaction to this change in the visual environment is in the direction of a change in that relationship between accommodation and convergence. As the impact of this environmental change continues, physical modification of existing structures must occur. We readily agree that structure will modify function, but it is more difficult to conceive of the converse relationship that *function must modify structure.*

Julian Huxley states:

> *Most biologists do not seem to realize the extent to which functional modification occurs in the normal vertebrate body. It appears to be true, not only that the size of every muscle in the body depends on function, but the size, direction and structure of every tendon and bone; the detailed configuration of the blood system depends largely, or perhaps wholly, on hydrodynamic considerations; the size of every gland is regulated by function and even the nervous system does not escape. It is only in the earliest development that structure precedes function; later, structure is the resultant of function.*

Edward Hartmann reports on the effect of functional modification *(Psychosomatic Phenomena In Ophthalmology. Br J Ophthmol 1949;33:461)* that:

> *Every physician knows that a sudden emotion can cause functional symptoms, such as a sharp rise in the systemic blood pressure. We ophthalmologists have often seen one of the most perfect examples of psychosomatic disease; a woman receives a wire bringing bad news, or is afflicted by the death of someone dear to her, and an acute attack of glaucoma sets in; the intraocular pressure shoots right up to 100 mm. Hg. or more. This is the functional stage, and if it does not last too long, it is reversible. . . If, however, the high pressure lasts, the functional disturbances become irreversible and, should surgery be delayed, structural changes familiar to all of us will ensue.*

Ian Stevenson in writing on "Why Medicine is Not a Science" *(Harper's magazine, April, 1949)* describes three stages in this process:

> *There are three stages of ill health. The first is a functional impairment or misuse which is often impossible to detect and may not be noticed by the patient or his physician; the second brings definite symptoms of illness: the third brings structural changes.*

Darrell Boyd Harmon has found three stages in the physical changes that occur when the child is under stress. These are: (a) *neural-highly-* reversible, leaving no symptoms; (b) *neuro-muscular-* still reversible, but now showing symptoms; (e) *muscular-* changes in supporting structures, reversible if accessible, leaving definite symptoms.

The same three stages are present in the development of visual problems (see Figure 4):

(a) *neural*—when the person acts "as if" he were a product of altered behavior, that is, he acts as if he were a myopic, astigmat, strabismic, anisometrope, etc. The performance is characteristic, but there are no measurements of this altered performance. This is the complete *functional stage.* At this point, merely altering certain environmental factors will readily reverse this altered behavior and return it to normal.

(b) *neural-muscular*—when we have characteristic changes in our refractive measurements, but the case is still in a fluid, amenable state, highly reversible, susceptible to all corrective procedures.

(c) *muscular*—considerable distortion is now present in the refractive measurements. The distortion is now embedded or structured and is extremely difficult to reverse. This distortion may be in the eye itself, in its attachments or in the central nervous system.

We readily concede the effect of growth, metabolic changes and senility upon the refractive condition of the patient, but we neglect the most important influence of all, *the environment.* The importance of environment in the total development of the child has been summarized by Darell Boyd Harmon *(The Coordinated Classroom. Grand Rapids, MI: American Seating Co., 1953:19)* as follows:

> *The organic child has just so much energy to expend. This energy must go towards satisfying his basic need in staying alive; converting his food into usable chemical forms; protecting him against infection and other disease threats; growing; and furnishing the energy for all the activities and adjustments demanded by his environment. Only a limited amount of his energies is really free for activity. When environmental demands exceed the energy free and available for meeting them, the environmental demand is met by depriving some other vital need of its energy. Growth suffers first in most cases. Continued stresses induced by poorly designed furniture, by poor distribution of light or by visual performance demands, inconsistent with basic visual performance patterns, might readily use energy needed for growth, for body function, for protection against*

The Stages of Organismic Impairment				
Stage	Type	Medical (Stevenson)	Postural (Harmon)	Visual
1	Neural	Functional Impairment	Highly reversible Leaving no symptoms	Acts as if he were myopic, amblyopic, etc.
2	Neuro-Muscular	Definite Symptoms of Illness	Still reversible now shows some symptoms	Refractive changes present; changes are still revers-ible to a con-siderable extent
3	Muscular	Structural Modification	Changes in supporting struct-ure, reversible if accessible,leaving definite symptoms	Embedded struct-ure; modification in eyeball, adnexa, and/or cortex; ex-tremely difficult to reverse

Figure 4.

> *infection, or for overcoming other adverse factors in a child's total surroundings.*
>
> *Bodily growth is inherently a balanced process. But a study of growth shows that its centers, at any given time, are always at the center of the greatest bodily activity. In other words, the child's body(or body systems) tends to grow along the lines of stress induced by various activities in order to reduce those stresses. If the environment sets up centers or lines of stress not fitting the alignment of inherent and normal growth forms, the result is structural warping. As the child continues to grow and function in such surroundings, the final result is asymmetrical or unbalanced body structures, deviating performances or physical or psychological lesions and disabilities.*

These induced stresses finally cause structural modifications in the organism. These structural modifications involve not only skeletal structures, but also muscle and sensory structures. In this group so modified, we find the eyeball.

It should not be a surprise that stress situations, which force organismic posture changes, will also cause modifications in the eyeball, adnexa or cortex. *(Duke-Elder, v. 1:242)*, "When vertebrates appeared . . . the visual impulses were primarily photo-static (light-balancing), and they were conducted to the roof of the midbrain which provided an automatic mechanism for promoting appropriate posture-movements. . . . The most salient factor in the evolution of man was the ousting of smell as the dominant sense and its replacement by vision *(Elliot Smith, 1927)*; and to equip the eyes with the power to form the basis of man's physical dexterity and intellectual supremacy the whole central nervous system has been reorganized . . . (however), *when the neopallium (higher brain centers) appeared the mid-brain certainly retained its phoo-static functions; . . ."* Further, he states *(pages 247- 248)* "The fibers from the retina end in two masses of grey matter; the *Lateral geniculate body,* which is phylogenetically part of the optic thalamus, and the *Superior Colliculus,* which is part of the *mid-brain. . .* The visual fibers (in man) find a (relay) station in the lateral geniculate body. . . 80% of the retinal fibers find their way here. . . . The (retinal) fibers which run to (the superior colliculus), however, are undoubtedly the most primitive phylogenetically. . . , and in *man they are associated with the primitive photo-static (light and posture) rather than the higher sensory functions of vision."* We can thus estimate that at least twenty percent of the retinal fibers end up in neurological centers involving organismic posture.

A comparison of the visual acuity of the school children in the Becker School, Austin, Texas, in November, 1942, revealed that 53.3% of the children failed a distant acuity test. The school environment was modified according to the specifications of Harmon. Of the same children six months later, 18.6% failed a distant acuity test. These results dramatically reveal the reversibility possible when proper environmental changes have been made. These changes were: the elimination of high contrasts; proper illumination without glare; proper color dynamics; and posture control of children.

In the light of these reversible changes, it is difficult to consider the visual mechanism as a *static* structure. It is a *dynamic* mechanism capable of making tremendous changes in its refractive status, depending upon environmental demand. These factors which influence vision are object size, shape, color, working distance, time, illumination intensity, glare, peripheral field contrasts, vertical/lateral working areas and the postural requirements of the operation. If we control these factors we can hold visual problems down to an absolute minimum.

Summary

(a) Vision is a process that involves the whole person, not merely the optical sensory structures.

(b) The profession of optometry is primarily interested in *preventing* visual problems and *enhancing* visual skills so that people can perform their jobs easier, faster and with greater accuracy. Lenses are prescribed as prosthetic devices only as a last resort. Lenses are used primarily as a means of preventing visual distortions and of stabilizing an adequate visual pattern.

(c) The visual process entails a visual mechanism which is *dynamic* in nature and is capable of making dramatic changes in its refractive status. These changes proceed through three stages: (1) *neural;* (2) *neuromuscular; (3) muscular.*

(d) Emmetropia can only refer to an individual who possesses standard acuity without the use of concave lenses and who rejects plus lenses.

(e) Orthophoria is a state of equilibrium in which the eyes under dissociation maintain the same posture as the eyes have when they are in the normal fused condition.

(f) Emmetropia and orthophoria are not ideal conditions for the visual mechanism. The presence of these conditions usually is indicative of the existence of a visual problem. Hyperopia and exophoria are found in normal individuals.

Two criticisms have been leveled against the functional viewpoint. These are:

(1) this method of analysis tends to make visual problems seem more complicated than they are, dramatically stated by Morgan, ". . . simple cases are made complicated, and the optometrist made into a Don Quixote charging a windmill."

(2) New terms are used or nebulous meanings are given to old terms.

In response to the first charge, the adherents to the functional viewpoint admit that this method of analysis is more complicated than any of the others. Therefore, what are the justifications for its use? I believe these are as follows:

(1) The concept of the effect of *time* upon the visual pattern, as shown in the deteriorations of the B-type case.

(2) The concept of the effect of *disorganization* and *organization* in handling the visual problem as far as administering visual training or the application of lenses.

(3) The concept of applying lenses as a preventive measure or to enhance visual abilities, rather than as a prosthetic device.

(4) The concept that a high percentage of visual problems arise from near-point activity and, therefore, the problem must be attacked from that area.

(5) The ability to follow the progress of the case so that the optometrist can determine if the remedial procedures followed are aiding the patient.

In response to the second charge, we must plead guilty. In establishing a new philosophical approach to visual problems, we have been guilty of using a term, then dropping it and using a different term to cover the same area of discussion. For example, the terms "embedded," "structured" and "organized" mean the same thing. Our semantics will improve with age. Hartmann in the preface to his book, *"Gestalt Psychology,"* answers the same question from the standpoint of psychology, but it applies equally well to the optometric profession. He states, "Nevertheless, the difficulties which even well-trained psychologists with different experimental backgrounds experience in comprehending the basic contributions of configurationism lie largely in the intentional and violent break which it makes with the past. It is like some sudden forward leap disturbing the continuity of scientific development. The revolution which has occurred in physics within the last quarter-century presents an analogous situation, for a few laymen, and perhaps few physicists are fully at home in the new realm of relativity." On page 289 of his book, Hartmann further states, "There is little doubt that psychology is constantly waging a battle with language and never quite expressing that which it intends."

In proceeding from the sole consideration that eye and vision are synonymous to the functional concept that the eye is merely the starting point of the process and vision does not start until the electronic pattern initiated by the eye reaches the cortex where it is matched with previous experience and a portion of this pattern is fed back to the eyeball in order to maintain control, this whole process is what we are measuring and analyzing when we consider the functional concept of vision. This jump from eyeball to brain patterns is like the jump from mechanistic physics (Newton) to quantum physics. Dyson *(Sci Am 1958 Sept:75)* describes the experience that his students go through when exposed to quantum mechanics. "They begin by learning the tricks of the trade. He learns how to make calculations in quantum mechanics and get the right answers, how to calculate the scattering of neurons by protons and so forth. To learn the mathematics of the subject and to learn how to use it takes about six months. This is the first stage in learning quantum mechanics and it is comparatively easy and painless. The second stage comes when the student begins to worry because he does not understand what he is doing. He begins to worry because he has no clear physical picture in his head. He gets confused in trying to arrive at a physical explanation for each of the mathematical tricks he has been taught. He works very hard and gets discouraged because he does not seem able to think clearly. This second stage often lasts six months or longer, and it is strenuous and unpleasant. Then, quite un-expectedly, the third stage begins. The student suddenly says to himself, "I understand quantum mechanics," or rather he says, "I understand now that there isn't anything to be understood." The difficulties which seemed so formidable have mysteriously vanished. What has happened is that he has learned to think directly and unconsciously in quantum mechanics language and is no longer trying to explain everything in terms of pre-quantum conceptions." It is the purpose of this book to lead the student quickly through this second stage so that he will be able to think directly in terms of functional vision.

References

1. *Betts EA. The Study of Reading Needs. Lectures delivered at the 44th Congress of the American Optometric Association, June 29, 1941:10.*
2. *Goldstein K. The Organism. New York: American Book Co.,1940:7-17.*

CHAPTER II
The Visual Pattern

Very early in the development of the primary concepts regarding functional optometry, it became evident that a visual problem could not be defined in terms of refractive error. It has been common clinical experience that a group of individuals could all possess the same refractive error, but some in this group could have no visual problem and the remainder of the group could have all degrees of visual problems. It soon became evident that the refractive error was the end result of some type of activity. This activity was related to the behavior pattern of the individual.

Tiffin in his vocational research, (*Industrial Psychology:*153-54) found a relationship between refractive change and months of experience on the job for hosiery loopers. The impact of the environment upon the individual is capable of causing a change in the eyeball. *Editors' note: The relationship of nearpoint work and changes in refractive status has more recently been researched by many including: Angle and Wissman, Sato, Hirsch, and Young.*

Visual problems do not seem to relate very well to the amount of muscle effort that might be involved. That is, a group of hyperopes of the same refractive error may need no plus lenses, or may need plus in excess of the amount of refractive error. Optometrists have all had the experience of a 1.50D hyperope with discomfort who becomes completely comfortable and efficient by the application of a plus 0.50D lens. He is now equivalent to a one diopter hyperope.

By the same token, we have found many one diopter hyperopes who have serious visual problems and need aid. We cannot account for visual problems on the basis of units of muscle effort involved in the environmental activity. The conclusion drawn is that vision is not an isolated function (involving eyeball alone) of the human organism, but it is a complex function of many action systems of the body. To understand vision, we must first understand the visual behavior pattern.

1. Behavior Pattern

The reaction of an individual to his environment is called behavior. Through the researches of Coghill, Carmichael, Gesell, (*Editors' note: more recently, Selye, Pribram)*, and many others, it has been shown that the individual makes a defined response of his neuro-motor system to a specific situation. This response is the result of maturation and experience, and is the authentic end product of a total developmental process which works with orderly sequence; a neurological pattern of organization. It has been defined as an enormously complex action in the central nervous system which brings about certain activity desirable to the organism. As the organism proceeds from birth towards death, a countless emerging, shuffling, merging and integration of these patterns is occurring. *Those neurological patterns which are of survival value to the organism are never relinquished, short of death.*

All behavior patterns are motor patterns; they always result in the activity of muscles and glands. The walking pattern of the child has been built upon the crawling pattern of the baby. In the initial stages of development of a behavior pattern, the movements are spastic, slow, and performed on a cortical level of activity. As maturation and experience continues, the efficiency of the pattern improves and soon its activity pattern is relegated to a subcortical level. These efficient movements are called ballistiform movements. If any change in the external environment ensues, immediately the pattern is performed at a cortical level with its stilted, inefficient spastic movements.

A favorite example is: an individual walking along a path who suddenly is confronted by a narrow bridge that crosses a small stream. Immediately his walking pattern changes from a smooth, effortless performance to a stilted, slow and spastic pattern. The effort in crossing this small bridge is more fatiguing than walking a mile along the path. What has happened to cause such an abrupt change in efficiency?

As long as walking conditions were normal for that individual, the motor activity was performed smoothly, efficiently, at sub-cortical levels. The change in the external environment to the *restricted* field of the bridge with its added *hazard* feature meant a radical change to the organism. Under these conditions, the walking pattern immediately comes under conscious executive control resulting in spastic, inefficient movement. *Whenever the external, internal or mental environment of the individual changes, behavior patterns which have been functioning efficiently on a subcortical level with ballistiform movements are lifted to conscious executive levels which will result in inefficient, spastic movements.*

We can postulate some of the possible reactions of individuals to this bridge situation and compare them with a visual counterpart.

(1) The individual when confronted by the bridge decides that he has walked far enough and turns about and leaves. He doesn't even try to cross the bridge. His visual counterpart is found in the millions of workers

and school children who decide to leave their job or school and seek some other task. These types of individuals are the cause of high labor turnover and school dropouts.

(2) The individual when confronted by the bridge decides to take a running start, so he can get enough momentum to carry him across the obstacle. He usually manages to get part way across and then, since he lacks sufficient motor skill, falls off the bridge into the water below. He may try this many times before giving up. The number of tries he will take before giving up the task will depend upon social and economic pressures. We have the same visual counterpart in the millions of visually inefficient producers both in our schools and industries. The economic cost of this group to the nation totals billions of dollars each year. These individuals can use their eyes for short periods of time, but then they become fatigued and must rest their eyes before they can again repeat the cycle.

(3) The individual when confronted by the bridge decides that the safest way to get across is to get down on his hands and knees and inch his way across the obstacle. He finally reaches the other side, but only after an enormous expenditure of energy. We have this visual counterpart in the disabled reader. He can read *if* the material is well below his grade level and at a slow rate. He finally finishes his assignment, but only after long periods of study.

(4) The individual when confronted by the bridge restricts his field of view to his feet and a small portion of the bridge, and thus walks across to the other side. We have this visual counterpart in the myope.

(5) The individual when confronted by the bridge, evaluates the situation as being the same as walking down the road and proceeds rapidly, keeping his gaze upon the distant horizon and not on his feet. He is the rarity. His visual counterpart also is very rare. He is the individual who has sufficient visual reserves so that he can adequately meet any visual situation.

All behavior is based on the integrative activity of numerous neurological patterns. All behavior involves motor activity. This all-inclusive statement includes mental activity, since any psychic state must involve bodily tension. *Therefore, all behavior is motor.*

2. Visual Pattern

Psychologists estimate that 80% of the information we obtain from our external environment is by means of our visual pattern. It is the most important portion of the behavior pattern. It is understood that the visual pattern is not separate from the behavior pattern, but rather that it is an important integrated section of its activity. The importance of the visual pattern to the survival of the organism is obvious when we compare the behavior of a person with his eyes closed with his behavior when his eyes are open. It is the dominant sense given to man.

In referring to the visual pattern, we are considering something much more complex than the eyes of the organism. The eyes are only the external receptors for the visual mechanism. The photic stimulus in the eye is converted by means of a photochemical reaction into electrical impulses in the rods and cones. These electrical impulses proceed to the mid-brain where integration of visual, auditory, kinesthetic and auricular impulses occur. It must be noted that all of these electrical impulses are the same. This galaxy of impulses proceeds to the occiptal lobe where an electrical field is established. This field acts as a means of stimulating the accommodative and convergence mechanisms where additional action must occur before a true visual response is obtained by the organism.

Modification of the visual impulses occurs at three levels. First, it may occur as the integrative action of the retina. Polyak has declared that the retina is as complex an integrative center as the brain itself. Second, integrative action occurs between the various types of receptor impulses at the mid-brain level. Third, modification of the visual pattern by past experience and emotion of the organism can take place at the cortical level.

Sherrington's description of the complexity of the visual pattern has become a classic (*Man On His Nature:*121), "The chief wonder of all we have not touched on yet. Wonder of wonders, though familiar even to boredom. So much with us that we forget it all our time. The eye sends, as we saw, into the cell-and-fiber forest of the brain throughout the waking day continual rhythmic streams of tiny, individually evanescent, electrical potentials. This throbbing streaming crowd of electrified shifting points, in the spongework of the brain, bears no obvious semblance in space-pattern; and even in temporal relation it resembles but a little remotely the tiny two-dimensional upside-down picture of the outside world which the eyeball paints on the beginnings of its nerve-fibers to the brain. But that little picture sets up an electrical storm. And that electrical storm so set up is one which affects a whole population of brain-cells. Electrical charges having in themselves not the faintest elements of the visual - having, for instance, nothing of 'distance,' 'right-side upness,' nor 'vertical,' nor 'horizontal,' nor 'color,' nor 'brightness, nor 'shadow,' nor 'roundness,' nor 'squareness,' nor 'contour,' nor 'transparency,' nor 'opacity,' nor 'near,' nor 'far,' nor visual anything- yet conjures up all these. A shower of little electrical leaks conjures up for me, when I look, the landscape; the castle on the height, or, when I look at him, my friend's face, and how distant he is from me they tell me. Taking their word for it, I go forward and my other senses confirm that he is there."

Two of the most important components of the visual pattern are the accommodative and convergence patterns. These segments of the visual pattern control the organism's need for single and for clear vision. These two patterns are so vitally an integral part of the visual pattern that the complete visual examination is devoted to investigating the extent, degree and intensity of the relationship between these two patterns by means of lenses and prisms.

3. Accommodative Pattern

The visual pattern controls a dynamic refracting system capable of adjusting its power so that spatial objects at different distances can be clearly discerned. This ability of the visual pattern is called accommodation. Accommodation is the mechanism of focusing, designated in its postural set-up by the measurable light value brought to a focus congenial to interpretation. Accommodation is a lenticular-retinal-cortical process which is used by the organism to obtain clear vision.

Kepler (1611) had observed the ability of the eye to change focus and attributed the change to a forward and backward movement of the lens. Descartes (1637) wrote of the ability of the eye to change focus. Sturm (1697) explained accommodation on the basis that the eyeball is able to elongate. Listing (1851) came to the same conclusion as Sturm. Young (1801) showed that accommodation was not due to the change in curvature of the cornea or elongation of the eyeball.

In 1848, the ciliary muscle was discovered. Langenbach (1849) showed that the Purkinje images resulting from the foremost surface of the lens changed most in size with accommodation. Donders (1864) developed the method of designating accommodative effort in diopters by conversion of the focus distance. The theory of Helmholtz is most widely accepted as the explanation of the mechanism of lenticular accommodation. His description of the process is as follows (Helmholtz H. *Physiological Optics,* English Translation;1:151).

"In the passive far-seeing state of the eye, the lens is stretched by the zonule attached to its edge. The folds of the zonule pass outward and backward from their insertion on the capsule of the lens, thereby forming sheaths for the ciliary processes, and are attached to the posterior extremities of these processes and to the ciliary muscle, where they finally coalesce with the hyaloid membrane, retina and choroid. On contraction, the ciliary muscle could pull the posterior end of the zonule forward nearer the lens and reduce the tension of the zonule. But the effect of the tense zonule is to exert a pull on the lens, and thus shorten its axis and make its surfaces flatter. If the pull of the zonule is relaxed in accommodation for near vision, the equatorial diameter of the lens will diminish, and the lens will get thicker in the middle, both surfaces becoming more curved. If the pressure of the iris is super-added, the equatorial plane of the lens will bulge forward, increasing the curvature of the anterior surface and decreasing that of the posterior surface, so that the latter may be approximately equal to its original amount when the lens is accommodated for far vision.

This theory only accounts for the lenticular accommodative action, but other accommodative changes occur which Pech has designated as chromatic and interpretive accommodation. Pech (*Arch Ophthmol 1930;*47:) reports: "When a human eye looks at a black object on a white background, it never sees it distinctly at any distance, but it always sees a white contour bounded by a distinct line of variable colors and dimensions. Thus, without the intervention of the crystalline accommodation (lenticular accommodation) the human eye possesses a chromatic accommodation which allows it, if it is normal, to see with the same distinctness polychromatic objects located a few centimeters from the eye (blue conjugate focus) and on to infinity (red conjugate focus)."

"This phenomenon has considerable physiologic value, for it is this that assures the depth of our field of distinct vision. It allows us to perceive simultaneously with the usual distinctness of the sash bars of a window (object at finite distance) and the moon or the stars (objects practically at infinity)."

Dr. DeJean (quoted by Pech) states, "A subject is functionally myopic only when he becomes myopic for red; that a subject begins to be functionally hyperopic or presbyopic only when his green-blue proximum withdraws beyond the minimal distance of distinct vision of which he has need."

Dr. H. Embert (quoted by Pech) has shown by means of his Duochrome test, "Chromatic accommodation is a factor possessing functional importance, since, on account of it, a subject unprovided with a crystalline lens, without irregular astigmatism, keeps a considerable accommodation (5.50 D.) in a particular fortunate case."

It can be observed (by utilizing mono-chromatic illumination) that lenticular accommodation functions slowly; this would be expected since smooth muscle fibers function slowly. We are never aware of the slow functioning of the lenticular accommodative mechanism because of what Pech calls the "accommodation of interpretation." Therefore, if we are to consider all phases of this mechanism, we must consider accommodation as being a lenticular-retinal-cortical process whose functioning is under control of the accommodative pattern. Accommodation is a part of the great visceral nervous system of the body, operating characteristically through smooth muscle and having to do almost exclusively with the internal environment. Visceral muscle action is relatively slow, practically inexhaustible and is part of the great internal process.

It is always assumed that the distance between the target and the eye determines the amount of accommodation in effect. Elmsley (*Visual Optics;* 166-167) points out the difficulty of this assumption:

> *. . . It is not an easy matter to determine precisely the state of accommodation of an eye. The brain is apparently capable of seeing an object distinctly when the eye's optical system is focused on some point nearer or further away than the object. . . . But it is to be noted that although the test object may be seen with apparent distinctness by the subject, the eyes may be accommodated for a point further away. If that is the case, the actual accommodation exerted has been less than it seems.*

Developmental research reveals that binocular vision develops in the following sequence: (1) fixation; (2) coordinated vertical movements; (3) convergence; (4) monocular accommodation; (5) binocular accommodation. Phylogenetic and embryologic considerations reveal that accommodation is more ancient and developed prior to convergence.

Accommodation changes with the age of the patient. Table 1 is the average accommodation found at each age level.

TABLE 1.

Age	Accommodation
10 yrs.	14.00 D.
15	12.00
20	10.00
25	8.50
30	7.00
35	5.50
40	4.50
45	3.50
50	2.50
55	1.75
60	1.00
65	0.50
70	0.00

The patient is assumed to have sufficient accommodative ability when his amplitude of accommodation is twice his dioptric working distance.

The act of accommodation is a complex pattern which is made up of many subpatterns. Some of these subpatterns can be identified. They are: tonic accommodation, aberrational accommodation, convergence accommodation and psychic accommodation. Thus, for the same subject and same test distance the total accommodation will be the same; but the amounts of the various subpatterns will vary. Tonic accommodation is the lenticular poise under the conditions of far-point fixation with maximum inhibition to activity.Aberrational accommodation is the range of performance in the accommodative pattern due to the modification in the flux conoid because of spherical and chromatic aberration.

Convergence accommodation is the effect of convergence upon the accommodative pattern. Its magnitude is equal to that of accommodative convergence. There is thus an innervational flow between accommodation and convergence which helps to stabilize the accommodative poise and the convergence poise at any moment.

Psychic accommodation is the amount of lenticular accommodation in action due to the emotional and psychological reaction of the subject to the surrounding environment.

Table 2 compares the subpatterns of accommodation and convergence.

TABLE 2.

A COMPARISON OF THE SUBPATTERNS OF ACCOMMODATION AND CONVERGENCE

	Accommodation		**Convergence**
1.	Tonic Accommodation	1.	Tonic Convergence
2.	Aberrational Accommodation	2.	Fusional (Aberrational) Convergence
3.	Convergence~Accommodation	3.	Accommodation~Convergence
4.	Psychic Accommodation	4.	Psychic Convergence

Note: For diagnostic purposes it is often desirable to measure the amounts of these components; but it should always be borne in mind that these are purely an arbitrary segmentation of a single complex act to provide clear and single vision.

4. Convergence Pattern

Another primary portion of the visual pattern is the convergence pattern. It provides the mechanism with maintaining single vision. The convergence pattern controls the posturing of the eyes in their orbits and the centering of the total organism in its total environment. This control of the posturing of the eye-globes is by means of the skeletal nervous system which innervates the extra-ocular muscles. The convergence pattern is of survival value to the organism. The presence of diplopia would be catastrophic in our efforts to survive.

If an object approaches the eye of an observer and if attention is demanded, the two eyes will converge upon the target so that single vision is maintained. Eventually, the object will approach so near to the observer that he can no longer maintain singleness of the object. This nearest point of single vision is called the nearpoint of convergence. The nearpoint of convergence is usually expressed in inches or diopters. Its average value is three inches or 13 meter angles. Its value does not change with age, as is the case with amplitude of accommodation.

The convergence pattern activates a striated musculature mechanism. Striated muscles are rapid in comparison with smooth muscles. Therefore, we find that convergence is a rapid acting mechanism. Lancaster has concluded (Certain Anatomical and Physiological Considerations Bearing on Heterophoria. *Southern Medical J* 1923:16) that very little effort is involved in moving the eye-globes. He states, "The four rectus muscles are a little over 40 mm. long. If the length of the tendon is deducted from the total muscle length, all of the recti muscles have the same length of about 36 mm. Physiologists estimate that the muscles can contract one-third of their length at maximum effort. This gives about 12 mm. as the maximum excursion in any direction. Now 12 mm. is just the radius of the eyeball. Since the radius is one-sixth the circumference, it must subtend 60°. The maximum rotation of the eyeball has been variously estimated at 45° to 50° degrees. The reason the eyes do not rotate the full amount of 60° is due to the presence of check ligaments. These must prevent greater rotations which would pull unduly on the optic nerve, ciliary nerves and arteries, the vortex veins, etc."

". . . The area of the extra-ocular muscles are from 17 to 12 sq. mm. Physiologists estimate the contractile power of striated muscle at 62.5 gm. per sq. mm. (Weber, Haughton.) At this rate the ocular muscles have a contractile strength of from 750 to 1000 gms. (12 x 62.5; 17 x 62.5). Now, the eyeball weighs less than eight gms. and so it would seem as though these muscles were amply strong to move so light a body which moves so easily. Neglecting friction and the resistance of the antagonists, a force of less than two gms. suffices to rotate the eye (Kennelly). Making liberal allowances for friction, for the drag of the optic and ciliary nerves, arteries, etc., we have say five gms. as a rough estimate of the force required to rotate the eyeball."

Using this data as a basis for calculation, we can say that the extrinsic muscles are about 150 to 200 times larger than they have to be in order to move the eyeball (750/5; 1000/.5). The mechanism of convergence is constructed on a sufficient magnitude to allow it to function for pro-longed periods of time with minimum expenditure of energy.

Convergence is a complex pattern which consists of many subpatterns. They are: tonic convergence, fusional convergence, accommodative convergence and psychic convergence. The obvious similarities between the subpatterns of convergence and accommodation can be seen in Table 2. Tonic convergence is the position of the visual axes under conditions of dissociation with farpoint fixation. These are the maximum conditions for inhibition to convergence.

Fusional convergence is the range of performance in the convergence pattern due to Panum's area. It is a psycho-physiological range in the convergence pattern.

Accommodative convergence is that amount of convergence in action due to the innervation from accommodation.

Psychic convergence is that amount of convergence stimulated, because of the emotional and psychological reaction of the subject, to the surrounding environment.

5. Accommodation-Convergence Pattern

In the previous sections, accommodation and convergence patterns were discussed as if they operate in isolation. This is not the case, however, for these two patterns always are associated. In fact, it is more than just an association. These two patterns of behavior are integrated, the extent and degree of this integration depending upon the learned relationships existing within the total response pattern and to the fundamental matrix of behavior in the organism. This integration of the two patterns assures single binocular and clear vision for the environmental activities of the organism. When this integration is not adequate for the environmental demands upon the organism (internal or external), blurred or double vision will result.

The mere fact that this integration exists is of the utmost importance. But, of more interest from a refraction standpoint is that this integration forces the coordination of the autonomic nervous system (operating without conscious guidance) and the voluntary nervous system (operating with conscious guidance). It is only in the visual pattern motor system that we find that these two great sections of the central nervous system must integrate their activity. In all other sections of the behavior pattern we find that these portions of the central nervous system must coordinate their activities in *sequence* for the survival of the organism. That is, one nervous system will perform one part of the activity and the other nervous system will follow and finish the activity. For example, in eating, the mastication of our food is under the guidance of the voluntary system while the digestive action is under the guidance of the autonomic nervous system. *Only in the case of the visual pattern do we find that these two nervous systems must integrate their activity simultaneously in order to maintain clear and single vision for the organism.*

This poses a special problem for the organism. These two nervous systems must integrate their efforts in order to maintain proper stimulation to the accommodative and convergence patterns so that single and clear vision will always be available. This, in itself, would demand that each nervous system function with extreme accuracy in order to maintain the proper stimulative balance to these patterns. Unfortunately, we usually find that these two nervous systems are not at the same level of electrical activity, but that one of the nervous systems is in a dominant role.

At certain periods of the day, the autonomic nervous system is dominant and the skeletal nervous system is at minimum level of activity. At other times, the skeletal nervous system is at a dominant level and the autonomic system is at a low level of activity. The fluctuation in dominance of these two nervous systems demands that the organism create some sort of a buffer area to absorb the increased stimulation when one system becomes dominant. This buffer area in the central nervous system would absorb excessive stimulation and, thereby, preserve single binocular and clear vision, regardless of which nervous system is in the ascendancy.

The buffer area in the accommodative pattern is called *hyperopia*. The buffer area in the convergence pattern is called *exophoria*. *Hyperopia is thus a relationship between the patterns of accommodation and convergence to protect the integrity of the accommodative performance.* Hyperopia operates to protect the mechanism of accommodation against changes taking place between the patterns of accommodation and convergence. Hyperopia exists in the central nervous system. It is measured by the change in the accommodative mechanism induced by a plus lens which does not create an undesirable change in the pattern of convergence. Hyperopia is an expendable item, from an organism's viewpoint, in order to maintain clear vision in spite of the exigencies of the environment.

Exophoria is a relationship between the patterns of accommodation and convergence, operating to protect the integrity of the convergence performance. Exophoria exists in the central nervous system. It is measured by the amount of prism base-in required to align two dissociated images. Exophoria is a developmental or maturational relationship within the visual behavior pattern to protect convergence performance.

Any increased dominance in the voluntary (skeletal) or autonomic nervous system will cause increased stimulation proceeding to the accommodative and convergence patterns. This is absorbed by the buffer areas in these patterns so that the normal relationship between accommodation and convergence will be maintained. This will be noted by a decrease in the amount of exophoria and hyperopia.

Excessive conditions of dominance will tend to absorb all the buffer area which has been developed by the organism. This would be the condition of emmetropia and orthophoria. This is an undesirable condition since the individuals with these visual conditions no longer possess the necessary buffer areas to take care of increased stimulation due to shifts in pattern dominance. If increased stimulation is maintained despite the complete absorption of the existing buffer areas (exophoria and hyperopia), the organism must *actively inhibit* this stimulation. This is an emergency condition to cope with this problem since clear and single binocular vision must be maintained for organismic survival.

This active state of inhibition in the convergence pattern is called *esophoria.* It exists in the central nervous system and is measured by removing the need for the inhibition by means of a dissociating prism - the excessive stimuli proceed to the convergence mechanism and the non- dominant eye swings in. The amount of this turning in of the non-dominant eye is measured by the amount of prism base-out needed to align the two images. Esophoria functions on a high cortical level; it is inefficient and the organism attempts to eliminate this condition as quickly as possible by re-establishing an exophoric buffer. If the re-establishment of exophoria is impossible because of the continued dominance of the voluntary system or environmental demands, it will attempt to lower the esophoria to subcortical levels. This type of esophoria -structured esophoria- is a sign of a long-established visual problem. This is the type of esophoria that does not respond readily to treatment by plus lenses.

If the excessive stimulation proceeding to the visual pattern is due to autonomic dominance, lowered hyperopia will result. This lower hyperopia at near, combined with the nearpoint exophoria, will result in the nearpoint cross-cylinder net projecting into minus. This "minus projection" is an active state of inhibition between the patterns of convergence and accommodation to prevent blurring. Minus projection is found at near when the cross-cylinder gross findings are plano or in plus, but the cross-cylinder net values are in minus. Similarly, the hyperopia at far will start decreasing and an active state of inhibition will be found at this spatial area when the static retinoscopy test value is in minus, but the distant subjective finding is plano or in plus.

The organism utilizes these areas of tolerance (exophoria and hyperopia) to preserve the status quo of the visual pattern. If they are not sufficient to absorb the shock of the imposed stress upon the accommodative and convergence patterns, then the organism will actively inhibit (cortical level) this excessive stimulation, since single and clear vision is of survival value. If these inhibitions cannot be maintained, the organism either must discontinue the environmental occupation or radically alter its output or quality.

6. Exophoria and Hyperopia.

The question arises, "Where is the location of exophoria and hyperopia?" Before we can answer this question, we must recall the following basic physiological facts: Muscles and glands respond only when they have received efferent impulses from the central nervous system. Contraction or shortening of a muscle group can occur only when the proper innervational command has been forwarded from the central nervous system. Therefore, the overt movement of the eyes which we objectively observe when the patient has been dissociated must be due to the innervational pattern issuing from the central nervous system. It can, therefore, be said that exophoria and hyperopia exist in the central nervous system.

a. Exophoria is *measured* by the amount of prism base-in required to align the dissociated images.

b. Exophoria *exists* in the central nervous system.

c. Exophoria *operates* to protect the integrity of the mechanism of convergence against changes taking place between the components of the visual pattern.

We can state similarly for hyperopia:

a. Hyperopia is *measured* by the change in accommodation produced by means of plus lenses without producing an undesirable change in the pattern of convergence.

b. Hyperopia *exists* in the central nervous system.

c. Hyperopia *operates* to protect the mechanism of accommodation against changes taking place between the components of the visual pattern.

As long as single and clear binocular vision is being maintained by the organism, the buffer areas in the brain of exophoria and hyperopia will function solely as a means for compensating for the shifts in dominance between the skeletal and visceral nervous systems. Whenever we interfere with the existence of single binocular or clear vision with our probe bodies (lenses and prisms), these innervational patterns are no longer locked up within the central nervous system. These impulses will proceed to the exteroceptors and cause the overt action which we measure as exophoria (with base-in prism) or hyperopia (with plus lenses).

If the organism is forced to maintain concentration for prolonged periods within a restricted area at near, the size of these buffer areas will gradually decrease. When these buffer areas have been completely utilized, we will have the condition of emmetropia and orthophoria. If this intensified activity is continued, some sort of active inhibition must be established to preserve the survival skills of clear and single binocular vision. These stages of active inhibition are called esophoria and minus projection. These changes are summarized in Figure 5.

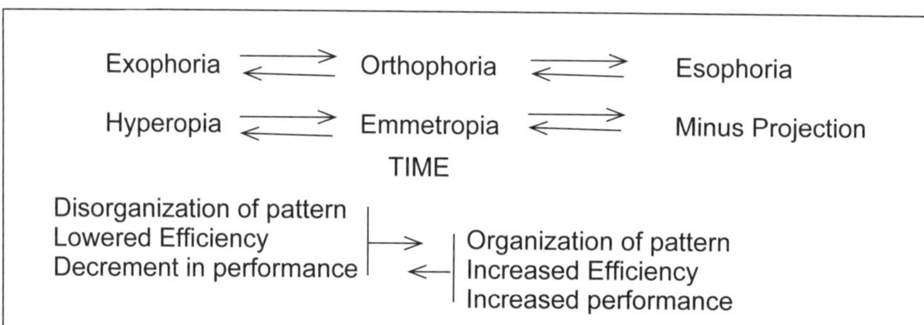

Figure 5.

Orthophoria is not merely the lack of exophoria; it is also a condition of equilibrium. Orthophoria is a dynamic condition which can be reached by a visual problem because of the absorption of the original maturational developed exophoria, or the organism has just managed to eliminate an existing condition of esophoria. Orthophoria, thus, is an indication of a downward trend or an upward trend, depending on the direction of the movement in the cycle occupied by the organism.

Similarly, emmetropia is not merely a passive stage, but rather a dynamic pivot condition. It can represent the inefficient downward progression from hyperopia, or it can represent the recovery from a condition of minus projection. Since there is no latitude of performance available, these equilibrium states of orthophoria and emmetropia, are undesirable conditions. Optometrically, we desire to shift the trend toward adequate development of hyperopia and exophoria.

In considering Figure 5, the changes shown in the convergence pattern and in the accommodative pattern, one must be careful not to insert parallel comparisons of exophoria with hyperopia, or orthophoria with emmetropia, or esophoria with minus projection. The time shifts in the convergence pattern will usually be different than the time shift in the accommodative pattern so we may frequently find exophoria associated with emmetropia or with minus projection. Similarly, we may have orthophoria associated with emmetropia or hyperopia. We can have esophoria associated with hyperopia, emmetropia or minus projection (only if the esophoria is found at far and the case has exophoria at near). In addition, we must be aware that while moderate amounts of exophoria are highly desirable and indicate a more efficient operation of the convergence mechanism, when the organism has been exposed to continual visual stress it may create quantities of exophoria of such magnitude that it may lead to suppression or even to the development of intermittent exotropia. In Figure 6 this is graphically shown with the range of from 4 to 9 exophoria indicating the maximum efficient operation of the convergence pattern, whereas higher exophoria

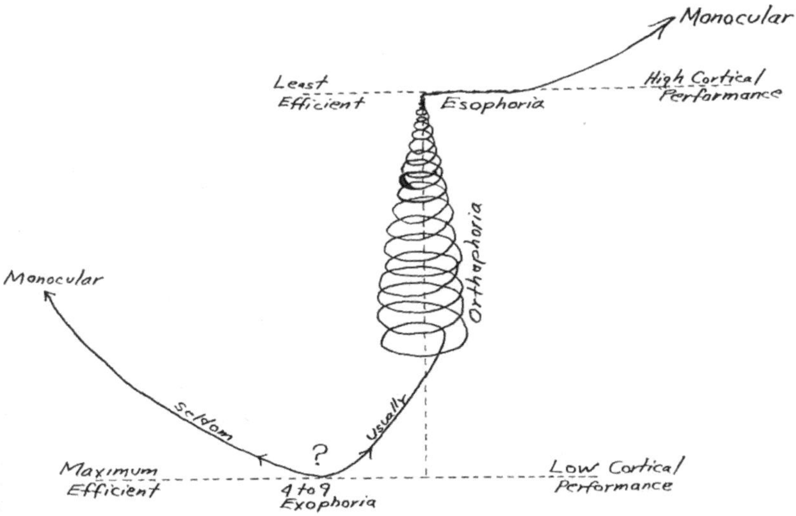

Figure 6.

indicates a decrease in efficiency (from the standpoint that monocular patterns tend to develop) and orthophoria shown as an ascending spiral indicates that we are now reaching a higher cortical level adaptation which is less efficient. Similarly, another construction could be made for the accommodative pattern to indicate that moderate hyperopia (one to one-half diopter) is highly efficient. If we build much higher magnitudes of hyperopia, it indicates a less efficient development since these also tend to lead to monocular adaptations. Emmetropia, in this diagram, would also be an ascending spiral indicating that it leads to a higher cortical level performance with a drop in efficiencies.

What Is It? Where Is It?

We have discussed accommodation and convergence as mere events that occur in the central nervous system. However, what are the events that trigger the overt patterns of accommodation and convergence? Is it the desire of the organism to determine what it is, or where it is, that stimulates the accommodative and convergence patterns? It is not an easy task to determine, what is it? In order to make this determination we must separate figure from ground. This requires motor activity on the part of the organism. He must either touch it, walk toward it or name it in order to maintain the isolation of the figure from the ground. The smaller the target, the dimmer the illumination upon the target; the lower the contrast of the target and the greater the unfamiliarity with the target the more vigorous the motor activity becomes.

At the same time we must locate where it is. This requires that the organism initiate a search pattern to scan the incoming visual stimuli and to make the necessary corrective movements to maintain an incoming pattern of maximum intensity. Again this is a motor activity.

What is it? This question requires that we identify the target and it is the covert pattern of identification which triggers the overt pattern of accommodation. Similarly, the "where is it?" requires the covert pattern of centering which activates the overt pattern of convergence.

Process	Covert Pattern	Overt Pattern
What is it?	Identification	Accommodation
Where is it?	Centering	Convergence

The greater the demand for precise identification of the target, i.e., smaller the print, the more difficult the vocabulary and/or the subjects unfamiliarity with the material, the greater the amount of accommodation that will be stimulated. This is easily observed by means of book retinoscopy, wherein we observe the retinoscopic reflex as the patient reads material at various grade levels. If we give a child with a reading level of the third grade second grade reading material, we will observe a “with” motion by means of the retinoscope. If we now require the same child to read third grade material, we will find a “neutral” motion. However, if we frustrate the child by presenting fifth grade material we will now observe an “against” motion. At all times in this experiment we are utilizing the same test distance. Therefore, these changes in retinoscopic motion are not due to any other variation of experimental conditions except the level of the reading material.

Similarly, if we present demands for increased centering, we will find that the patient will progress from exophoria with the easy material, orthophoria with material at grade level, and esophoria with very difficult material. Thus increased centering demands are observed through the overt pattern of convergence.

Thus, centering and identification are the processes in the central nervous system which involve the naming and location of the source of stimulation. Accommodation and convergence are the mechanisms in the central nervous system which involve these activities of the organism.

CHAPTER III
The Visual Problem

Two assumptions regarding visual problems commonly encountered are: that all visual problems are problems of acuity; and that when the refractive error is corrected, all visual problems must cease.

The proof that the first assumption is not adequate to explain visual problems consists of evidence that has been gathered in occupational vision programs. If industry were to select the worker on the basis of distant visual acuity, it would be selecting the individuals with the poorest near-point efficiency.

The inadequacy of the second assumption is based on clinical research which has shown that the most uncomfortable cases and those least amenable are either emmetropic or orthophoric, or both. A visual problem is caused by erroneous visual behavior that arises from the stresses imposed upon man because of the socially compulsive, near-centered task.

A visual problem is a decrement in visual performance which is not acceptable to the patient or to his social-economic environment. Thus, a visual problem does not live in isolation from its environment. Where there are two subjects with the same visual measurements, one working in an environment with limited demand and the other in an environment of intensive demand, the former would not have a visual problem, while the latter would have a visual problem. Thus, measurement by itself is not sufficient for the diagnosis of a visual problem. A careful and complete case history must be taken in order to determine the environmental demand factor. It is for this reason that we frequently will have a subject with grotesque distortions in his visual measurements who will have no subjective complaints; another individual with slight deviation from the normal measurements will have serious complaints. *A visual problem cannot exist in isolation; it can only be measured in relationship to the environmental demand.*

The problem of efficient vision is further complicated in that we have both efficient monocular vision and efficient binocular vision. Here, we are considering efficiency in terms of achievement in reading symbols on a flat surface. Many of these monocular cases are thus surprised when they find out that they are using only one eye. The visually uncomfortable are those individuals who were unable to make a complete monocular adaptation. It is for this reason that the monocular case, who is going to receive visual training, should be informed that he is going to have a period of

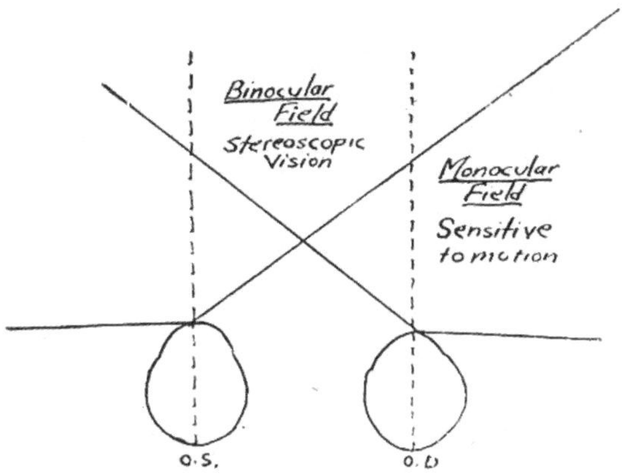

Figure 7. Distant vision.

uncomfortable vision while he is making the transition from this adaptation to efficient binocular vision.

The caveman's environment placed dependence upon his ability to achieve at far. He had to be able to see at a distance to kill enough game for survival and so he could detect danger at the earliest possible moment and then could prepare for fight or flight. The complex environment of modern civilization places increasing demands upon the human organism, placing a premium upon adequately conquering a nearpoint world of 13 inches. *Editors' note: Dr. Manas used 13 inches.* Nearpoint visual demands are constantly increasing. The reading load in our educational institutions has increased 150% in the past 10 years. (Any citation for this or should we make editors note of when this is referring to?) An analysis of all persons gainfully employed revealed that somewhere between 80% and 90% of these individuals are required to perform more near work than far work.

This shift in environmental emphasis from distance to near has necessitated a shift in the type of visual pattern necessary for survival of the organism. Binocular vision was developed by the species because of the benefits of wider form fields and stereoscopic vision. The increased peripheral fields were a sensitive indicator of any motion and, therefore, warned man of approaching danger. Stereoscopic vision gave man a means for the precise location of objects in space.

The shrinkage of our visual environment to 13" has nullified the benefits we receive from the increased peripheral field and stereoscopic vision. The sensitivity of the peripheral field to motion disturbs us when we are concentrating upon a constricted area at a distance of 13". In the same manner, stereoscopic vision has little benefit when we are concentrating

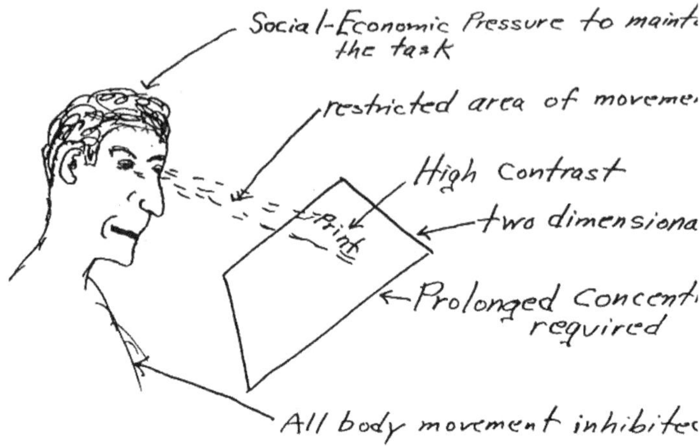

Figure 8.

upon a flat surface at 13". Is it any wonder that visual problems have multiplied when we consider that modern civilization has placed a premium upon neglecting or suppressing the two great benefits given to our species in obtaining single binocular vision? (See Figure 7.)

The original use of our visual sense was for the purpose of discriminating size, space, position and movement of objects at a great distance. The modern use of our visual sense requires a maintained visual concentration within a restricted area of movement, over a protracted period of time, at a close working distance (Figure 8.) This abnormal situation produces a distortion in the visual behavior pattern which produces a visual problem. A visual problem is accompanied by lowered visual achievement. This lowered achievement may be in acuity rather than in interpretation, or the reverse.

1. Types of Visual Problems.

All visual problems can be placed into one or more of the following categories:

a. Those who have lost acuity:
   (1) distant (myope, amblyope, absolute hyperope, astigmat, squinter).
   (2) near (presbyope).
b. Those who have uncomfortable vision (anisometrope, emmetrope, orthophore, minus projection).
c. Those who have unsatisfactory achievement (retarded reader, non-reader, unsatisfactory industrial producers).
   d. Cosmetic reasons (squinter).

These varieties of visual problems arise from a common etiological factor - *the effect of environmental stress upon the biochemical makeup of the individual.* Thus, a group of children, all exposed to the same environmental stress, will develop a spectrum in variety and degree of various visual problems. The following factors can cause one child to make the myopic adaptation, and another child to develop anisometropia: (a) dietary factors; (b) hereditary predispositions; (c) type of previous environmental exposure; (d) the home demand upon the child. Thus, the resulting visual syndrome will be quite different despite the fundamental sameness of the applied stress. Selye *(The Story of the Adaptation Syndrome.* p. 105), discusses how a common stressor agent may cause a variety of effects, "The same stressor may cause a variety of diseases by selectively conditioning or deconditioning some parts of the stress response. Actually, this situation is not without precedent in medicine. It is known that the same, well identified pathogen, the tuberculosis bacillus, may produce: pulmonary phthisis, meningitis, peritonitis, Pott's disease, military tuberculosis or tuberculosis lupus of the skin. Before it had been shown that all these conditions could be reproduced by infection with tuberculosis bacilli; it would have seemed quite unreasonable to think of them as being in any way related to each other. A list of more dissimilar maladies could hardly have been made up. Yet, we are certain now that all these are diseases produced by the same micro-organism. Their polymorphic nature must be ascribed to conditioning circumstances, such as: differences in hereditary, traumatic, nutritional, serologic factors, the portal of infection, and many other agents which selectively render certain tissues "loci minoris resistentiae (a place of less resistance)."

2. The Development of the Visual Problem

Nearpoint tasks do not create visual problems because of the task distance. It is not the increased muscle effort at this near distance that is imposing stresses upon accommodation and convergence. Nearpoint tasks have become synonymous with the existence of visual problems. It is the continuous concentration within a restricted area of movement, in a two-dimensional plane, that creates visual problems at nearpoint. When the same conditions exist at some other distance, we will have visual problems arise from that activity. For example, many patients became aware of unsatisfactory achievement when they started observing television.

The change in visual achievement of the worker as he continues at the visual task (that requires continuous concentration) is graphed in Figure 9. You will note that the maximum change in visual achievement occurs within a relatively short time. The organism then starts the process of reor-

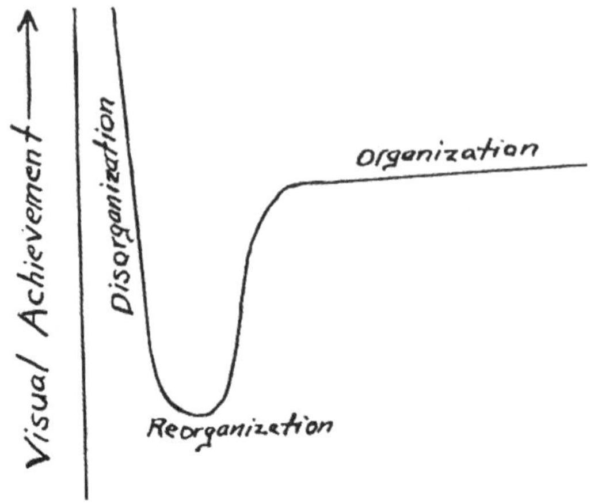

Figure 9. The impact of time upon visual achievement.

ganization in order to recover some of its original achievement ability. The individual will do this by making certain adaptations or concessions. Usually, it will be found that he has succeeded in organizing his pattern to the visual task, but that his achievement will not be as high as that in his original, unimpaired condition.

The curve shown in Figure 9 is typical of the change in magnitude of many physical and physiological measurements when a system has been placed under a constraint. If, for instance, we take a liquid and place it within a thermostatically controlled vessel, so that the temperature of the liquid can be slowly lowered, we obtain a curve which is very similar to that shown in Figure 9. We first obtain a gradual lowering in temperature of the liquid. Then the process of crystallization occurs, and when the heat liberates, we obtain an increase in temperature. The result is a leveling off of the cooling curve as long as solidification occurs. This would be the typical cooling curve.

Not all liquids will give the typical response. In fact, some liquids will give either the typical or an atypical response, depending upon test conditions. This atypical response, of a liquid under cooling conditions, is the formation of a frozen-oil rather than the formation of a crystalline solid. We also have this atypical response with our visual data. Figure 10 illustrates the normal change in phoria values under the typical response and also the time-change curve for the two atypical situations. The normal exophoric child, upon impact of the visual task, will show a sudden decrease in the magnitude of the exophoria and finally the change into orthophoria and esophoria. With this lowering into esophoria, which is an emergency condition, the organism starts building into exophoria.

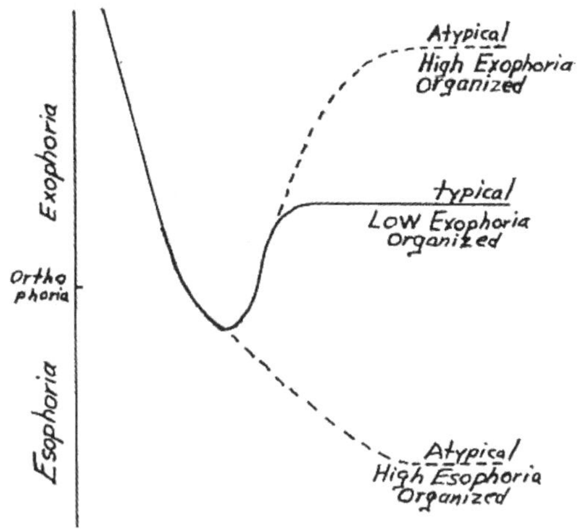

Figure 10. The typical and atypical responses as found in the phoria test values.

This is the typical response shown by the organism. Sometimes, when the organism makes the dip into esophoria, it finds it is unable to make the transition into exophoria. The individual will structure into high esophoria, which is an atypical response. We have other subjects who, when making the transition from esophoria into exophoria, are not able to level off at a nominal amount of exophoria. In this exophoric, atypical response, the organism will keep on building exophoria in the amount of from 15 to 20D before it levels off. Thus, the two atypical responses, are on opposite ends of the spectrum of possible phoria test values. The atypical, high exophoric individual, with his organized adaptation, will absorb minus sphere stimulus like a sponge. This individual will come into the office with nearpoint complaints, and he will have 15D of exophoria through plano. Minus one sphere is prescribed, and the patient is dismissed for a progress report. He will usually return at the end of one month with comfort at near. After he has had this correction for several months, he will have a return of his original complaint. If a phoria is now taken, the subject will reveal the same amount of phoria through the minus sphere as he originally had through the plano lens. In other words, there is a difference in the immediate response to the minus sphere, as to its effect upon the convergence pattern, when compared to the effect upon the convergence pattern after it has been continually worn for some time.

Similarly, the patient who exhibits the atypical, high esophoric response will also give this same rebound to the application of plus sphere for near-point wear. The following case illustrates the changes in phoria value

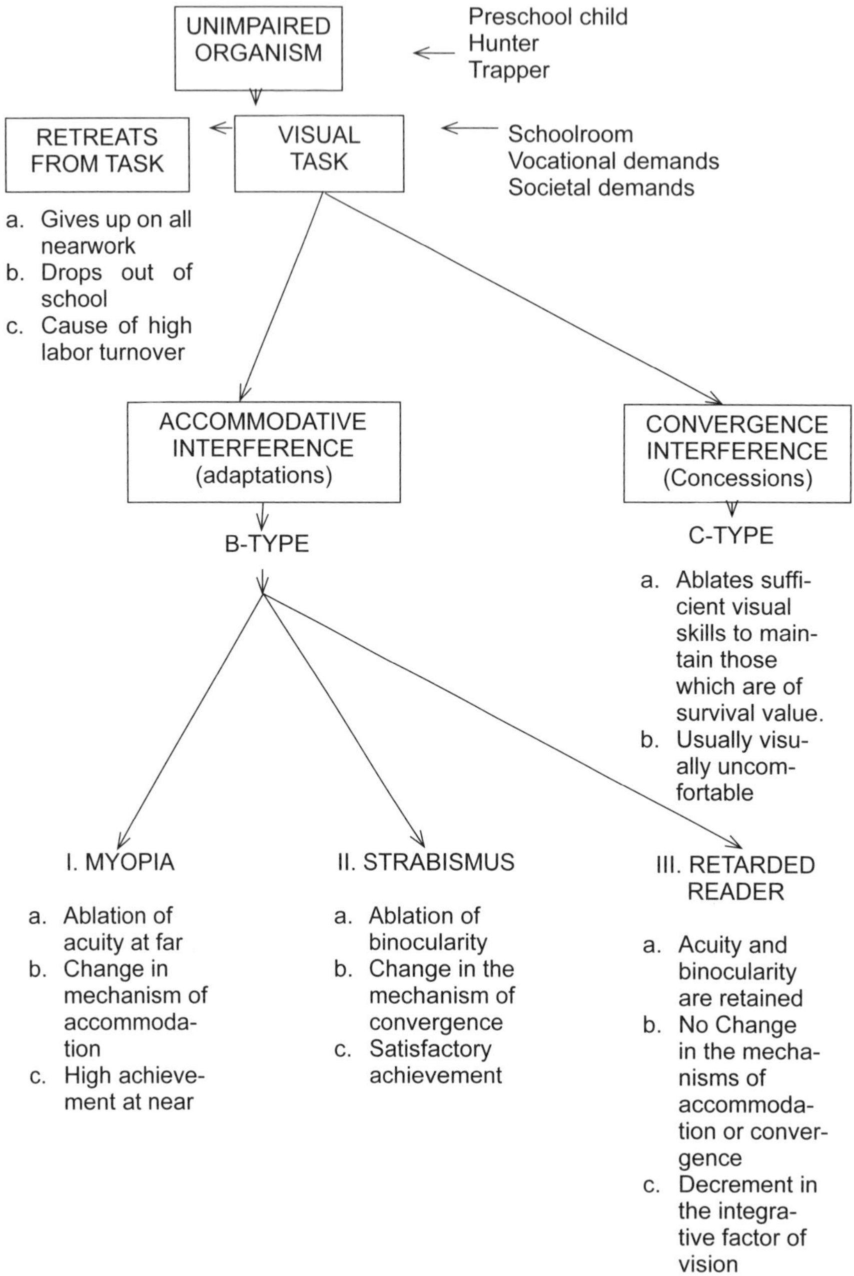

NOTE: Most adaptations are not clear cut, but are combinations of the above.

Figure 11. The reaction of the unimpaired organism to a visual task.

with plus lens application at near. The patient was a beginning presbyope; distant prescription remained stable.

	Induced Phoria At Far (#8)	Nearpoint Add	Induced Phoria at Near (#15A)
3/10/47	12 Esophoria	+0.50 D.	10 Esophoria
11/7/50	12 Esophoria	+1.25 D.	12 Esophoria
9/14/51	16 Esophoria	+1.25 D.	10 Esophoria
8/16/52	12 Esophoria	+1.50 D.	15 Esophoria
4/16/53	18 Esophoria	+2.00 D.	13 Esophoria

Thus, contrary to normal expectations, we found that the nearpoint phoria test value remained in high esophoria in spite of increased plus sphere application at nearpoint. Simple lens application was not adequate for the visual problem that was exhibiting an atypical response. For this case visual training, as well as lens application, was used in order to re-establish a normal visual pattern.

What causes one individual to give one type of response and another individual of the same age to give an atypical response depends upon many factors. Some of these factors are: heredity, growth, diet, previous infection, injury, and emotional and environmental demands. The important environmental demands are: intensity of demand, area of concentration, intensity of illumination, contrast, and body posture required.

Every portion of the visual pattern will give either the typical or atypical response when exposed to the environment. Thus, it becomes very important to determine not only the magnitude of the various visual tests, but also the organizational status of the visual pattern as well. The patient exhib-

8/7/51 Tilts head when she reads. Eyes tear after wathcing TV	5/9/52 Misses words when she reads	10/11/53 School system: Reading way below class level. Trouble with spelling. Eyes water when she reads. Mother-"Child seem very nervous.
#3 1 Eso	#3 4 Eso	#3 1 Eso
#13A 2 Exo		#13A 3 Eso
#4 -1.25 -0.75	#4 +.50 -.50 x 180° +.50 -.50 x 180°	#4 +.25 +.25
#7 -0.75 20/20 -0.25 20/30	#7 +.50 -.50 x 180° +.50 -.50 x 180° 20/20	#7 plano plano 20/20
#8 3 Eso	#8 6 Eso	#8 1 Eso
Rx: +1.00 D. O.U. for Near	Rx: Continue wearing glasses	

iting the measurements of disorganization (disembedding) can be handled much easier as far as lens application is concerned. The patient exhibiting the measurements of organization (embedding), cannot be handled properly by lens application alone. Visual training is needed for these cases.

Upon receiving the impact of the visual task, the organism tends to retreat or narrow the visual environment to such an extent that it can function effectively in this restricted area. Three types of functional visual changes can result from this impact between visual task and organism, namely, adventitious myopia, adventitious strabismus, or low achievement (retarded reader).

1. The adventitious myope: (a) ablates acuity at far; (b) changes the mechanism of accommodation; (c) attains a high order of achievement at near.

2. The adventitious strabismic: (a) ablates binocularity; (b) changes the mechanism of convergence; (c) attains a satisfactory visual adaptation.

3. The low achiever: (a) retains acuity and binocularity; (b) does not change in the accommodative or convergence mechanism; (c) remains on a low level of visual achievement.

See Figure 11 for the reaction of the unimpaired organism to a visual task.

It is not to be construed from Figure 11 that the organism will make a clear cut choice of one of the three basic adaptations of myopia, strabismus or poor achievement. Very often the organism will explore one type of adaptation, and it will then retreat and start a second type of adaptation. Thus, we have many poor readers or poor achievers who, because of parental pressure, will put in many hours on their school assignments and pass their courses. These individuals will very often develop low degrees of myopia as an auxiliary adaptation.

Sometimes the lens application of the practitioner may cause the blocking of a particular organismic adaptation, and the patient will start on another pathway of adaptation. The following case illustrates this situation:

Initially, the child was exploring the myopic adaptation. The +1.00D spheres prescribed by the practitioner to block the myopia were successful, for at 5/9/52 the myopia was no longer present. The myopia was gone, but now the child was dropping in achievement. By 10/11/53 the child was a reading poorly. One adaptation had been stopped; a new one had taken its place. Perhaps the cure was worse than the disease. This could have been prevented by applying visual training simultaneously with the application of the plus spheres.

The characteristic response of a biological system is its ability to adapt. The process of adaptation allows the biological system to shift its equilibrium in such a way as to minimize the impact of the environmental stress. If the environmental stress is of such a magnitude that it exceeds the adaptability of the organism, then death will ensue. Thus, the human organism cannot live above a certain altitude because of the decreased oxygen content of the air. The various body systems have a certain flexibility of operation which allows them to function in spite of an external change in the environment. The various body systems have a certain *latitude of performance* which will allow adaptation to occur so that the effect of the change in the environment can be minimized. Of course, if the environmental change is of such a magnitude that it exceeds the *latitude of performance,* very serious consequences will ensue. The visual system, with its extreme importance for the survival of man, also has certain latitudes of performance available. Just as the respiratory and circulatory systems of man will undergo adaptation to environmental changes, so will the visual system adapt to environmental changes. If the adaptation occurs in the accommodative pattern, the result is the development of myopia (or, less hyperopia; or greater change in one sensory structure than the other with resultant anisometropia). If the adaptation occurs in the convergence pattern, the result is the development of strabismus (or convergence instability). If the adaptation occurs in the symbolic pattern, the result is the development of the poor reader (or poor achiever).

3. Which Adaptation?

The primary characteristic of any living system is its ability to adapt to changes in environmental demands. It is these adaptive changes which modify the organism. These adaptations must serve a useful purpose in that they allow the organism to function optimally through a restricted range. There are two basic areas in which visual adaptations may occur. These are accommodation or convergence. The adaptation may be primarily in one of these areas, or we may have a mixture type of adaptation in which both areas have been utilized. We also have the individual that will maintain the accommodative and convergence status quo but make a cortical adaptation which leads to the problem of the poor reader. The five basic changes to visual stress are illustrated in Figure 12. One visual reaction is not given in this figure since the subject makes the decision not to adapt by retreating from the task. He quits school or his job rather than try to make some type of survival adaptation.

You will note in Figure 12 that which visual adaptation the organism will make depends upon the age at which environmental demands are encountered. If they occur early in life (prior to four years of age), they will lead to esotropia (or high esophoria) or to the development of high hyperopia. If the impact of environmental demand occurs later in life (four years of age or later), we have the adaptations of exotropia or myopia. The adapta-

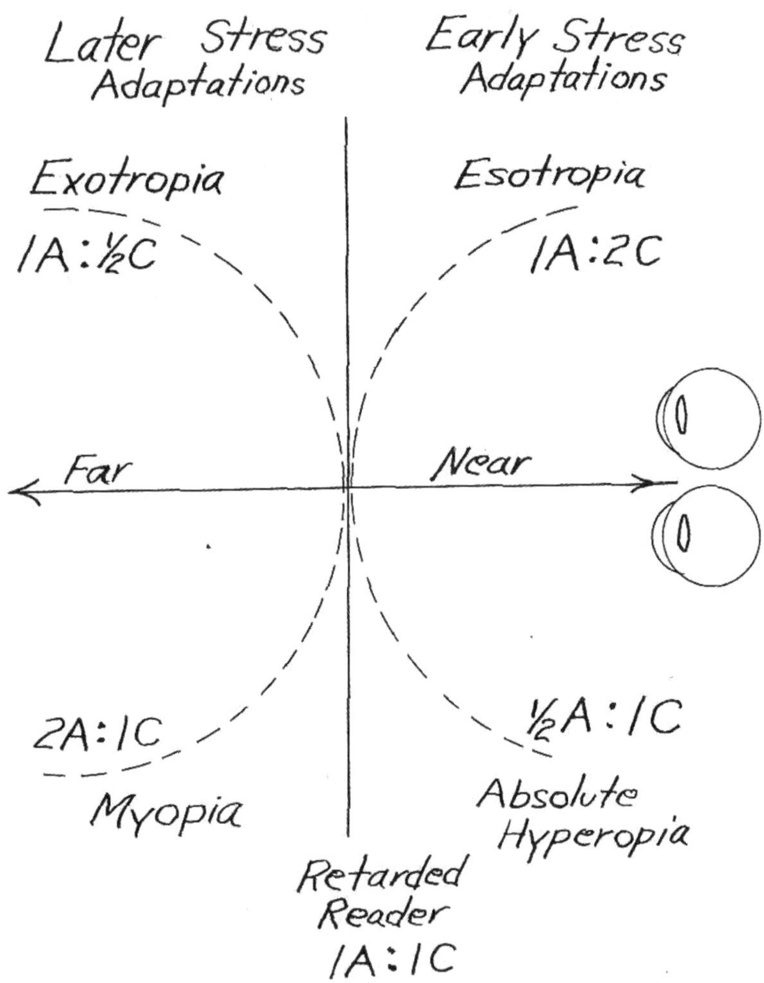

Figure 12.

tion of the poor reader occurs at that age when the organism must learn the vicarious interpretation of symbols.

In interpreting Figure 12, the numerical designations used for each of the adaptations does not indicate prism diopters or lens diopters but merely is a code to indicate whether the associated pattern is inadequate, adequate, or excessive for the demand situation. Thus:

lA: 1C Adequate pattern of accommodation associated with an adequate pattern of convergence.

½/A: 1C Inadequate pattern of accommodation associated with an adequate pattern of convergence.

2A: 1C excessive patterning of accommodation associated with an adequate pattern of convergence.

4. The Adventitious Myope

The adventitious myope is the individual who has acquired myopia at about the age of eight, and thus differs from the congenital myope.

The myope no longer has a lowered visual achievement at the point where visual achievement is of vital importance- at nearpoint. The existence of such myopia is a sign that a visual problem was present and that the cause of it still is present. It is well-known that the myope can reorganize his visual behavior pattern for efficient performance at near. This reorganization will spread to the whole visual behavior pattern and result in lower distant acuity.

The comment of Giles (*The Practice of Orthoptics*, 2nd ed:19) regarding the development of anisometropia: ". . . The child is born with hypermetropia. Myopia is seldom developed under ages 10 to 12 except in very special cases. Less hypermetropia in one eye can be regarded as an arrested tendency towards myopia."

Tiffin's data *(Industrial Psychology:*153) for the silk looping job, shows a decreased number of employees were able to pass a distance acuity test with experience on the job. The steady increase in the percent of myopes in each class, as we proceed from the first to the eighth grades, is indicative of the effect of the increased nearpoint demand upon the visual pattern of these students. It is almost a maxim with the teacher that the best students are wearing minus lenses.

The adventitious myope is an individual who had standard acuity at far, and lost it, but to whom it can be restored by means of a minus lens. The cyclic steps of adaptation leading to adventitious myopes are: (a) a daily recurrent vocational myope; (b) a "fixed" myope with loss of distant vision, but still having a plus net in the cross cylinder test values; (c) increased myopia at far, minus projection at near; (d) equal amounts of myopia at far and near (stabilized).

In the first developmental stage of myopia, the prescription of plus lenses for near work will reverse the tendency of going through the complete myopic cycle.

In the second stage, it is much more difficult to create reversed conditions. It is best corrected by means of acceptable plus at near and the minimum minus at far to meet distant visual acuity requirements. Visual training will aid in these cases.

The third stage in the myopic cycle is more difficult because it is necessary to establish plus acceptance at near through training before plus can be given at near. It would be difficult to prescribe for these cases without visual training. A lens prescription by itself will usually speed up the progression through the myopic cycle.

When the myope has reached the fourth stage, he is completely stabilized and he can wear his distant correction for both far and near work with efficiency and comfort. In these cases, changes in distant correction will usually be very small. If the stabilized myope is brought into a different environment that requires increased efficiency at near, the myopic cycle may be repeated. The myope has taken this pathway of adaptation in order to achieve increased efficiency at near.

The adventitious myope, in almost all cases, characteristically will show a better production rate, less wastage, and less time lost from the job than his hyperopic counterpart. The indiscriminate application of minus lenses to industrial nearpoint workers has often resulted in worse performance on the production line. The myopic worker must be given his appropriate lens at near which may and often will differ from his far-point requirements if we are to avoid a decreased performance of the myopic worker.

5. The Adventitious Strabismic

The adventitious squinter has made an extreme adaptation in binocularity in order to obtain increased efficiency at near. These individuals will usually have excellent reading rates and comprehension and seldom complain of discomfort, but are usually brought to the optometric office because of the cosmetic defect. Contrary to expectations, very few of these strabismics ever complain of diplopia. They may note some diplopia for a few moments at some new task, but it is readily kept under control. Single vision is of survival value; therefore, when binocularity is given up, the transition to monocularity is rapid. That is, suppression occurs and many of these cases have amblyopia. The action of turning one eye in or out moves the stimulus patch away from the macular region into the peripheral retina area, thereby finding it easier to suppress the visual activity of the eye.

The cycle of adaptation for the adventitious divergent strabismic is: (a) intermittent squint at far, none at near; (b) increased squint at far, intermittent squint at near; (c) increased squint at far, slight squint at near; (d) equal degree of squint at far and near.

The cycle of adaptation for the adventitious convergent strabismic is: (a) intermittent squint at near, none at far; (b) fixed squint at near, intermittent at far; (c) increased squint at near, fixed squint at far; (d) equal amount of squint at far and near.

6. The Poor Reader (poor achiever)

The contraction of the environment on the part of the myope and the strabismic is easily seen. In one case, we have loss of distant vision; for the strabismic, we have the cosmetic appearance, as well as the elimination of one eye from normal use. Less obvious is the idea that the poor reader has likewise contracted his environment by an avoidance procedure. The distortion of the visual behavior pattern that lowers visual achievement results in a lessened ability to interpret or get meaning from the printed page. This lowered ability to extract meaning from "symbols" will make for poor reading performance. The poor reader in the schools is the socially undisciplined prototype of the visually ineffective person throughout life.

These individuals usually have no symptoms of visual discomfort, for *discomfort occurs when the level of achievement is unsatisfactory to the organism*. The only yardstick of measurement that remains is the achievement in the given situation in which the patient is found, as compared with that of others in comparable levels of intelligence and instruction.

It is this group which creates the largest economic loss to society. They have the intelligence to be creators, but because of the lowered visual achievement are environmental failures. *It is this group which offers the greatest challenge to our profession.*

7. Ocular Fatigue

The majority of the patients seeking optometric assistance do so because of the subjective complaint of visual discomfort. Attempts to account for this phenomenon have been made on the basis that the eye muscles get "tired."

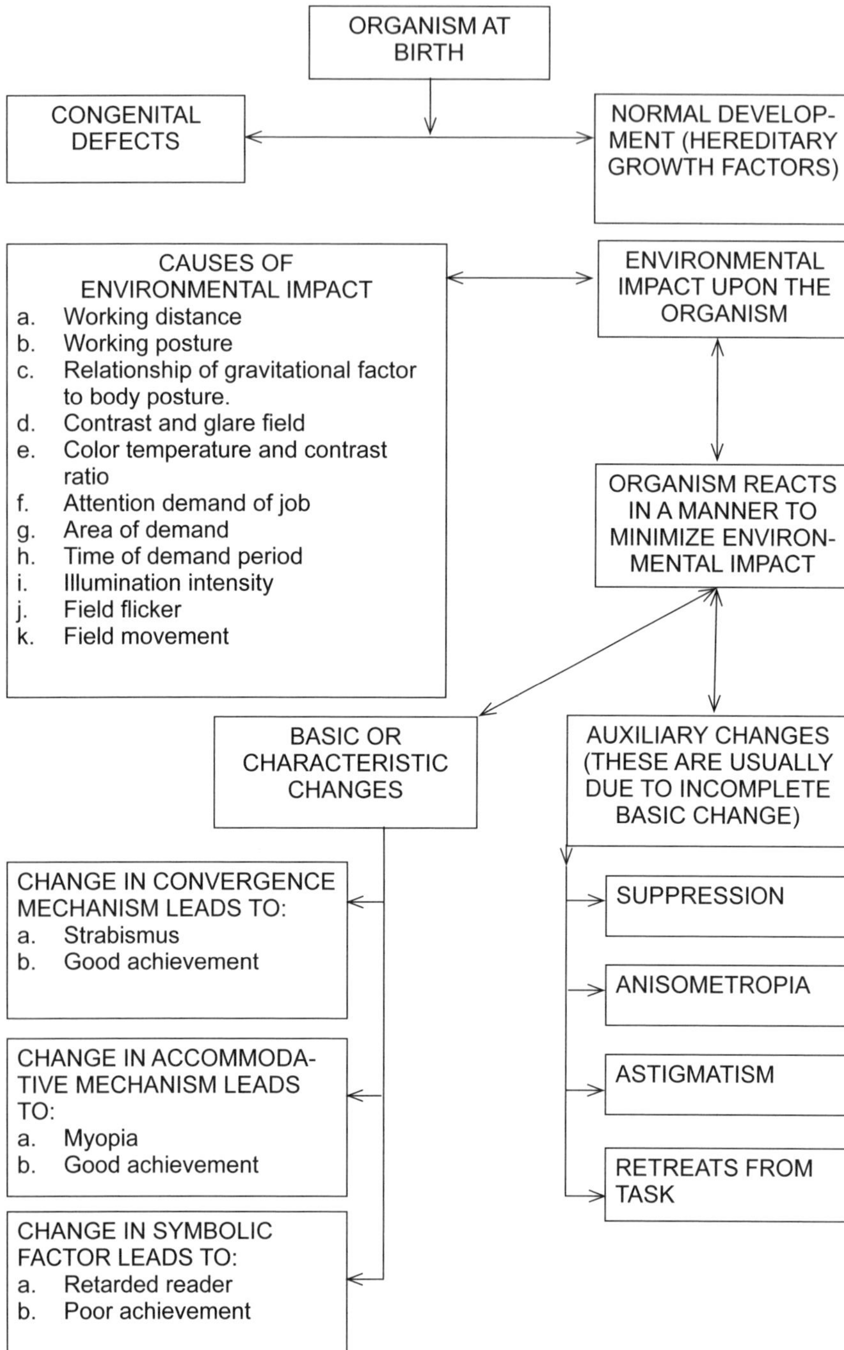

Figure 13. The development of a visual problem

This is seemingly borne out by the usual physiological demonstration of muscle fatigue. A muscle-nerve preparation is made and mounted in such a manner that when the nerve is stimulated and the contraction occurs it will move a lever which will magnify the amount of movement and record same on a rotating drum. As the muscle continues to receive stimulations, the amount of contraction decreases until finally a time is reached when stimulation of the nerve-muscle preparation results in no movement of the muscle. The muscle is now said to be in a state of fatigue. This would seem to lend credence to the idea that the patient using his eyes all day would finally reach this condition and he would experience ocular fatigue.

A closer examination of the problem of ocular fatigue reveals the inadequacy of this simple physiological explanation. Targast, in 1873, counted the fibers in nerve and muscle. He made the important observation that in the extra-ocular muscles of sheep, the ratio was one nerve fiber to three muscle fibers; whereas, the corresponding ratio in the muscle of the limb was one nerve fiber to 80 muscle fibers.

Lancaster calculated that the total force needed to move the eyeball 10 degrees in 0.03 seconds is less than 10 grams. He also found that the extra-ocular muscles were individually capable of exerting a force of from 500 to 1,000 grams. This means that the eye muscles are from 50 to 100 times larger than necessary to perform their function. It is therefore, necessary for only a small fraction of the total muscle fibers to contract at any one moment in order to move the eyeball. *The physiological arrangement is organized for prolonged activity without fatigue.* It is difficult on the basis of the existing eye mechanism to say that the muscles get tired and, therefore, the patient experiences those symptoms which we have labeled as asthenopia. We must look elsewhere for the meaning of the subjective patient expression, "My eyes feel tired."

Fatigue is one of those common words which seem so familiar to us until we attempt to define it. The literature is replete with definitions of fatigue.

"Fatigue is the decreased capacity for doing work as a direct result of having worked; the amount of decrement varies with the duration, rate and intensity of the work, and with the initial strength or capacity of the organic mechanisms involved." Spaeth (*The Problem of Fatigue. J Ind Hyg 1919;*1:22).

"Fatigue is a comprehensive term which in its widest application embraces all those immediate and temporary changes, whether of a functional or organic character, which take place within an organism or any of its constituent parts as a direct result of its own exertions and which tend to interfere with or inhibit the organism's future activity." - Ash *(Fatigue And Its Effects Upon Control. Arch Psych 1914;4(3).*

"In the total organic pattern, the activity of striped muscle modifies the efferent impulses from these muscles to the central nervous system. These efferent impulses change the functions of the central nervous system, the central nervous system influences the efferent impulses to the muscles, and these impulses alter the conditions and activities of the muscles."- Cason *(The Organic Nature of Fatigue. Am J Psychol 1935;47:337).*

"Fatigue is characterized by: (a) a decreased capacity for work, known as work decrement; (b) modification in the physiological state of the individual; (c) a feeling of weariness." - Guilford (*Fields of Psychology:498).*

"Fatigue really has two components, one is the feeling of fatigue, the subjective experience which makes the person feel as though he must slow down or stop work. The second is the actual incapacity of the organism to function efficiently." - Gilliland, Morgan, and Stevens (*General Psychology:462).*

Regarding ocular discomfort, Bartley states, "It has been supposed that discomfort localized in the eyes must originate there. Evidence suggests that the localized discomfort is a function of the organism as a whole, becoming thus localized when visual achievement becomes unsatisfactory." - *(Psychosomatic Medicine J.,* Oct., 1942)

Murroughs and Manas (*Optometric Wkly 1944;35:1189)* point out, "The sensation of pain (ocular discomfort), therefore, is protective in nature, giving warning of the injurious nature of the stimulus. These impulses are imperative and pre-potent, other stimuli being ignored for the time being. The sensation of fatigue warns the organism of future danger if the particular function is not stopped."

We can enumerate the following regarding visual discomfort: (a) It involves the whole organism; (b) it is the product of the central nervous system; (c) it protects the organism against impairment of vital processes. Both the organism and the environment are contributory factors in creating visual discomfort. From the environment, we have the pressure of environmental demand. The organism provides a certain visual performance. If environmental demand exceeds the visual performance ability of the individual, he will experience visual discomfort. If his visual performance ability exceeds his environmental demand, the patient will have visual comfort. If at any time the environmental demand should exceed the limits of visual performance ability, the organism must send out some kind of distress signal, a warning to itself, that visual curtailment or functioning in the environment must occur. This warning, or distress signal, is *visual discomfort*. For the purpose of comparison, we can state that visual discomfort is analogous to the knocking noise of a gasoline engine. When the demand (or load) upon the gasoline engine exceeds the performance ability of the motor, a knocking noise is heard. This knocking sound is a warning that if the driver doesn't do something to correct the situation, eventual motor failure will occur. Visual discomfort serves the same function for the human organism.

The term "visual performance" refers to the totality of visual abilities possessed by the organism. At birth, visual performance is very poor. It rapidly improves with age and is at its peak value in the early teens. Thereafter, a gradual decline in visual performance occurs. At birth, environmental demand is zero. As growth continues, this gradually increases. With the entry of the child into the school system, environmental demand starts increasing rapidly. Thereafter, environmental demand is constantly increasing since it is the composite of the demands of school, recreation, vocation and social life upon the organism. When the curve of visual performance intersects the curve for environmental demand, active visual discomfort starts. This is graphically illustrated in Figure 14.

The actual shape of these curves for a particular individual would vary, depending upon his environment and the efficiency of his visual pattern. The visual performance curve for a farmer would reach its peak in the early teens and then taper off very gradually. The environmental demand curve for this farmer would reach its peak while in school and would decrease rapidly. Therefore, for this farmer the visual performance curve and the environmental demand curve would cross very late in life. Contrast this with the case of the accountant; his visual performance curve would reach its peak in the teens and, thereafter, drop at an ever-increasing speed because of the economic, social, and vocational demands. In the case of the accountant, these two curves will cross at a much earlier age.

Unless death intervenes, at some point in his life cycle every individual will need visual rehabilitation, regardless of social, recreational, or vocational demands.

Figure 14 illustrates how careful we must be in evaluating patient response. Many patients will testify that they have no discomfort and that they enjoy reading. Yet, your case study will indicate the presence of extensive adaptations and visual concessions. It is obvious that the patient does not do

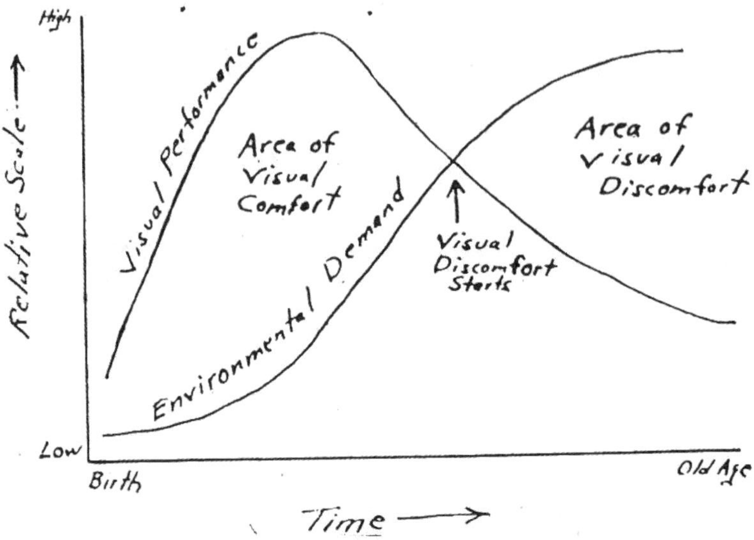

Figure 14. The relationship between visual performance and environmental demand.

any near work. Usually, extensive questioning will reveal that the patient likes to read, but that somehow he is unable to find the time to do any reading.

The statement is often made that diplopia is intolerable to the organism. It would surely be intolerable to anyone who attempts to function at the normal achievement level in his environment - the visual performance level is at zero. How can comfort exist at such low visual level? The organism can just lower environmental demand to the same level. The following case illustrates such a condition.

A youngster of eight was an alternating strabismic. He was operated upon to correct this condition. The operation was a success with perfect cosmetic results. The difficulty was constant diplopia. This was never reported to either the parents or the surgeon because the youngster thought this was normal. The operation was performed at the end of the school year and the child had a very happy three month vacation at home. He did no reading or other activities requiring fine concentration. His outdoor play required gross visual adjustments. He even reported that he enjoyed the movies, but he would watch one picture part of the time and the other picture the remaining time. He thought it amusing that sometimes if his distance from his playmates was just right, they would seem to have three eyes and two noses. When did this youngster finally report visual difficulty? He finally told his parents that his eyes were bothering him when he returned to the school in the fall. It was the increased environmental demand of the classroom that finally brought him to the optometrist for visual rehabilitation.

Figure 14 illustrates how every individual can avoid visual discomfort. There are two possibilities: visual performance level can be increased by proper optometric services or the individual can restrict his visual environment and, thereby, decrease environmental demand. It is this second group which offers the greatest challenge to our profession. They are the failures, the poor readers, the visually inefficient, and the behavior problems. If we consider the population as a group, we can state that very little change has occurred in the visual performance curve, but a very considerable change has occurred in the environmental demand curve. The slope of the environmental demand curve is increasing. The reading load in our schools has tripled. Production accuracy has doubled in the past 10 years. Television viewing is a daily habit. It is obvious that if we are to avoid visual discomfort and still maintain a high environmental demand, we must increase our visual performance ability. This can be done by means of lenses or visual training or a combination of both.

Regardless of the degree of visual deterioration, we can expect visual discomfort when the environmental demand exceeds the visual performance ability of the patient. This explains the paradox of a patient with a B-1 deterioration complaining of visual discomfort; while a second patient who has a B-6 deterioration states his eyes never bother him. The B-1 is still trying to function in his normal environment; the B-6 has long given up and has contracted or simplified his environmental demands. *Whenever a person with a deteriorated visual pattern testifies that he has none of the symptoms of visual discomfort, we can be positive that he has restricted his visual environment.*

The comments of Cobb upon eye fatigue are of interest. "An organism such as the human being is infinitely more complex than any inanimate agent we can think of. As it begins to exhaust its supplies, it does not run at top speed, like an automobile engine, only to stop suddenly when the last drop of gas is burned. Nor does it show in its activity a gradual loss of power, as does a dry battery, with the using up of its active material. It would seem rather that with moderate depletion the human organism begins tentatively to anticipate further drains, and to protect itself by reducing its activity without, however, being incapable of reproducing its original efficiency when demand arises. Such unconscious protection might take the form of mere indisposition or reluctance toward effort." (*Trans. "Ill. Eng. Soc.," 22, 426, 1927)*

8. Measuring the Visual Problem

The amount of refractive error does not correlate well with either the degree of visual problem or the amount of visual discomfort. The elimination of the discomfort may require that only a portion of the existing refractive error be occupied by a lens. In concentrating upon measuring the refractive error, we assumed that we were measuring the visual problem. To measure the patient's estimate of his visual problem, a five-stage grading system was set up for headaches (frequency and intensity), blurred vision (far and near), ocular pain (frequency and intensity), diplopia (far and near). A portion of this data is given in Table 3 for 10 emmetropes selected at random.

There is a considerable variation in the intensity and amount of visual complaint for the same refractive error. Our analytical examination consists of many measurements of the relationship between accommodation and convergence at both near and far. It is these measurements which inform us as to the degree and intensity of the visual adaptations made by the patient. Since we are investigating a behavior pattern whose end organ (eyeball) utilizes the services of striated muscles (convergence) to maintain single vision and smooth muscle (accommodation) to maintain clear vision, it is obvious that we can have only two types of visual problems, namely, accommodative or convergence visual problems. This excludes the congenital and pathological cases for obvious reasons.

TABLE 3.
Subjective Complaint Summary (Emmetropes

Case No.	Headache Factor	Blurred Vision Factor	Ocular Pain Factor	Diplopia Factor	Total Subjective Complaint
1	15	0	0	0	15
2	2	0	0	0	2
3	1	0	2	1	4
4	0	2	0	0	2
5	6	2	0	0	8
6	8	0	0	0	8
7	1	0	0	0	1
8	9	0	0	0	9
9	1	2	0	1	4
10	0	0	0	0	0

The analytical examination consists of:

1. Ophthalmoscopy.
2. Ophthalmometry.
3. Habitual phoria at distance.
4. Static retinoscopy.
5. Dynamic retinoscopy at 20 inches.
6. Dynamic retinoscopy at 40 inches.
7. Subjective finding (basic finding).
8. Induced phoria at distance.
9. True adduction at distance.
10. Convergence at distance.
11. Abduction at distance.
12. Vertical phorias and ductions at distance.

13A. Habitual phoria at near.

13B. Induced phoria at near.

14A. Cross-cylinder, dissociated.

14B. Cross-cylinder, fused.

15A. Induced phoria through dissociated cross-cylinder.

15B. Induced phoria through cross-cylinder.

16A. Positive relative convergence.

16B. Positive fusional reserve.

17A. Negative relative convergence.

17B Negative fusional reserve.

18. Vertical phorias and ductions at near.
19. Amplitude of accommodation.
20. Positive relative accommodation.
21. Negative relative accommodation.

CHAPTER IV
Case History

Introduction

All authorities agree, regardless of differences in the methods of analysis of visual problems, the most important portion of our case study is the *case history.* Why the patient came in for a visual examination will enable us to determine what loss of visual ability was of importance to the patient. The patient may complain of *tired eyes* and the examination may reveal reduced acuity at both far and near. If glasses are essential for constant wear, the patient must be carefully indoctrinated in the loss of vision that he has tolerated for so long. He must be given a demonstration as to the gain in vision he will have with the glasses. He must be informed as to the value of his new correction for his tired eyes. This factor is of importance to *him* and it *must be satisfied* in order to assure proper patient control. This complaint of *tired eyes* must be successfully dealt with even if it requires other services besides glasses. The patient must be fully informed concerning the necessity of these services.

The nature of the complaint will aid us in diagnosis. The occurrence of sudden blindness may be due to retinal detachment, hemorrhage, embolism, multiple sclerosis or trauma; whereas gradual blindness may be due to cataract, chronic glaucoma, retinal degeneration, choroiditis or presbyopia. By questioning the patient it is possible to differentiate between possible causes of the visual complaint. Each visual complaint should be considered from a dual viewpoint:

1. Does this symptom arise from inefficiencies or inadequacy of the visual system?
2. Does this symptom arise because of the environmental conditions?

An employed tailor may have the visual complaint of not being able to do fine stitching when working on dark clothes. His glasses and visual skills may be adequate. The solution to his complaint may be to increase the intensity of illumination on his sewing task at the workplace. This does not mean that new lights must be purchased since, in many instances, merely moving the lamp closer to the task will produce the desired increase in intensity. In one case it was found that the light, at a particular lathe operation, had never been cleaned or the bulb replaced. When the worker was instructed to polish the reflector and replace the bulb in his light, his visual complaint disappeared.

Vision should never be evaluated in terms of excellent or poor. The visual status of the patient is either adequate or inadequate for the environmental demands present. The danger of merely providing the mechanical correction of refractive error, without considering the environmental factors, is illustrated by the following case given by Kuhn (Kuhn HS. *Industrial Ophthalmology.* St. Louis: Mosby, 1944:70):

> *The president of a large industrial company, seeking to give its employees the best eye advice possible, hired an ophthalmologist to refract (in his office) 200 employees. Most of these workers, ranging between 17 and 20 years of age, were nearsighted and many had never worn glasses before their examination. They were refracted and their prescriptions were filled. They were also told to be sure to wear their glasses on the job. Their work distance, about which no inquiry was made, was a short 8 inches straight ahead, not down. The minus lenses prescribed threw most of them into a real tail-spin. In others, moderate degrees of phorias shot into excessive brackets at that abnormal distance. The many repercussions of this incident could have been avoided had the refractionist been familiar with the mechanics and operations of the jobs for which he was attempting to equip his employee-patients.*

Therefore, in order to evaluate the visual status of the patient in these terms, we must have complete information as to the economic-social-recreational history of the patient. Contrast the environmental demands of the accountant and the farmer upon vision. The difference is obvious. But consider the differences in environmental demands of two farmers. The first farmer lives on an electrified ranch, views television, operates various mechanical devices. The second farmer lives on a farm which does not have electricity, plowing is done by a horse; he has very few mechanical devices. Obviously, the visual needs of the second farmer are quite different from those of the first farmer. With the advent of three dimensional movies, color television, and the increased reading loads in our educational institutions, the critical evaluation of the environmental needs of our patients will aid us in deciding whether lenses alone, lenses and visual training, or visual training alone shall be prescribed.

Another important function of the case history is the mutual evaluation that occurs. That is, while we are recording the data given by the patient and determining possible avenues of attack on his problem, the patient is simultaneously evaluating the practitioner. The economic advantages to the practitioner, in establishing rapport with his subject and creating in his mind that he is vitally interested in restoring him to maximum visual ability, is extremely important. This is professional public relations at its maximum effectiveness.

In the interrogation of the patient, changes in phraseology will often be necessary depending upon the age, educational background and intelligence of the patient. A very young patient will not be able to understand what the doctor means by blurred vision, but he will understand if he is asked, "Do you ever have any difficulty seeing what the teacher writes on the blackboard?" Kronfeld *(J Am Optom Assoc 1950;21:484)* believes that words like "rainbow" or "halo" are not meaningful to patients when inquiring as to the possibility of glaucoma. He prefers to ask, "Do you have any spells during which your vision isn't quite as clear as usual?" Therefore, whenever the patient hesitates in responding to the question, the practitioner should immediately rephrase the question into simpler terms. He will note that in each of the particular sections of the case history exact questions are used; but the practitioner must be able to rephrase these questions depending upon the response of the patient. Certain sections of the case history may be omitted or modified, depending upon the type of patient. For example, in interrogating an advanced presbyope, the section on educational history could very well be eliminated.

A case history is never completed or finished. As additional information becomes available during the examination, dispensing, or the four week progress report, the case history should be revised and kept up-to-date accordingly. The case history can be divided into the following sections:

1. External Observations
2. Age, Chief Complaint
3. Ocular History
4. Health History
5. Educational History
6. Occupational History
7. Developmental History
8. Familial History

Each is presented in some detail in the following sections. Specific attention is also given to investigating hobbies, and considering symptoms of asthenopia and headache.

1. External Observations

These are observations to be made upon meeting the patient and while obtaining case history information. Observe the walking movements, posture of body and head, as patient enters the consultation office:

(a) Are his walking movements normal?
(b) Does he exhibit any possible motor paralysis?

(c) Does he meet your hand clasp with a smooth coordinative movement?

(d) Does the patient seem shy and hesitant in his first meeting with you?

(e) Does he have difficulty in seating himself? (This may indicate poor body coordination or the impairment of spatial judgment.)

(f) Does he have a head tilt? If so, does it remain constant? (This may indicate vertical phoria, cyclophoria or ocular paralysis.)

(g) What is his head posture? Normal, high or low? (Persons with a high head posture should be fitted with a lower bifocal segment; if they have a low head posture the bifocal segment should be positioned higher.)

(h) Does he favor head movements or eye movements in observing various objects about the office? (The head mover can use a smaller bifocal segment. The head mover, since he utilizes the central area of his lenses, is less sensitive to large changes in lens powers.)

(i) What is his seated posture - erect or slouched? (This is important in prescribing bifocals.)

(j) Does he have a hand tremor?

(k) Does he have a tic?

(l) How does he hold his reading material, close to him and in his lap, or up and out? Careful observations of his nearpoint posture will enable the practitioner to prescribe ophthalmic materials that will ensure optimum visual performance.

2. Age

The exact age of the patient must be recorded. We can expect certain physiological changes to occur with age. The amplitude of accommodation decreases with age. Farpoint and nearpoint visual acuity vary with age. Color sensitivity seems to decline with age. Depth perception ability is lower at early age levels, reaches its maximum level at from 25 to 45 years of age, and after 45 years of age it starts to decline. From the age of the patient we can expect certain performance norms for the various visual skills tests.

The age of the patient is a determining factor in the type of treatment which may be used. A younger patient might receive lens application and a program of visual training for a particular visual difficulty; whereas an older patient might receive a lens application incorporating a relieving prism addition. A very old patient suffering from the same visual condition might receive a monocular lens application.

The age of a patient often decides whether a full or modified correction will be prescribed. This is particularly true in cases having high degrees of anisometropia, uncorrected myopia or hyperopia, astigmia (particularly at an oblique axis), and tolerance for prismatic corrections. The younger patient adapts rapidly to large changes in his prescription; the older patient finds it difficult to establish new visual habits.

3. Chief Complaint

The chief complaint is the explanation given by the patient as to why he is seeking visual care at this time. The statement by the patient must be recorded in his own words. Occasionally, the patient may have more than one chief complaint. If so, they should all be recorded. The chief complaint informs the practitioner what the patient thinks or is willing to admit is wrong and, therefore, what the patient expects to have remedied. For patient satisfaction, the complaint must be cared for and the patient carefully and thoroughly informed about the diagnosis and prognosis regarding his chief complaint. It is so very important to record the patient's chief complaint or complaints in his own words that many practitioners use disc recorders that they file with the case records. Proper patient control dictates that this complaint be recalled to the patient at the progress report examination, four weeks after remedial work has been completed.

A statistical analysis of chief complaints exhibited by patients seeking optometric care included:

1. Periodic checkup (a healthy practice has many of these.)
2. Pain
   (a) ocular
   (b) orbital
   (c) headaches
3. Conjunctivitis and blepharitis
4. Cosmetic
   (a) appearance of glasses
   (b) broken glasses
   (c) strabismus
5. Glasses are uncomfortable
   (a) size
   (b) fit
6. Disturbances of vision
   (a) diplopia
   (b) tearing
   (c) poor achievement on job or at school.

(d) blur at far or near
(e) asthenopia
(f) photophobia
(g) holds things close when he reads
(h) failed school screening
(i) sits too close when he watches TV

4. Ocular History

This is interrogation regarding previous eyecare received by the patient, the benefits received for such care, and an inventory of visual complaints.

A) Previous Eyecare

Has the patient ever received any previous eyecare? If so, how long ago was this examination? Was the examination performed by a medical or optometric practitioner? If the previous examination was medical were drops used? What were the results of the examination? What was the patient told was wrong with his or her eyes? Why did the patient have his eyes examined at that time? What were the benefits derived from the examination? Has the patient been having his eyes examined at regular intervals, and how frequent are these examinations?

The purpose of these questions is to determine the following facts:

1. What concept of eye health does the patient exhibit?
2. Does the patient have any idea that there are different kinds of vision specialists?
3. Is the patient aware of what was wrong with his eyes at the time of the previous examination?
4. Did the previous visual examination have any meaning for the patient?

B) Benefits of Previous Eyecare

Is the patient wearing glasses at the present time? If so, how old are they? When are the glasses worn? Are they worn constantly, for driving, on the job, television viewing, movies, reading, etc.? Why were the glasses prescribed? Did the glasses eliminate the visual complaints? How often were the glasses changed? Have the present glasses been comfortable, and are they now comfortable?

If the patient is presbyopic and wearing bifocals, further questioning on this point will often elicit valuable information. Did he have any difficulty adjusting to his bifocals? Can he hold his head in a natural position when he does his near work? Is there any particular near task that causes him difficulty?

At this point, the following items regarding the patient's old glasses should be carefully observed and recorded. Is the lens size adequate, too large or perhaps too small for his face? Is the bifocal height correct? Are the glasses properly centered for distance and for near vision? Is the bridge size correct? Are the glasses straight on his face? Are the lenses scratched? Is the frame bent?

If he isn't wearing glasses at the present time, has he ever worn glasses? If so, why were they prescribed? How long did he wear them? Were they of any help, or did they aggravate the initial complaint?

C) Eye History Inventory

1. Can you clearly see the print in your books? (Adults: Do you have any difficulty with your reading?)
2. Can you see clearly what is written on the blackboard? (Adults: Do you have any difficulty seeing at a distance?)
3. Do your eyes bother you when you go to the movies?
4. Where do you sit in the movies?
5. Do three dimensional movies bother your eyes?
6. Can you view television with comfort?
7. How far do you sit from your television set?
8. Do you lie down on a couch when you view TV?
9. Do you lie down on the floor when you view TV?
10. . Do your eyes tire when you read?
11. . Do you ever shade your eyes when you read?
12. . Do you ever see two things when you know there is only one?
13. . Do you have headaches very often? If so, what are they like? (Describe them.)
14. . Do the lights at school or at home hurt your eyes? (Adults: Do the lights at the office or plant hurt your eyes?)
15. . Does outdoor light bother you? If so, in what way?
16. . Do your eyes ever burn, water or tear?
17. . Do your eyes ever hurt? Do you rub your eyes a lot?
18. . Do you ever become dizzy?
19. . Do you ever see spots before your eyes?

Textor[5] states that certain symptoms are associated with heterophoria. Occasional diplopia when physically tired is the most obvious.

Diplopia might also become apparent to the patient when the peripheral stimuli to fusion have been diminished. The patient may report diplopia when hanging clothes on a line, or while watching an airplane in the sky, or when reading. Vertigo, severe headache or nausea may occur when the patient is subjected to an environment where there is considerable motion. This is peculiar to heterophorias. In such cases, the patient will report dizziness, headaches or gastro-intestinal disturbances when shopping in a crowded area, or when riding in a car, train or ship; (car-train-sea sickness). Other symptoms in heterophoria cases are fatigue, pain in the eyes, tearing, and blurred vision. These latter symptoms are usually associated with close work.

5. Health History

Wick[4] states that the value of a complete case history increases with the age of the patient. As age increases, the chances are greatly increased for the accidents of living to take their toll from the patient. The importance of general health to the entire visual mechanism cannot be over emphasized, and it is obvious that more detailed questions must be asked of the older group on this important matter.

The visual mechanism, with its rich connections with all of the systems of the body, is affected by many of the general diseases which are common in childhood and also by the geriatric changes common to later life. Obviously, a slight infection does not leave the ravage of more serious or extensive infections. Therefore, it is important to inquire not only if the patient had any of the following diseases, but also the intensity, the duration and frequency of attack. (See Table 4.)

It should be determined whether the patient has ever had any injuries to his head or eyes. These injuries should be listed in the order of occurrence, together with the type of medical treatment received. If serious head injury ever occurred ask, "Was a head X-ray or scan of any kind taken? If so, what did it reveal? Has hospitalization been required during the past year? If so, for what reason?"

The dental health of the patient is an important portion of the health history since any oral infection may cause fusional and motility difficulties. Secure answers to such questions as: Does the patient have regular dental care? Has he ever had a mouth X-ray? Does the patient have any non-vital teeth? Does he have gum disease? Does he have frequent toothaches?

Table 4.

General Disease	Possible Ocular Manifestation
Measles, Mumps, Scarlet Fever, Chicken Pox, Influenza, Typhoid	Conjunctivitis, sensitivity to light, weakness of accommodation, tropia
Diptheria	Conjunctivitis, accommodative paresis
Arteriosclerosis	Asthenopia, reduced acuity
Hypertension	Fluctuations in refractive error, vascular retinopathy
Nephritis	Reduction in acuity, edema of lids
Diabetes	Fluctuations in refractive error with variations in sugar concentration of the urine and blood. Diabetic cataract, diabetic retinopathy
Allergy	Conjunctivitis, blepharitis
Pregnancy	Radical changes in refractive error may occur. Periods of diplopia may develop.

What is the condition of the general health of the patient at this time? Is the patient taking any medication at the present time? Does the patient have sufficient sleep? Does he have an adequate or a balanced diet? Is his consumption of tobacco, alcohol, tea or coffee excessive?

Does the patient consider himself a nervous individual or does he take things calmly throughout the day's activities?

6. Educational History

This information should be obtained from all grade and college students:

1. Did the child attend kindergarten? If so, how long did he attend kindergarten? The child who attended one year of kindergarten is usually better prepared to start reading.
2. At what age did the patient enter first grade? If entrance to grade school was delayed, what was the cause of the delay?
3. Did the patient attend school regularly, or were there frequent absences? If there were frequent absences, what was the cause?
4. Did the patient change schools frequently? If so, what was the reason for the changes?

Determine which subjects presented difficulties. Ask the child:

1. Which subject do you like the best?
2. Which subject do you like the least?

3. What grade did you get in the subject you like the best?
4. What grade did you get in the subject you like the least?
5. Do you have any trouble copying work from the blackboard?
6. How far are you from the blackboard?
7. Do you have any difficulty seeing the words in your book?
8. Does this happen often or only occasionally?
9. Do the words in your book ever double?
10. Do you lose your place easily when you are reading?
11. Do you find yourself reading on the wrong line?
12. Do you consider yourself a below average, average, or above average reader?
13. Do you understand easily what you have read, or must you do frequent re-reading in order to obtain meaning?
14. Do you have any difficulty in hearing your teacher?

The child's present scholastic grade is recorded. If the child or parents feel that difficulty with reading is present, a visual skills efficiency report should be forwarded to the present teacher. A form for the Teacher's Report of her observations should be included with a request for her aid.

It is important to observe both the child and the parents while they are answering the various questions of the case history in order to determine the attitude of the child toward his school, reading and teacher. It is also advisable to note the attitude of the parents toward the child's difficulty. The cooperation of both parents is extremely important for the success of a visual care program. The foregoing information is never to be obtained by direct questioning.

7. Occupational History

Proper visual habits and visual aids are the most important implements a workman can bring to his daily work. The occupational case history should be taken on every gainfully employed person.

Company Name: Address:

Department:

Operation Name:

Type of Machine:

Working Distances: Average Maximum ______ Minimum ______

Multiple Working Distances Required: (Sometimes) (Usually) (Continuously)

Size of Working Area: Critical Concentration Required: (Yes) (No)

Illumination: Intensity_______________ Type of_____________

Glare present (Yes or No)

Infrared Exposure. Ultraviolet Exposure.

Exposure to Variable Light Intensity: (Rare) (Usually) (Continuously)

Color Perception: (None) (Average Need) (Critically Needed)

Work in Motion: (Yes) (No) Other Motion in the Field of View: (Yes) (No)

Working Posture: Standing ___ Seated ___ Uses Ladder ___ Scaffold___

Is Coordination of Hand & Eye Important? (Yes) (No)

Do you have to look upward when you work? (Yes) (No)

Do you have to tilt your head to the (Right) (Left)?

Remarks:

Contrast Ratio: Central Area: (Low) (Normal) (High)

Peripheral Area: (Low) (Normal) (High)

Fume Hazard: (Yes) (No) Splash Hazard: (Yes) (No) Dust Hazard: (Yes) (No)

What are the visual acuity requirements at Far? (Low) (Average) (High)

What are the visual acuity requirements at Near? (Low) (Average) (High)

What are the stereopsis requirements? (Low) (Average) (High)

Does your plant have a visual program? (Yes) (No) If so, did you ever fail the plant visual tests? (Yes) (No). If you did fail, when was it?

Do any workers at the same job wear bifocals? (Yes) (No)

Do any workers at the same job wear trifocals? (Yes) (No)

Do you feel that your production has suffered because of your eyes?

Do you have visual discomfort at your job? (Yes) (No). If yes, do you have this discomfort: (Sometimes) (Usually) (Continuously)?

Do you visit your first aid department frequently? (Yes) (No)

8. Developmental History

Gesell has made several points in regard to child and vision development:

> *The concept of development adds a new dimension to all problems of visual care - diagnosis, supervision, prevention, education, training, and re-education. . . .*
>
> *The concept of development applies with equal force to the normal and to the visually disadvantaged child.*
>
> *A developmental approach gives conjoint consideration both to intrinsic and to environmental factors. . . .*
>
> *A developmental hygiene of the child's vision must naturally take into count the stages and the cycle of the growth process. In terms of systematic supervision, this would entail periodic appraisals of the child's visual economy, with special attention to the trends and the needs of his total development.*
>
> *Deviations of visual development make their appearance in various ways: (a) An essential trait or pattern may manifest itself with excessive or subnormal intensity. (b) It may appear too early or too late in the growth cycle. (c) It may remain too briefly or too long.*

Gesell also stated a few general principles which apply to all developmental phenomena:

1. Behavior development usually tends toward an optimal realization.
2. Developmental organization does not advance on an even front. There is a fluctuation of dominance in counterbalanced functions. the principle of reciprocal interweaving.
3. The growth action system and its constituent organ system are in a state of formative instability, combined with a progressive movement toward stability.
4. The course of development resembles a spiral more than it does a trajectory. General patterns of organization repeat at ascending levels, with increasing complexity.
5. Every child has a distinctive ground plan of growth, determined primarily by innate, constitutional factors in interaction with extrinsic influences.

Betts[10] gives the following performance norms for children:

Performance	Norm
I. Locomotion	
A. Sits momentarily alone	8 mos.
B. Crawls alone	9 mos.
C. Stands alone	14 mos.
D. Walks alone	15 mos.
II. Teething	
A. Eruption of temporary teeth	
2 lower central incisors	6-9 mos.
4 upper incisors	8-12 mos.
B. First permanent teeth	5-6 yrs.
III. Elimination	
A. Established bowel control	12-24 mos.
B. Established bladder control	2-3 yrs.
IV. Dressing	
A. Buttons clothes	4 yrs.
B. Laces shoes	5 yrs.
V. Speech	
A. Sounds	
1. Syllables	6 mos.
2. Da-da, etc.	9 mos.
B. Words	
2 Words	12 mos.
4 Words	15 mos.
C. Sentences	
Short sentences	24 mos.
D. Gives full name	30 mos.

The expanded horizon and activities of the child fluctuate with his age. The following descriptions of the child from four to nine are from a consolidated study of the young child, by the Chicago Public School System, in 1953, under the direction of Benjamin C. Willis.[11]

> *Four Years - He is verbally assertive and dogmatic; he shows the urge to speak out, to create, to produce; he constantly questions why, and how, but often fails to wait for explanations. He practices the mechanics of speech freely and is fluent in associative thinking. He is able to reproduce eight- or nine-word sentences, as well as a series of three or four digits; but he does not like to repeat. He can name many common-pictured objects and identify these pictures in terms of use. He can understand and answer questions, such as, 'Why do we have books?' by answering, 'To read.' He can follow*

multiple directions of simple vocabulary and context. His proficiency in self-help includes not only feeding and toileting, but also washing his face and hands, dressing himself, including buttoning and lacing, but not tying, and going about his residential block alone. He can correctly name the colors of his shirts and pencils if of primary hue, that is red, green, blue, or yellow.

He can match simple geometrical shapes on cards and can place similar wooden cutouts in form boards. He can count to four by rote; but he is apt to describe numbers of things as one, two, or many. He can copy a circle and a cross, and he can trace a path between lines. His drawing of a man is frequently restricted to a Humpty Dumpty like figure. He can build vertically and horizontally with blocks and can make a 'gate' with five blocks. He can run, break his stride, and make standing and running broad jumps; he can skip, balance on one foot, throw strongly overhand, and thrust a spear into a small hole.

In contrast to his increasing abilities the four-year-old may have many fears, such as fear of the dark. He may be expert in fashioning alibis and may fabricate, not readily distinguishing truth from fable. He is handicapped in his beginning independence by his lack of knowledge and by his limited experience.

Five Years - Five is learning to get along well with strangers and to enjoy them. He is beginning to play with, not beside, other children. He can recognize his own outdoor clothing and can dress himself completely with knot-tying. He can brush his teeth and comb his hair with little supervision. He asks meaningful questions and waits for information. His definitions are in terms of use: A ball is to throw; a hat is to wear. He knows his age, his name, and his home address. He can repeat a ten-word sentence. He may distinguish his right from his left hand and probably shows preference for one or the other. He can draw a man complete with all extremities and can copy a square and a triangle; he is able to trace and cut out a pumpkin or turkey, and color it appropriately. He does not destroy work materials and will put his possessions away without constant urging. He can count four times and knows the difference between big and little, heavy and light, and other opposites. He enjoys listening to a short story; he is able to sit quietly, giving fairly steady attention to short stories, radio and television.

Five is dependable, obedient, social, and even polite and relatively truthful. His interests have widened to the environment outside his home, and he is adjusting to this fuller life.

Six Years - Active, impulsive, curious, eager and inconsistent, he flits from one exciting experience to another. He is mobile, even when standing or sitting wriggles and moves constantly. Although his eyes are incompletely developed and are often inadequate for close work under formal instruction, he is ready for instruction in reading, writing, and arithmetic through association with creative activities. He profits from a rest period each half-day for he tires readily from the intensity of his 'work' and his anxiety to start new things. He can handle crayons, paint, clay, and simple carpentry tools. He is also interested in letters, numbers, and word symbols and can use a pencil for printing simple words. He enjoys talking about himself and the proficiency of his accomplishments, but failure is difficult for him to face. He may attempt to avoid school by playing ill because of an unpleasant school experience.

Six can express himself in an increasingly exact vocabulary; he can define words and can select as many as seven or nine objects; he can identify the missing part of a pictured object. He is able to determine the shortest path between two points and can identify a different symbol among similar ones; he can perceive the alternating pattern of a bead string (&&*&*&*&*) for reproduction.*

Six, learning by leaps and bounds, is leaping and bounding while so employed. Often nearly frantic with haste, anger, or frustration, he needs wise guidance and sympathetic supervision. Rewards are cheap at this age; for example, a gold star is more valuable than a coin.

These descriptions of the four-, five- and six-year old child illustrate the gradual developmental changes which occur with time. Gesell,[9] in discussing the importance of developmental morphology to the study of human vision, states:

In the study of human vision, and doubly so in the study of child vision, one cannot escape problems of pattern and form. Morphology is the science of form. It is equally applicable to physical and to functional phenomena. It applies to behavior as well as to skulls and bones. Behavior grows, and as it grows it assumes characteristic forms. As a process, vision is so complex and inclusive that it needs all possible elucidation from the chemical, physical, and physiological sciences. But vision also comes within the scope of embryological science; . . postnatally as a growing complex of reaction patterns. . . Vision always remains a process, but the process is a manifestation of an action system which has structured form, and which is subject at all ages to maturational mechanisms of form regulation. . . . A developmental approach broadens the scope and the goal of visual hygiene. It shifts the emphasis from acuity and refraction to the total visual economy and developmental welfare of the child. Such a shift in emphasis can be made only by taking into account the growth status and the growth trends of the total organism."

The slowly developing child will usually exhibit a slower schedule in the development of his visual skills. It thus becomes possible to differentiate between the slow learner and the disabled learner.

9. Family and Birth History

1. Birth History-Normal Time: Premature: Overtime:
   a. Any complications before, during or immediately after delivery?
   b. Instrument delivery:
   c. Caesarian section:
   d. Birth Injury:
2. Family Ocular History
   Is there any family history of:
   a. Color Blindness
   b. Strabismus
   c. Myopia
   d. Cataract
   e. Glaucom

Strauss and Lehtinen[12] classify the factors that may produce brain injury:

1. During Prenatal Period
   a. German Measles
   b. X-Ray Treatment
   c. Serious Heart and Kidney Infections
   d. Serious Intoxications
   e. Vitamin Deficiencies
2. During Birth
   a. Prebirth Conditions
      i. Premature birth
      ii. Caesarean birth
      iii. Prolonged pregnancy
   b. Birth Conditions

        i. Long and difficult birth
        ii. Dry birth
        iii. Precipitate delivery
    c. Maternal Conditions
        i. Eclampsia
        ii. Pelvic malformation
        iii. Antepartum hemorrhage
    d. Fetal Conditions
        i. Anomalies in presentation
        ii. Twisting of the umbilical cord
    e. Medical Conditions
        i. Use of forceps
        ii. Improper use of anesthetic or drugs

3. After Birth
    a. During the first few months:
        i. Whooping cough
        ii. Measles
        iii. Scarlet Fever
        iv. Pneumonia
    b. Encephalitis and Meningitis
    c. Skull fractures or Concussions

Strauss and Lehtinen define the brain-injured child thus - "A child who before, during, or after birth has received an injury to or suffered an infection of the brain. As a result of such organic impairment, defects of the neuromotor system may be present or absent; however, such a child may show disturbances in perception, thinking, and emotional behavior, either separately or in combination. . . . These disturbances prevent or impede a normal learning process.

Additional considerations in taking the case history

A. Hobbies

The adequacy of the visual care obtained by the patient may often be gauged not at his daily visual tasks, but by his visual efficiency when he is engaged at his hobby. It is not sufficient merely to record the name of the hobby; we must ascertain the particular aspect of the hobby which is of primary interest to the patient. As Wick states, "To record fishing as a man's hobby is not sufficient. Fly fishing, for example, requires the use of the eyes at frequent intervals at about thirteen inches. Bifocals for such cases should be set several millimeters lower than the average because of the amount and kind of walking required. All patients should be informed of the need for different types of lenses for various visual tasks. They will then feel free to consult the optometrist as these problems arise."

B. Asthenopia

This is one of the common complaints of patients who seek visual care. They may describe their symptoms as: ocular pain, headaches following the use of the eyes, visual fatigue or discomfort following the use of the eyes, drowsiness when near work is attempted, lacrimation after short use of the eyes, photophobia, congestion, puffiness, itching or irritation of the lids, vertigo, or nausea. Asthenopia literally means "weak eyes", and applies to any symptoms expressed by the patient resulting from use of the eyes. They are symptoms of discomfort following nearpoint or concentrated visual activity. Shepard[13] determined by the method of statistical analysis of clinic records the significant difference between those persons having no visual complaint and those having a visual complaint. (See Table 5.)

The amount of visual discomfort experienced by a patient depends not only on the status of the visual pattern but also upon the general health of the patient. The amount of discomfort is usually pronounced in delicate, anemic and neurasthenic subjects. Therefore, in order to obtain visual comfort with these persons, the general health picture must be improved simultaneously or previously to applying visual care.

The value of careful questioning is illustrated by the following case reported by Bannon.[6] "I remember the case of a school teacher, referred by her physician for an aniseikonic examination, whose chief complaint was that of one-sided headaches lasting for several hours for the past two years and occurring nearly every week. She had seen three eye specialists, worn five different refractive corrections, and had four months of orthoptics for convergence insufficiency. Although her eye doctor had not referred her to a physician, the patient had consulted one because her headaches were continuing, and she had lost faith in the various eye treatments. Although some aniseikonia could be measured, I hesitated to prescribe a correction for her because of the complete lack of relief from her former glasses and because of certain details in the case history. The patient related that she did not have headaches while at summer school, where she used her eyes more than during the winter months. One point that stood out was that the headaches usually occurred on Fridays during the regular school year. Further questioning revealed that in the past two years she had roomed and boarded with a certain family; but while at summer school, in a different city, she and some other girls had a small apartment where they did their own cooking. When asked if she were allergic to anything the patient

Table 5.

Test	No Complaint	Complaint
Age	Over 30	Under 27
N.P.C.	No diplopia or within 3 inches	Diplopia and beyond 4 1/2 inches
#4	Over +0.50	
#4-#7		Minus
#7 Cylinder	None	Over 0.12 diopter
#7 Anisometropia	None or over 1.50 diopters	Over 0.50 diopters or under 1.50 diopters
#10 Break		Under 22 pd
#12		Over 1/2 pd hyperopia
#14A-#7		Over +2.00 diopters
#15A		Over 9 pd
#15B		Over 5 pd
#16 Break	Over 32 pd	Under 25 pd
#16 Recovery		Under 9 pd
#17 Break	Under 16 Break	Over 27 pd or over 16B Break
#18		Over 1 pd hyperopia
Visual Pattern	Monocular	Binocular
Glasses worn	Constantly	Part time

replied, "Oh, no, of course not. I think that allergy business is a lot of foolishness." However, when I asked her if the summer diet (when she had her own choice) differed from her boarding house meals, she did recall that she would never cook fish for herself. Later, she remembered that they always had fish on Fridays at the boarding house. She mentioned that she had been brought up to eat whatever was served. However, she did admit that when she lived at home, prior to the beginning of her headaches, her mother rarely served fish because her father did not like the smell of fish being cooked.

When I reported these details to her physician, as well as my own findings, he felt, as I did, that it would be worthwhile and certainly less expensive than aniseikonic glasses to have the patient abstain from fish for a month. If her headaches continued, we were going to prescribe the correction for aniseikonia. The patient, as well as her physician and I, was very pleased when at the end of a month the report was, "no headaches".

Atkinson[14] describes the symptom complex of asthenopia: "An inability to sustain a steady or prolonged use of the eyes, and more or less pain and discomfort when this is attempted. The pain may be of any degree of severity, even to an agonizing neuralgia. At times there is not actual pain at all; but after prolonged use of the eyes the vision becomes blurred and the patient is obliged to rest. If, in spite of the inconvenience the patient forces himself to continue his work, he will presently begin to develop positive signs of inflammation, such as photophobia, conjunctivitis, etc. Headache is a prominent symptom of asthenopia, and assumes various forms. . . . Dizziness is always a more or less accompaniment of eye strain."

C. Headaches

Of all of the visual complaints presented by patients, blur and headaches are the most frequent. The lay person seems to associate headaches with eyestrain, thus, we are often the first professional person consulted. There seems to be considerable disagreement as to the degree of relationship between headaches and vision. Elmstrom[2] states the situation as follows: "While one authority may state that most headaches are *not* of an eye origin, equally capable investigators will state quite emphatically that the great majority of headaches *are* of ocular origin. The true picture of origin, therefore, is between these extremes with the very likely condition that most headaches are so obscure that a multitude of causes may be postulated. The psychosomatic basis of many headaches has been entirely overlooked by many refractionists as well as many physicians. Volumes have been prepared upon the psychogenic origin of symptoms, with particular emphasis on headaches. The familiar trend of disorders has been observed in functional and organic diseases and abnormalities, with headaches, again, coming to the forefront."

Blumenthal,[3] in discussing headache diagnosis, states, "It is important to remember in the differential diagnosis of headache that a careful and detailed history, and at least a superficial exploration of the patient's personality pattern, are usually more helpful than the physical or neurological examination which is often entirely negative. To the experienced observer, the perfectionistic, worrisome migraine victim, the anxious, tremulous sufferer from a tension headache, and the blandly histrionic hysteric will be readily identifiable. The social and economic background, which makes up the life situation of the patient, will frequently offer a more cogent explanation of a headache than a battery of laboratory procedures."

The etiology of the headache can only be determined when the questioning has covered the following areas:

1. Character -- The headache may be sharp or dull, it may have a throbbing or continuous pain, a sense of fullness or pressure; it may be diffused or localized.
2. Location - Headaches may be located frontally, temporally, occipitally, parietally or back of the neck. The headache may be located superficially or deep; it may be in the eyeglobes or in the surrounding area; it may be unilateral or symmetrical.
3. Frequency How often do the headaches occur - daily, weekly or occasionally?
4. Intensity - How bad are your headaches? Are they just a dull ache? Is the pain so bad that you can not read, watch television, or go to work?
5. Onset - Is the onset of the headaches gradual or sudden? Do you experience these headaches in the morning, afternoon or evening? Do you wake up with the headache? Do you get these headaches during school days (working days) or on weekends? Do these headaches occur during the night?
6. Duration - How long do the headaches last? Are they of short duration, an hour or so; do they last all day or do they last over a period of several days?
7. Associated symptoms - Simultaneously, with the headache we may have nausea, vomiting, blurred vision, flashes of light, pain, auditory disturbances, loss of coordination, dizziness or increased sensitivity to light.
8. Factors which relieve or aggravate the headache - - The factors which relieve or aggravate the headache will aid in its diagnosis. What is the effect of rest, sleep, exertion, hunger, darkness, altitude, climate, or season of the year upon the headache?

Headaches may be classified in various ways. For our purpose we can consider the following categories: ocular, intracranial disease, psychogenic, migraine, vascular, neuralgias and sinusitis.

Ocular Headaches - Rabben[1] describes the ocular headache thus: "The typical ocular headache is not an occasional one; it occurs daily or several times a week, and it has a regular incidence. . . . It is frequent, regular and annoying, as long as the patient pursues his normal activities. The type of pain is also characteristic. It is not usually severe enough to incapacitate the patient. It is almost always a dull pain that is steady and persistent. Sometimes the pain is severe enough for the patient to view it as his primary symptom and to seek relief for it alone; but this is not the rule. Most often the patient's comment on his headache is that he has it frequently.

In many cases the patient is not at all vague about the part of his head that hurts, or first begins to hurt. In at least 80% of these cases the headaches are first noted in the frontal area, usually just over the brows, and they seldom extend higher than the frontal eminences. The pain is frequently reported as being centered in the space between the eyeball and the brows.

Occasionally, the pain either radiates to or is initially located at the temples, and infrequently it is limited to this area. Also, in decreasing order of frequency, the pain may be lateral parietal, usually radiating there after long frontal duration. It may be occipital initially and reflect down over the back of the neck and shoulders.

As a rule, the headache is bilateral; in cases where it is monolateral, or more severe on one side or the other, it is wise to be suspicious that while refractive error may be contributing to the headache, it is not solely responsible for it. However, it has been found that a primary monolateral headache, which otherwise corresponds to the course and characteristics of non-pathological ocular headaches, may be relieved by lenses and/or orthoptics.

Ocular headache is almost never present on arising. It usually does not manifest itself until midmorning or early afternoon, or sometimes not until early evening. But it usually appears at an accustomed time, unless the patient in some way makes unaccustomed use of his eyes. There also seems to be a relationship between the extent of the refractive error and the time of onset of the headache; the higher the error, the earlier in the day the pain appears. For instance, it is not uncommon to find a two diopter hyperope, about 25 years old, who will start to get his headache at about eleven o'clock in the morning. If he is exceptionally vigorous and his work is manual labor, his headache may hold off until two in the afternoon, that is if he has headaches at all. Similarly, an emmetrope who becomes presbyopic, and who requires perhaps a one-and one-half diopter reading addition, and who is about 48 years old, gets his headaches about 10 in the morning, if he works at a desk, or at about one in the afternoon, if he is a pipe fitter. An astigmat, who suddenly develops ocular headaches, often has them within one hour after arising; a myope is usually untroubled."

Ruedmann,[8] in discussing ocular headaches, states:

> *Nearsighted persons do not have headaches or head pain unless the nearsightedness is unequal, or severe, or unless they are abusing their eyes. It is true that persons with myopia have difficulty looking long distances when they are outside, or when in bright lights. This exposure may produce headaches. Those who watch air races, and either forget to wear dark glasses while peering skyward, or deem it unnecessary, may get severe headaches, nausea, vomiting, or they may collapse. Nearsightedness, in combination with a muscle error, may cause trouble. This is true of farsightedness as well."*
>
> *Farsighted people are apt to have frontal headaches which are moderate to severe in character and are present almost daily in the afternoon or evening. If there is an inequality in the amount of error in the two eyes the pain may be more severe over one eye; this is a common cause of headache."*
>
> *Errors in refraction usually produce frontal, vertical or bi-temporal pain, which may be associated with slight dizziness. Nausea is usually relieved by going to bed or resting, or taking a single tablet of acetylsalicylic acid. It is made worse by sewing, playing cards, and other close application. An error of refraction associated with a muscle error is almost certain to produce symptoms of headache, such as pain or nervousness, irritability, exhaustion, nausea (rarely vomiting, except in extreme cases), and loss of weight.*

Neck pain is more frequently due to ocular muscle imbalance than to anything else. The neck muscles function primarily to move the head so that the eyes will be in position to see. There is a definite periodic increase in head pain of muscle origin. It usually becomes more frequent in October, and it is well on its way in December; it reaches a peak in January, and falls off in the spring when the days become longer and outdoor exercise becomes the custom.

Elmstrom[2] places ocular headaches into six types or syndromes none if which is exclusive in all details from the others. They are:

1. Presbyopia: headache is generally frontal or mid-orbital, increasing in duration and in severity as the day goes by. Excessive near work may result in a residual headache lasting through the evening and into the following morning.
2. Astigmatic: headache generally is mid-orbital, but in some cases may be frontal. The condition commences earlier in the day than presbyopic headache, but resembles it closely.

3. Vertical Phoria: headache over brow with a tension and pulling effect. It may be a unilateral radiating headache.
4. Esophoria: headache coming on with near work; very similar to the headaches of hyperopia. Headache is often associated with toxemia or internal malfunction requiring medical attention.
5. High Exophoria: usually occipital headache, but may extend to frontal region.
6. Hyperopia: Frontal or/and mid-orbital headaches, along with a series of symptoms, such as watery secretions and burning sensations. Not usually headache alone.

Intracranial Disease Headaches. The pain is constant, more or less severe, and of a deep, steady boring character. It is fit at the top or front of the head, or in the occipital or cervical region, depending on the location of the inflammatory or mechanical irritation of the dural nerve endings.

The headache associated with brain tumor characteristically occurs as recurrent episodes of bursting pain, usually worse in the morning, and often associated with vomiting and evidences of localized neurological dysfunction. Paroxysmal headache, suddenly appearing or disappearing with changes in the position of the head, is characteristic of ventricle tumor.

Psychogenic Headaches. Psychogenic headaches can be divided into two groups, the tension-anxiety and the conversion-hysteria. The conversion-hysteria represents an attempt on the part of the patient to relieve an emotional tension. In the tension-anxiety headache the symptoms are not a substitute expression of the emotion, but they are the result of its normal physiologic concomitants, an anxiety equivalent. Thus, in the restless, dammed-up individual suffering from an anxiety state, part of the effect of his chronic emotional tension is to cause spasm and contraction of the cervical and scalp musculature, thus producing the usual tension-anxiety headache.

Migraine Headaches. The typical migraine attack is occasionally preceded by the occurrence of visual phenomena, such as scotoma or field defects. It is followed in 15 or 20 minutes by a throbbing headache on one side (unilateral) of the head which lasts for hours or days, and it is often associated with nausea and vomiting. Migraine tends to occur in individuals of a certain type of personality which has been described as being indecisive, insecure, perfectionistic, compulsive, sensitive, anxious, and easily discouraged. In many respects migraine is akin to psychoneuroses, and the importance of emotional conflicts and problems in the genesis of attacks cannot be overestimated.

Vascular Headache. The typical hypertensive headache is dull or throbbing, often predominantly frontal or fronto-temporal, and is present on awakening, or awakens the patient in the early morning. Nausea and occasionally vomiting may be associated with this type of headache. Headaches which result from exertion are usually indicative of hypotension or hypertension.

Neuralgias. The pain of neuralgia is characteristically sudden, violent and paroxysmal, usually lasting for a matter of seconds. It is usually described by the patient as a tearing, knife-like or stabbing pain. The attacks can often be precipitated by pressure on a trigger area, at the supraorbital foramen or in the lateral neck area.

Sinusitis. The sinus headache is dull, deep aching and non-pulsatile in quality. It is felt usually in the frontal and maxillary regions and less often in the occipital region. It is characteristically more severe in the morning, diminishing later in the day, except for the maxillary sinusitis, in which the pain often begins in the early afternoon and is relieved by recumbence.

For diagnostic purposes, a very careful headache history covering at least four weeks of the patient's activities must be taken. Information regarding every headache should be recorded as to date and time of onset, location of headache, how long the headache lasted, and activities engaged in by the patient just prior to the start of the headache.

Headaches Accompanying Changes in Lens Prescription or Visual Training. A patient may experience headaches when he starts wearing a new correction. In order to eliminate the possibility of incorrect optics, the following characteristics of the glasses should be carefully checked: Distant interpupillary setting, near interpupillary setting, base curve of the new lenses different from the patient's old glasses, absence of a tint or a different tint used than that incorporated in the patient's old glasses, different style of bifocal prescribed, vertical height of one bifocal different from its mate, vertical centering of the lenses different from the patient's old glasses, incorrect anisometropic correction, incorrect amount or axis of astigmia, and vertical prism, if present, is not correct.

Professional judgment must be exercised when a patient has gone without an Rx for many years, and finally his discomfort or inability to see brings him to the optometric office for a visual examination. This examination may reveal large amounts of anisometropia, astigmia, oblique astigmatic axes or presence of antimetropia. A complete correction, particularly if the patient is an adult, may evoke a considerable period of discomfort while he is now learning the new visual tricks of binocularity. It is advisable, therefore, to prepare the patient for this period of discomfort by calling the glasses dispensed as a "*temporary,*" "*treatment,*" or "*rehabilitation*" correction. Visual training, either office or home, prescribed for these patients will aid in quickly establishing the new binocular pattern.

Similarly, in administering visual training to a patient with a structured visual pattern of monocular or binocular nature, we may have some visual discomfort in the initial phases of the training. This is due to the shift in the visual pattern that is occurring because of the disorganizing phases of the training routine. The older the patient the more discomfort we may expect in developing a normal binocular pattern. Thus, it is wise to prepare the visual training case for this initial discomfort before it is actually experienced.

Conclusion

The diagnostic importance of the case history cannot be overestimated. It is often the primary clue as to the type of visual care to be administered. *The case history is never finished.* It proceeds during the initial interview, while we are performing the visual tests and dispensing, and during the progress examination. You can never have too much information about your patient.

REFERENCES

1. *Rabhen EL. Headaches of Refractive Origin. Opt J Rev 1950 Dec:33.*
2. *Elmstrom GP. The Symptom of Headache. Optom Wkly 1953 Oct 22:1772.*
3. *Blumenthal LS.: Headache: Diagnosis And Treatment. Am Acad Optom 1950;27:611.*
4. *Wick RE. Visual Examination Of The Patient Past Forty. Am Acad Optom 1950;27:226.*
5. *Textor RR. Clinical Indications For Prescribing Prisms. Am J Optom 1949;26:519.*
6. *Bannon RE. Symptoms And Case History-The Patient As A Person. Am J Optom 1952;29:275.*
7. *Lebensohn J E. Photophobia Am J Ophthalmol 1951;34:1294.*
8. *Ruedmann AD. Headache And Head Pain of Ocular Origin. J Am Med Assoc 1950; 144:517.*
9. *Gesell A, Ilg FL, Bullis GE. Vision Its Development In Infant And Child. Santa Ana, CA: Optometric Extension Program, 1999.*
10. *Betts E. Foundations of Reading Instruction. American Book Co., 1946:236.*
11. *Willis BC. Guide Posts For Kindergarten Primary Teachers. Chicago Public Schools, 1953.*
12. *Strauss AA, Lehtinen LE. Brain Injured Child, Vol. 1. Grune & Stratton, 1947:106.*
13. *Shepard C. Optometric Science in Practice, 1942:71.*
14. *Atkinson T. Oculo Refractive Cyclopedia & Dictionary. Chicago: Professional Press, 1944:44.*

CHAPTER V
Visual Skills

Introduction

A skill is an acquired or developed ability to perform a given act efficiently. Thus, a visual skill test is a measurement of the ability of the patient to perform a particular visual act efficiently. Visual skills are measures of neuro-muscular coordination involving either or both the convergence or accommodative mechanisms and the essential feedback circuiting. They are also measures of the performance ability of the central integrative factor. These skills can be simple, such as following a moving target with one eye open, or complex, when we measure such a skill as effective reading rate (reading rate x comprehension).

The visual process is extremely complex. From this neuro-complex a great number of visual skills tests have been isolated. Many of the skills tests have been given simple names such as fusion, stereopsis and color perception. These names are misleading, particularly for the neophyte. The neophyte concludes that a particular stereogram measures only this one variable and no other. For example, if a patient passes the test for fusion he can be said to possess normal fusion; if he fails this particular test he does not possess normal fusion. Unfortunately, it is very difficult to measure any degree of fusion as an isolated function. The Keystone fusion stereogram consists of four balls, two of which are exposed to each eye; one ball on each side is located on a common horizontal plane. [Editors note: The photos shown here are from the Keystone View series but similar tests are available from Bernell Corporation.] These colored balls are printed against a black background. Thus, we have common fusional elements with peripheral field consisting of an undifferentiated background. The patient possessing normal fusion should therefore, fuse the common horizontal balls, and report the presence of three balls all in the same vertical line. A patient who does not have second degree fusion will fail this test. It is equally true that a patient who has good second degree fusion in his normal environment, because of the stabilizing effect of the peripheral visual field, will also fail this test. He may not fail the test because of the absence of fusion, but rather because of a lateral or vertical phoria which may be present.

The statistical analysis of visual data obtained from workers on certain production lines has shown a significant correlation between environmental factors and color perception tests. This significant relationship, between production and color perception, is obtained in spite of the fact that the particular job does not require any color perception. It is obvious that the color test stereogram used must measure other visual factors besides that of color perception.

It is extremely difficult to isolate a single, simple visual skill out of a complex visual act. The usual visual skill stereogram is measuring several related skills or portions of these skills. Therefore, in applying visual skills tests in offices, schools, or in industry, we must use a group of tests if we are to isolate the visually ineffective and inefficient from the general population.

Many of the visual skills tests bear names which are similar to tests taken during the routine visual examination performed with the phoropter. The question is often asked, "Why should I waste time repeating these tests?" The phoria test is a typical example of this seeming duplication in testing. The question which must be answered is, "In what way does a phoria test taken during the regular optometric examination differ from a phoria test taken as a visual skill test?" The method of dissociating is one of the points of difference. A vertical dissociating prism is used in the phoropter technique. A patient experiences diplopia. He has visual awareness of a very peculiar sensation in that, whatever direction he gazes, everything is seen double. This is a disturbing condition. In fact, some patients will experience nausea and some will have ocular distress. When a phoria test is taken as a visual skill test, the patient has no clue that dissociation even exists. He experiences a normal perceptual field without distortion or any discomfort. It is true that he may wonder why the arrow keeps jumping about; but he has no visual clue as to the physical conditions of the testing situation.

Second, in taking a phoria test with the phoropter, we stop the lateral measuring prism as soon as the patient reports vertical alignment of the targets. The patient is told that the end of the test is reached when the targets are lined up one above the other. In psychological testing, it is agreed that it is better if the patient is not aware of the final answer. Therefore, since psychological factors are present, the knowledge of the final answer may call forth some mental effort on the part of the patient to align the targets. Whereas, in the visual skill test measuring the lateral phoria, the patient merely reports the number at which the arrow is pointing.

Third, in the phoropter test we record the patient's immediate response to the testing situation, while in the visual skills situation we are interested in the variations in the response of the patient with time. For example, a patient may show a normal amount of exophoria for a second, but the arrow may now move into the area of high exophoria or into esophoria as he continues to view the testing stereogram for a few seconds. At times, the patient may reveal instability in the convergence pattern in that he may report that the arrow is pointing at nine, now ten, back to nine and out to eleven, back to nine. All of this variation takes place over a matter of a few seconds of observation.

Fourth, in taking our visual skills tests, we try to give the patient full visual rein so that the projection of accommodation and convergence will more closely correspond to the manner in which he responds to stimuli in his normal environment. In the analytical tests, we try to hold accommodation fixed and vary the stimulus to the convergence pattern; or we fix convergence and vary the stimulus to the accommodative pattern. In spite of the similarity of many of the names of phoropter and analytical tests, they measure different phases of the same visual function. It is for this reason that correlation studies between the two types of testing methods are usually low.

Purpose

The advantages of having a visual skills profile on your patient are:

(1) *To the Practitioner* - The visual skills not only present a picture of the performance ability of the patient in terms of magnitude, but perhaps of greater importance, they tell us about the quality of his performance. They answer such important questions as: does he have convergence stability? Does he have fusion when only figural targets are present? What is his monocular acuity when he must maintain fusion? How does he perform when we present a tri-dimensional target which has a normal figure-ground relationship that demands precise fixation? What is his stereopsis when retinal disparity is the only clue? What are his abilities in performing the basic survival skills of rotations and fixations?

A visual skills profile informs us what the patient has done about his visual problem. What type of adaptation did he make in order to maintain survival in his visual environment? What did he do in order to simplify his binocular visual pattern? All of this important information is readily available when you observe the visual skills profile.

(2) *To the Patient* - The visual skills tests often reveal the absence, warping, or distortion of visual abilities to the patient for the first time. The patient may not understand what you mean when you tell him that he suppresses one eye. However, when you show the patient the second degree fusion test and he reports the presence of only two balls, and when you occlude

the other eye, he can see the other two balls, then you remove the occluder and again they disappear, it becomes obvious to him that he is not using both eyes. The skills battery has no equal in its value in indoctrinating the patient, not only to his visual inaptitudes, but to his need for visual training.

(3) To Pass Screening Tests - Visual skills tests are being used in our school systems, in industry, and by motor vehicle licensing departments. An increasing number of persons seeking visual care failed some type of screening routine which involved from seven to 15 visual skills tests. Therefore, the practitioner can no longer prescribe visual care without knowing what the effect of his prescription of lenses or visual training program has been on the visual abilities of the patient who was referred by one of these visual screening batteries.

Patient Indoctrination

In order to obtain consistent results with the visual skills tests, proper patient indoctrination must be practiced. Your instructions to the patient are particularly important. Psychologists learned a long time ago the danger of not standardizing instructions to the patient. That is why a psychologist, who may have administered a particular test hundreds of times, will not rely on memory, but each time he will carefully read the instructions to the patient. Since the visual skills are primarily psychometric measurements of visual performance, extreme care must be taken to inform the patient precisely as to what the testing situation will be, what the patient's attitude toward the test should be, and what type of response or judgment he must make. The following will illustrate the importance of proper patient instruction. A stereopsis test was being administered. The patient was asked, "Which of the five symbols on the top row is the clearest?" He replied that they all looked the same. The patient was told that he had no stereopsis. He was rechecked, and the instructions to the patient were, "Which of the five symbols in the top row seem the closest to you?" The patient now gave a normal response to the test.

Many of our tests are strange to the patient, and he should be given a short warm-up period before recording the observations. This is very important for the so-called motor skills of rotations, fixations, and accommodative rock. Usually, in an endeavor to follow instructions, the first attempts of the patient will be spastic and convulsive; but as he begins to understand what is expected of him he will settle into his natural performance pattern for that particular skill. Sometimes, when he first starts to follow the rotating target, the patient may use his head rather than his eyes. We again caution him that we are interested in his eye movements. As he once again follows the rotating target, he will settle in to his normal pattern for following a moving target using his eyes only. It is important that we repeat instructions several times to make certain that the patient understands precisely what we want him to do. It should be noted as to how many times the instructions were repeated.

Quality of Performance

In order to obtain the maximum information from our visual skills tests, it is important to record not only the quantity of the performance, but also the quality of the response. Two patients may both pass a fusional test, one performing the test easily and readily, while the second patient can only maintain the fused state with effort. It is obvious that the second patient has a different type of performance ability and that he will need some type of visual help. Many skills summaries have very little meaning because of lack of comments. Frequently, the only indication on the visual skill form may be just a check mark, "passed," "OK," or "normal." The response to a test may be "normal," but at what cost in mental effort?

What is the speed of the patient's response? Does he react slowly to the stimulus situation? Is his response at the normal speed? Are his reactions rapid? The reaction time of the patient has considerable bearing on the use of the visual apparatus in his normal environment where quick decisions must be made.

What is the stress reaction of the patient? Does it take considerable effort on his part to perform the visual task, or are his efforts certain, indicating that he performs the task easily?

What is the accuracy of the patient in performing the various skills tests? Are his movements accurate and precise? Are they good, with perhaps some little errors? Are his movements erratic and inaccurate? Does he start to perform, hesitate, and make several corrective movements before he finally finishes the task?

The careful evaluation of the speed, effort and accuracy of the patient's responses will aid us in diagnosing the degree and intensity of the anomalous visual adaptations made by the subject.

The following group of visual skills tests is not complete, but they are the tests most frequently used. Your professional judgment will dictate which of these should be used in any particular case.

Non-Stereoscopic Tests

These are the skills tests which are performed without the use of a stereoscopic instrument.

1. *Nearpoint of Convergence (Triangulation)*

A. Target: Wolff wands, pencil, pointer florist's pin, or small flashlight.

B. Procedure: The patient is seated comfortably, and the fixation target is gradually brought from a position at arm's length towards the patient's nose. The target must be in the median plane and about 20 to 30 degrees below the horizontal plane. The eyes must have a downward posture as the target is brought closer to the patient. Watch the movement and positioning of the patient's eyes. As soon as the patient reports diplopia, or you observe one eye deviating from the fixation target, record the distance from the target to the bridge of the nose.

C. Normal: one inch.

D. Instructions to patient: Please follow the top edge of this target which is moving toward your eyes and report when you see two of them.

E. Remarks: The subjective response (when the patient reports the target is doubled) and the objective response (when we see the eye deviate away from the fixation target) should be at the same distance. When we observe (objectively) that the patient breaks fusion at six inches, but he never reports diplopia (no subjective response), we can conclude that the patient is suppressing one eye. The dominant eye is usually the fixating eye therefore this test is also an eye dominancy test. The nearpoint of convergence does not vary with age; its expected value is constant.

F. Precautions:

a. Be sure that you are moving the target from a downward position so that the eyes of the patient have a downward posture.

b. Move the fixation target at a steady speed, neither too slowly or too rapidly.

c. One of the advantages of using a flashlight as a fixation target is that the objective response can readily be observed by noting the position of the Purkinje images.

d. Be sure that the patient understands the testing procedure. Verify this by repeating the test at least twice before taking an actual reading.

G. Record: record the objective and subjective nearpoint of convergence to the nearest inch.

2. *Donder's Amplitude of Accommodation (*Push-Up Amplitude)

A. Target: 20/20 reduced Snellen letters.

B. Procedure: The patient is seated comfortably and the target is presented at arm's length. The target is presented to him in the midline and slightly below the horizontal meridian. As the patient reads the letters aloud, the target is brought slowly and steadily toward the patient until he declares that the letters are blurred or difficult to read. The distance in centimeters, from the bridge of the nose to the plane of the target, is converted into diopters of accommodation by dividing it into 100.

C. Normal: as per age (Donder's Amplitude of Accommodation Table).

Age	Amp	Age	Amp
10	14	40	4.5
15	12	45	3.5
20	10	50	2.5
25	8.5	55	1.5
30	7.5	60	1.0
35	6.5	65	0.5

D. Instructions to patient: Please read these letters aloud as I move this card toward you. Please tell me when the letters are too blurred for you to read, or when you find them difficult to read.

E. Remarks: The Donder's Amplitude of Accommodation differs from the minus lens amplitude taken during the analytical examination, principally, because we have convergence aiding the accommodative reflex in the Donder's method. Thus, Donder's amplitude is the maximum available when the object of attention is moving towards the observer. It is a dynamic, full measure of accommodative ability.

F. Precautions:

a. Be sure that you are moving the reduced Snellen target from a downward position so that the eyes of the patient will have a downward posture.

b. Move the target at a steady speed, neither too slowly nor rapidly.

c. Keep the patient reading the letters from the start of the test until he states that the target is blurred; or have the patient read aloud until he falters.

d. Repeat the test at least twice to make certain that the patient understands the instructions.

G. Record: Record the binocular amplitude of accommodation in diopters.

3. *Monocular Rotations*

Editor's note: There are several other eye movements tests that have been developed since this book was published. Two of them that employ similar methods are: The NSUCO/Maples Oculomotor Test and the S. A. NOEL Eye Tracking and Locating Skill Test. Both are enhancements of Dr. Manas' testing. It was deemed appropriate to leave his original testing unchanged.

A. Target: Wolff wand, pencil tip, wand or small flashlight.

B. Procedure: The patient's dominant eye is occluded by a card (5 by 8 inches) or occluder. The angle of the occluder card with the face must be adjusted so that you can observe not only the non-occluded eye, but also the eye behind the occluder. The target is presented at about three feet from the open eye of the patient, and the target is rotated in a circle of about two feet in diameter. You can quickly judge whether the diameter of the rotation is too small or too large by watching the movements made by the eyes of the patient. An almost maximum rotational movement is desired. The rate of rotation should be about one rotation every three seconds. This test is performed in both a clockwise and counterclockwise direction. You must use several rotations, prior to starting your observations, for a warm-up period. After about five rotations clockwise, repeat with five rotations counter clockwise; the occluder is now shifted to the other eye and the observations repeated.

C. Normal: Smooth, ballistic rotations in the clockwise and counterclockwise directions.

D. Instructions to patient: "Look straight ahead and follow this moving target with your eyes. Don't move your head. Follow with your eyes *only.*"

E. Remarks: The movement of the rotational target must be smooth and performed at a regular speed. Any irregular movements of the eye of the patient must be recorded, and the portion of the rotational movement in which irregularities occur should be carefully recorded. The clock method is the easiest way in which to record these defects, i.e. irregular movement of O.D. from 3 to 6 o'clock. The hour positions are from the patient's view of the clock. Any substitution of head movement for eye movements must be noted. If these head movements persist, the patient should be cautioned to move only his eyes. If he still continues to move his head, rather than move his eyes, place his head in a headrest and note the type of eye movement pattern as he attempts to follow the rotating target. The posture of the head should he noted. Is the head held up? Is the head tilted down? Is the head tilted to one side?

With what effort is the patient following the moving target? Is the movement performed easily, or do you note signs of tension? All of these observations are important in order to evaluate the performance ability of the patient.

F. Precautions:

(1) Keep the speed of rotation constant and the magnitude of the rotation within the physiological limits of the eye rotation.

(2) Encourage your patient to move the eyes and *not* his head.

(3) The normal rotational movement should be free from flutter, jump or any spastic irregularities.

(4) Compare the movement of the eye behind the cover with that of the unoccluded eye.

(5) Give the patient an adequate warm-up period before you start your actual observations.

G. Record:

(1) Head posture of patient.

(2) Right eye occluded - left eye unoccluded - type of movement in both clockwise and counterclockwise directions.

(3) Left eye occluded - right eye unoccluded - type of movement in both clockwise and counterclockwise directions.

4. *Monocular Fixations*

A. Target: Wolff wand, pencil tip, wand, or small flashlight.

B. Procedure: The patient's dominant eye is occluded. The target is presented at about three feet from the open eye of the patient. The fixation target is now steadily and at a medium speed moved in the cardinal directions. The extent of these movements should be about two feet. Whether this fixation movement is too small or great can be readily determined by watching the movement of the eyeball. The movement must stay within the physiological limits of ocular movement. Allow the patient to make several fixation movements before recording the results of the test. Now reverse the position of the occluder and repeat the test for the other eye.

C. Normal: The fixation movements should be smooth and ballistiform, without any pauses at intermediate points. No regressions or over fixations should be present.

D. Instruction to patient: "I want you to look straight ahead. Keep your head in this position. Now follow this moving target with your eyes only." If patient tends to move his head caution him to move his eyes only.

E. Remarks: Any irregular movements of the eye should be noted. Does the patient substitute head movements for eye movements? Does he have more difficult in one meridian, or does he have this difficulty in several meridians?

F. Precautions:

(1) Target must be moved at a steady and uniform rate.

(2) Don't allow the patient to move his bead.

(3) Give your patient a warm-up period before starting your actual observations.

(4) Vertical movements do not have the magnitude of the lateral or oblique fixations.

G. Record:

(1) Head posture of patient.

(2) Fixation ability of right eye.

(3) Fixation ability of left eye.

5. *Binocular Rotations*

A. Target: Wolff wand, pencil tip, wand, or small flashlight.

B. Procedure: The fixation target is presented to the patient at a distance of about three feet; it is rotated in a spiral pattern starting with a small loop about one foot in diameter; and it gradually increases the diameter of the rotation, until after about five rotations the diameter of movement of the fixation target has been increased to three feet. Now reverse the direction of movement from clockwise to counterclockwise and repeat the procedure. The speed of rotation must be uniform and at about one revolution every three seconds. At all times concentrate on the eye movements of the patient, and be alert for the presence of saccadic or regression movements.

C. Normal: smooth and ballistic rotational ability.

D. Instructions to patient: "Please look straight ahead and follow this target with your eyes. Try to follow this target without moving your head. We want to see how well you can move your eyes without any head movement."

E. Remarks: Any irregular or correctional eye movements should be noted and carefully recorded. The clock method of designating sectors, where saccadic or regression movements occur, may be used. It is well to call the patient's attention to an area of difficulty and see if he can now do better when you repeat the rotation. Record if such instructions improve his performance.

F. Precautions:

(1) Target must be moved at a steady and regular speed.

(2) Keep cautioning patient to move his eyes only and hold his head still.

(3) Do not make the diameter of the rotation outside of the physiological limits of motility.

(4) Urge your patient to perform.

C. Record: (1) The sector in which patient exhibits difficulty.

(2) Whether it is found in one eye or in both.

(3) If the direction of rotation affects the difficulty exhibited by the patient.

6. *Hand and Eye Orientation test*

A. Target: Wolff wand, pencil, small wand, or small flashlight.

B. Procedure: The target is placed in the median plane at eye level and about 16 inches from patient. The patient occludes one of his eyes with an occluder or card (5 x 8 inches). The patient is told to place his forefinger of the other hand just at eye level before his open eye. For example, occlude his left eye and use his left hand to hold the occluder; use the forefinger of his right hand, just below his right eye, for the orientation test. He is to aim his forefinger at the target, and at your command of "touch" he is to stab at the target and touch it with his finger tip. Shift the position of the target a little and have the patient repeat the test. The patient now reverses the position of the occluder and repeats the orientation test using the forefinger of the other hand.

C. Normal: an accurate landing on the target with either eye and hand combination.

D. Instructions to patient: "I want you to use your forefinger as a pointer. Cover your left eye with this occluder, holding it with your left hand. Place your right forefinger right below your open eye, so that you are looking over the top of the finger, and line it up with the target. When your have your finger lined up with the target, quickly *stab* your finger forward and *quickly* touch the target." This is repeated for the other eye.

E. Remarks: The patient uses the hand corresponding to the open eye for the touching test. Allow the patient to line up his finger with the target before he makes his stab at the target. The movement must be done rapidly. If the patient tries to do this slowly, have him repeat the test. This is a monocular test for spatial-kinesthetic organization. If the subject has amblyopia or eccentric fixation, he will find it difficult to place his finger on the target. If his finger passes to one side of the target, it would indicate proprioceptive disorganization.

F. Precautions:

(1) Patient must not be allowed to move his finger slowly toward the target. The hand movement must be done quickly, as soon as the patient has his finger lined up with the target. Slow movements allow for corrections, and, therefore, it is difficult to pick up faulty orientation.

(2) Have patient do each fixation several times, but each time be sure and shift the position of the target a little.

(3) Have patient line up his forefinger with the target and with his hand very close to his face. When the patient is satisfied that he is '*on target*' he then completes the thrust toward the target.

(4) Have patient use the hand corresponding to his open eye.

(5) Emphasize to your patient that you want both accuracy and speed of movement.

G. Record: (1) Accuracy of fixation with right eye.

(2) Accuracy of fixation with left eve.

(3) Note any hesitations, and either subject tends to make errors on the left or right of the target.

7. *Saccadic Fixations (Monocular)*

A. Target: two dissimilar targets. You may use a red pencil and a blue pencil, a red pointer and a blue pointer or the gold and silver ends of the Wolff wands,

B. Procedure: Occlude the patient's dominant eye. The two fixation targets are placed in front of the open eye, at a distance of three feet and with a lateral separation of two feet. The two fixation targets are in the horizontal meridian. Upon command, the patient is to shift his gaze from one target to the other in one quick movement. At the rate of one fixation change per second repeat, "blue," "red," "blue," and etc. Allow the patient to make several fixation changes before starting your observations. Encourage the patient to make the fixation jump from one target to the other in one sweep and not in several small fixations. Now move the two fixation targets in the vertical meridian and repeat your observations. You can also vary the cadence of the command to see how the patient handles the change. Shift the occluder to the non-dominant eye, and repeat the test for saccadic fixation ability in the horizontal and vertical meridians.

C. Normal: a smooth jump of the eye from one target to the other without any corrective movements.

D. Instructions to patient: "I want you to look at the red target first. When I say 'blue,' I want you, as rapidly as possible, to look at the blue (second) target. Try to move your eye from one target to the other in one sweep. Listen to my count, and try to move your eyes from one target to the other as I say, 'red,' 'blue,' 'red,' and so on. We want you to make this change, in looking from one target to the other, without moving your head. We want your eyes to do all of the work."

E. Remarks: If the patient substitutes head movements for eye movements, he should be cautioned that he is to move his eyes only. In some cases, particularly with children, they may anticipate your fixation directions and start a saccadic fixation before you have asked for the fixation. It is important, in order to prevent this, to call at a regular rate and ask the patient to wait until he hears your direction before he starts his fixation. You can also vary the cadence of the command to keep the patient from moving their eyes too soon. Good fixation ability is important for any type of visual task. Be careful to watch for "under shooting" which requires two or more fixations to make the jump from one target to the other. He may overshoot the target and, therefore, he will have to make a regression movement to land on the target. Careful observation is required in order to observe the various abnormal fixation patterns which may be present.

F. Precautions:

(1) Make sure that the patient understands that we want him to change fixation from one target to the other in one continuous sweep.

(2) Allow the patient to make at least five fixation jumps before you start your observations.

(3) Be certain that the distance between the two fixation targets does not exceed the physiological limits of the eye.

G. Record: The quality of the saccadic fixations in the horizontal and vertical meridians for each eye.

H. This can also be done as a binocular procedure.

8. *Near-To-Far and Far-To-Near Fixations*

A. Target: The nearpoint fixation target is a reduced Snellen card. The farpoint fixation target is the regular distant Snellen chart.

B. Procedure: The patient is directed to read the nearpoint fixation target which he is holding in his hand at his regular reading distance. The farpoint Snellen target should be centered in front of the patient and at 20 feet away. In order to view the fixation change properly, the patient must be seated higher than the observer. The patient must be able to view the distant fixation target above the observer's head. The observer should be seated close to the patient so that by looking just above the nearpoint reading card he will be able to see the eye movement pattern of the patient. The patient is to read the nearpoint target at the command of "near." He is to look up and read the farpoint target at the command of "far." At the rate of about one fixation change per second you repeat the commands "near," "far," "near", and so on until the patient has had a warm up period of at least five complete changes in fixation. You now observe carefully the eye movement pattern of the patient as he changes fixation from near to far and back again to near.

C. Normal: no unsteadiness or corrective eye movements made by the patient in proceeding from far to near fixation or vice versa.

D. Instructions to patient: "You are to hold this reading card in your hand at your regular reading distance. When I say 'far,' I want you to look up and read the letters on the chart in front of you. When I say 'near,' I want you to look down at the card in your hand and read. I will continue this counting of 'far,' 'near,' 'far,' several times, and at each command look at the proper target. Please don't move your head. We want to see how well you can move your eyes.

E. Remarks: Watch for any irregular movements of the eye as the patient makes the fixation change from far-to-near or from near-to-far. Does the patient make this change in fixation in one continuous, rapid sweep; or does it take several small fixations to land on the target? Some patients may be able to perform this skill smoothly, when transferring attention from far-to-near; but they may have difficulty in going from near-to-far. Have the patient repeat a number of fixation cycles before you start your observations. Does one eye seem to lag behind the other when he performs a fixation? Check for proper pupillary changes, when subject looks at far, pupillary dilation; when subject looks at near, pupillary constriction. Do both pupils change simultaneously? Is the change in diameter of the pupils the same in both eyes? Is the pupillary opening always circular? Careful observation is essential.

F. Precautions:
   (1) Position yourself so that you can follow the complete eye movement of the patient.
   (2) Allow the patient to make several fixation changes before you start your observation.
   (3) Observe both the eye movements and the pupillary changes as well.

C. Record:
   (a) The quality of the fixation change from both far-to-near and near-to-far directions
   (b) Pupillary responses.

9. *Brock String Test* (see Figure 15)
   A. Target: a four foot piece of ordinary string.
   B. Procedure: The patient is told to hold one end of the string at the tip of his nose and the other end at his normal nearpoint working distance. He is to hold the string taut at all times. The string thus stretches in a straight line from his nose to the ordinary position

Patient Responses to Brock String

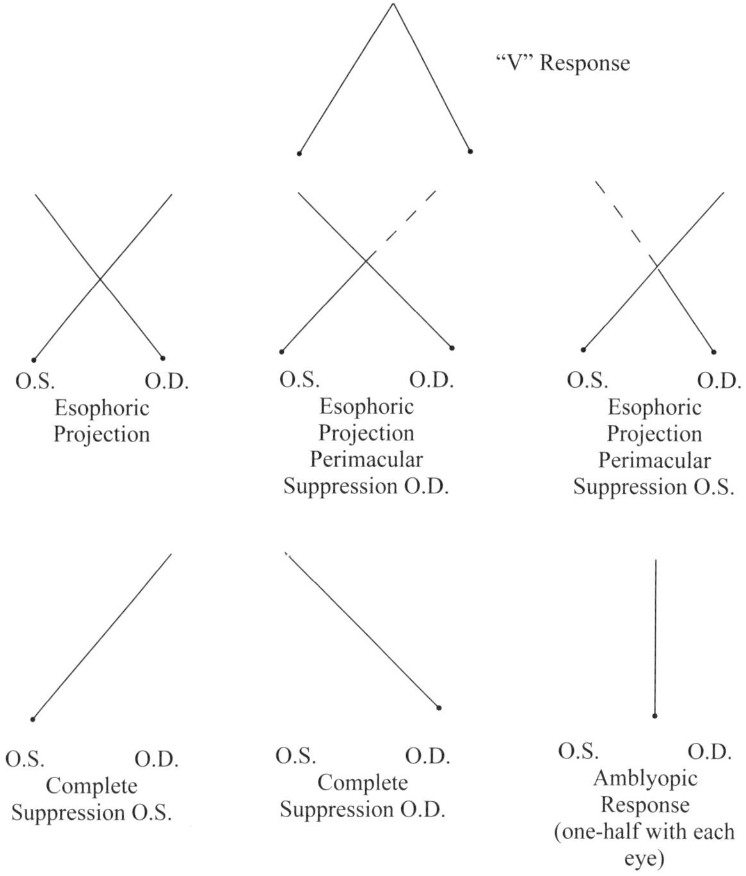

Figure 15.

of his nearpoint work. We ask the patient to fixate at the far end of the string. We now inquire as to the number of strings he sees emerging from his head and going to the far end of the string. The patient should report the presence of a "V" with the strings meeting at his far finger. The presence of a single string, or the two strings meeting as an "X," or the two strings meeting as a "Y" are anomalous responses. Since the idea of seeing two strings, when the subject knows there is only one, is a strange experience, it is important to aid the patient by means of alternate occlusion of the eyes to see the shift in the position of the string. Therefore, he will become aware of the presence of the two strings meeting at his finger. The patient is psychologically set to see one string and, therefore, he may deliberately ignore one of the images. This indoctrination training is important.

C. Normal: Seeing the two strings emerge from the side of the head and proceeding toward the distal finger and meeting there to make a "V."

D. Instructions to patient: "Please watch how I hold this String. You see that I hold one end of the string against my nose and the other end of the string at my normal reading distance. Now you take this string and do the same. Hold the string taut so that it goes from your nose to your other finger in a straight line. As you look at the end of the string how many strings do you see? Do you see only one string going to your finger, or do you see more than one string? What letter does it look like?"

E. Remarks: This test investigates the spatial output of the patient, and how he uses his eyes when he looks at near in a normal environment. Some of the points we can investigate are:

   (1) Does he use both eyes at the same time and project to the same point in space? If he does, he should see a "V" with both strings equally clear.

   (2) Does he use one eye only? If he does, he should see one string only.

   (3) Does he see one string most of the time, and the other string part of the time? If he does, this indicates an alternate suppression of one eye.

   (4) Does he see an "X" instead of a "V"? If he does, this indicates that he is using both eyes, but that he projects closer to himself than the actual location of the object of regard.

   (5) Does he see a "Y" instead of a "V"? If he does, this indicates closer projection than the object of regard. At the same time it indicates suppression of one eye in the spatial area between the touching of the two strings to the actual location of the object of regard.

   (6) Do the strings seem to emerge from the head on the same level, or is one string higher than the other? In what way does he have to tilt his head in order to get the strings on the same horizontal line? This indicates a hyperphoria posture. It is an excellent test for patient indoctrination since it measures how the patient sees at near under normal conditions.

F. Precautions:

(1) Demonstrate the proper technique in holding the string.

(2) If patient reports one string, give the patient a period of alternate occlusion so that he can detect the jump in the string.

(3) If the patient reports that he sees two strings meeting at his finger, it is still necessary to determine if he sees them both equally clear, or if one string seems to be much dimmer and nebulous in character. This latter response indicates a partial suppression of that eye.

(4) We have crossed projection of the images of the string, that is the right string is projected from the left eye, and the left string is projected from the right eye. This cross projection is the familiar physiological diplopia occurring when one looks at a distal object and at the same time a near object is in the field of view.

G. Record: (1) The projection pattern of the patient. Describe it in detail.

Stereoscopic Tests

These are the visual skills tests which are performed in a stereoscopic instrument.

1. *Simultaneous Perception* (first degree fusion)

A. Target: DB-10 (dog-Pig) stereogram; stereoscope is set at farpoint adjustment. (Figure 16)

B. Procedure: Since this is the first test performed in a stereoscope, it is important that you indoctrinate the patient as to the proper posture for this type of testing. The correct posture should be: (1) Both feet flat on the floor. (2) The instrument must be at eye level. (3) The plane of the target should be parallel to the plane of the face. (4) The patient should be in a balanced position, with forehead resting against the headrest. (5) Head must not be tilted. (6) For young children, have them stand while taking farpoint skills; adults may be seated, but hands should not be touching the instrument. Psychic convergence must be minimized when we are doing farpoint testing.

The target is at the farpoint setting of the instrument. The patient is asked to report what he sees. The normal response is that the patient reports the presence of both the dog and the pig. If the patient reports that he sees only one of the animals, or if one of the targets tends to fade, demonstrate the presence of both targets by occluding each eye in turn and asking the patient what he sees. Remove the occluder and see if he can now report the presence of both the dog and pig. This is a very important demonstration for proper patient control. It is an exceedingly gross visual test, and any anomalous responses at this level indicate extended adaptations. If the patient reports that the dog and pig are both present at the same time, we are now interested in the relative positions of the dog and the pig. Does the patient exhibit a crossed projection (pig to the right of the dog)? If so, the patient indicates exophoria. Does the patient exhibit uncrossed projection (pig to the left of the dog)? This response indicates esophoria. So far our questioning has covered whether or not both targets are present all the time, and the relative position of the targets. The third area of questioning investigates the relative stability of the positions assumed by the targets. Do the targets start in the normal position and then drift into an exophoria or esophoria projection? Does the opposite situation occur, with the patient initially reporting an exophoria or esophoria projection with the targets drifting into an orthophoria positioning? Does the position of the targets change slowly or rapidly? Since these are very gross targets any change in positioning indicates poor visual stability.

C. Normal: a whole dog and a whole pig lined up vertically.

D. Instructions to patient: "What do you see?" (The patient will probably report a dog and pig present.) "Do you see all of the dog and all of the pig all of the time?" "Is the dog above the pig or to one side?" "Do they stay this way all of the time or do they move about?" "Which way do they move?"

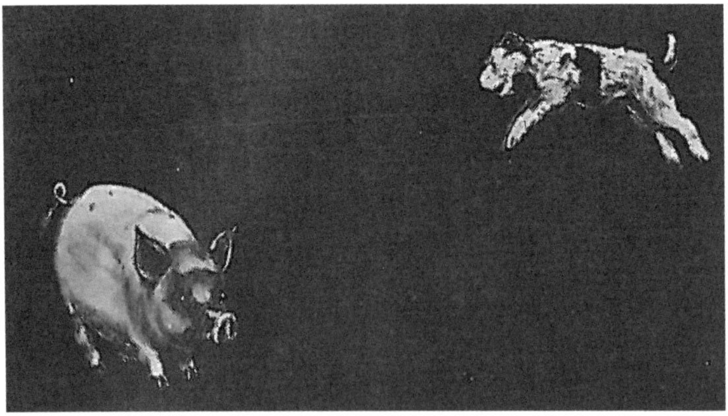

Figure 16. Simultaneous perception. DB 10A Keystone View Company.

E. Remarks: These targets are massive and they are seen against a nonfigural background. Therefore, suppression exhibited on these targets indicates a long standing adaptation. Unstable positioning exhibited here also indicates a long standing problem. The questioning must cover three aspects of the testing situation: (a) The presence of the complete targets, (b) The relative position of the two targets, and (c) The stability of the positioning of the targets. Each of these aspects of questioning is important for proper diagnosis. Thus, the test measures not only the presence or absence of simultaneous perception, but also spatial localization and the stability of this localization as well. If the patient exhibits suppression or shifting localization, it is important to the patient to demonstrate that the instrument is not causing this effect, but that this variation is happening in the visual system of the patient. This can be demonstrated by having the patient move his head from the instrument and assure himself that the targets are really there. In all of the stereoscope testing procedures to follow, always demonstrate to the patient that any anomalous response obtained is not due to variation in the instrument, but to how he is using his eyes.

F. Precautions:

(1) Instrument adjusted properly to minimize psychic convergence.

(2) Patient posture adjusted so as to minimize psychic convergence.

(3) Have patient keep his eyes closed until you have the target properly positioned, and then have him open his eyes and describe what he sees.

(4) Be sure that you obtain the immediate response to the stimulus target. Also question the patient as to what happens when he continues to observe the target for about 15 seconds.

(5) Explain the test to the patient in words that he can understand.

G. Record:

(1) Presence or absence of targets.

(2) Relative position of the targets to each other.

(3) The stability of the positioning.

2. *Visual Discrimination (Farpoint)*

A. Target: DB-1, 2, 3 stereograms; stereoscope adjusted at "farpoint." (Figure 17)

B. Procedure: This test consists of a series of three stereograms used to check the monocular ability to discriminate detail at far, and the binocular ability used to discriminate detail at far. We start the test with target DB-3 (right eye) which is inserted into the target holder. The patient and height of instrument are adjusted so that the patient posture is normal. The patient must be looking straight ahead into the instrument. He is told to report the position of the black dot in each of the signboards.

If the patient has diplopia on the target, note this on the report form. Proceed your testing with the monocular targets by occluding one eye.

If the patient is unable to report the correct location of the black dot through the ninth signboard (which is equivalent to 20/20), occlude one eye (the right eye on DB-2 and the left eye on DB-3) and the test is repeated. We will have two measurements of the visual discrimination of each eye; first, visual discrimination of one eye while exposed to binocular stimulus, second, visual discrimination of one eye with the other eye occluded.

The patient having normal visual ability should be able to reach the ninth signboard correctly which is scored as 100%. The test is repeated for the left eye (DB-2) and both eyes (DB-1).

C. Normal: 100% visual acuity O.D., O.S., and O.U.

D. Instructions to patient: "In this picture you will observe a series of signboards which are numbered from one to eleven. You will note that the first signboard is larger and closer to you, and the succeeding signboards become smaller and are further away. I want you to concentrate on the first signboard. You will see in this signboard five diamond shapes. In one of these diamonds you will observe a black dot. In this first signboard, in which diamond do you see the black dot in the upper, lower, right, left or center diamond?"

As soon as the correct response is obtained for the first signboard, you continue with the remaining targets in this stereogram. When the patient has reached the limit of his discrimination it is well to encourage the patient to try the next target. For example, the

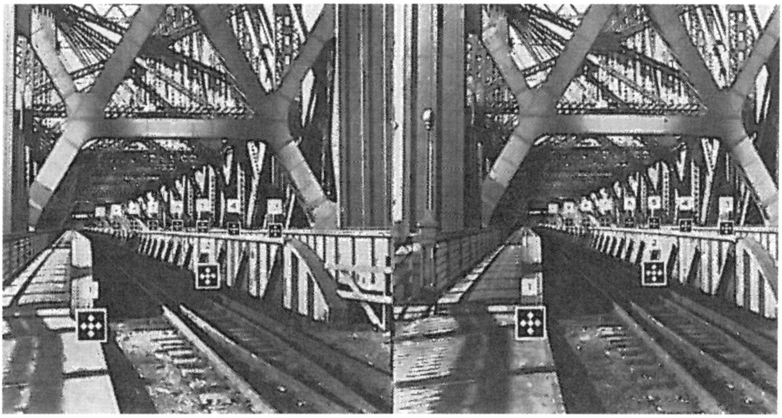

Figure 17. Visual discrimination (farpoint). DB 3D Keystone View Company

patient has reported correctly on the eighth signboard, but states that he does not see any dot in the ninth signboard. You might say: "Take another look at the ninth signboard. Is there something there that might be a small dot?" The same instructions are used with each of the remaining stereograms.

E. Remarks: This is an unusual discrimination test in that we can test monocular acuity while the patient is receiving binocular stimulation.

Thus, whenever the patient's response is less under binocular stimulation than when one eye is occluded, we can expect to find suspensions and suppressions present. For example, if on stereogram DB-3 the patient's maximum visual acuity is 80%, but after occlusion of the left eye, the patient has 100% visual acuity in his right eye, this would indicate that under conditions demanding fine discrimination, the subject is not using his right eye. Another example: patient reports 60% vision on DB-3. If we occlude his left eye the subject can still only show 60% acuity. In this case the patient is either amblyopic, or he is not wearing the proper correction.

F. Precautions:

(1) Adjust posture of patient and of the instrument to minimize psychic convergence.

(2) Be certain that the patient understands your instructions.

(3) Encourage the patient to continue to try to determine the position of the black dot to his ultimate resolution ability.

(4) If the patient does not show 100% acuity on this test, occlude one eye and note the change in acuity.

(5) If the patient has a low score be certain and determine if it is due to diplopia, suppression or possible amblyopia.

G. Record:

(1) record the maximum score obtained for each eye.

(2) Record the change in score upon occlusion.

3. *Lateral Phoria* (*Farpoint*)

A. Target: stereogram DB-9: (Figure 18) stereoscope adjusted for infinity.

B. Procedure: Since this is a farpoint phoria test it is important that every effort be taken to inhibit psychic convergence. Patient must be seated and erect with both feet flat on the floor. Head posture should be erect looking straight forward into the instrument. Hands must not be touching the instrument. The patient is directed to observe the target and is asked if he can see the arrow and numbers at the same time. Here again is verification of simultaneous perception. We now determine at what number the arrow is pointing as he continues to observe the target. We are concerned with three different aspects of this testing situation. (1) The initial position of the arrow. (2) The direction of movement of the arrow as he continues to observe the target. (3) The range of movement as he continues to observe the target.

C. Normal: arrow pointing between 8 and 9 with stability.

D. Instructions to patient: "What do you see?" (pause) If they don't respond appropriately then ask. "Do you see an arrow? Do you see a series of numbers? Do you see the arrow and numbers at the same time? I want you to close your eyes again and when I say, 'open' - open your eyes and tell me at what number the arrow is pointing."

After patient reports initial position of the arrow, continue questioning regarding position of arrow: "Where is the arrow now?" (5 sec. pause) "Where is the arrow now?"

E. Remarks: Intensive interrogation is a must. Even though we established simultaneous perception by another test, we must again determine the presence or absence of the visual quality at this time. The present target involves figures having less mass and, therefore, a patient may have passed B-1 and fail here. We have degrees

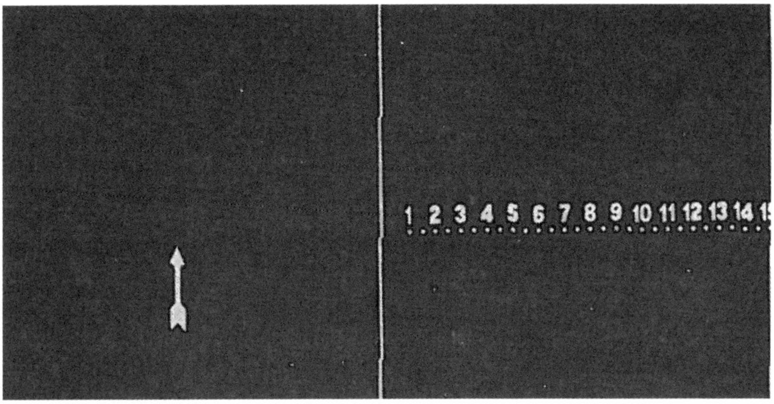

Figure 18. Lateral phoria (farpoint). DB 9 Keystone View Company

of simultaneous perception just as we have a range in quality of fusion and stereopsis. Similarly, the mere recording of the initial position of the arrow is not sufficient for accurate diagnosis. We are just as interested in what happens to the position of the arrow as the subject views the target. For example, some subjects will report an initial ortho position; but as they continue to observe the target they will report the arrow drifting out to higher or lower numbers. Instead of this slow drifting in the position of the arrow we may have a nystagmus type of movement of the arrow. The patient may report somewhat as follows: Arrow at 8, no it's at 10, no it's at 9, etc. This instability of convergence would surely be a handicap for someone having to do accurate fixations in his normal environment.

The arrow moving towards the higher numbers indicates exophoria (above 9.5). The arrow moving towards the lower numbers indicates esophoria (below 8.5). If the arrow or numbers disappear, it indicates a complete suppression of the appropriate eye.

F. Precautions:

(1) Adjust the position of the instrument and posture of patient for maximum inhibition to psychic convergence.

(2) Young patients may have difficulty following your instructions. For these cases, a pointer may be inserted, and the patient asked to report when the pointer is just above the tip of the arrow. Since you have inserted the pointer on the number side of the instrument, you can readily determine the position of the arrow

(3) Do you have the target at the infinity position?

G. Record:
   (1) The initial position of the arrow.
   (2) The direction the arrow tends to move.
   (3) The extent of the oscillation of the arrow.
   (4) The presence of any signs of suppression.

4. *Vertical Phoria* (*farpoint*)

   A. Target: stereoscope is adjusted for infinity, stereogram DB-8C (Figure 19).

   B. Procedure: Precautions must be taken to minimize psychic convergence; see directions previously given. The patient is directed to look at the target and to report what he can see. The usual response is the presence of a line and a series of symbols. The more careful observer will describe the stereogram as consisting of a green line and red symbols. The patient reporting the presence of both the line and symbols is exhibiting simultaneous perception. The patient is now asked to report which symbol the green line passes through. Once the initial position of the line through the symbols is ascertained, urge the patient to continue his observation for a few seconds so that any change in position due to sustained stimulus may be found.

   C. Normal: The patient reports the green line passing through the red ball.

   D. Instruction to the Patient: "What do you see?" (pause) If they don't respond appropriately then ask. "Do yon see a green line? Do you see the group of red symbols? Do you see the green line and the red symbols at the same time? Which symbol does the green line pass through?" (5 second pause) "Which symbol does the green line pass through now?"

   E. Remarks: The vertical phoria test, just as in the case of the lateral phoria test, presents a means of creating simultaneous monocular vision which has several advantages. Principally, these are: the patient is not aware of diplopia. He does not have any discomfort which is frequently exhibited by patients who have been dissociated by means of a vertical prism.

   The presence of a high lateral phoria may prevent the green line from passing through any portion of the red symbols. In this case, ask the patient, "If the green line was long enough, through which one of the red symbols would it pass?" If the patient reports the

Figure 19. Vertical phoria (farpoint). DB 8C Keystone View Company.

presence of either the green line or the red symbols, it indicates a suppression of the appropriate eye. If the patient reports the presence of the line and then the symbols, it indicates an alternate type of suppression.

The green line passing through a symbol above the red ball indicates right hyperphoria. The green line passing through a symbol below the red ball indicates left hyperphoria.

F. Precautions:

(1) Adjust the instrument for maximum inhibition to convergence.

(2) For young patients use a pointer as a probe to determine through which symbol the line is passing through.

(3) Head posture of patient is very important. Any head tilt may show up as a hyperphoria.

G. Record:

(1) The presence of any vertical deviation.

(2) The stability of the report.

(3) The presence of any suppression.

5. *Fusion (second degree fusion) farpoint*

A. Target: stereogram DB-4K; (Figure 20): stereoscope is adjusted for infinity.

B. Procedure: Since this is a farpoint test, every precaution must be taken to minimize psychic convergence (see previous instructions). The patient is directed to observe the target, and report what he sees as soon as the stimulus is presented. The possible responses to this test are the presence of two balls, an alteration of two balls, three balls, four balls, three balls becoming four balls, four balls becoming three balls, two balls becoming three balls or three balls becoming two balls. It is thus important that you continue to ask the patient to describe how many balls he sees as he continues to observe the binocular stimulus.

Figure 20. Fusion (second degree farpoint). DB 4K Keystone View Company.

C. Normal: The expected response is the presence of three balls which indicates normal fusional ability. Acceptable responses are three balls becoming four balls, or four balls becoming three balls.

D. Instructions to patient: "Tell me how many balls you see as soon as I turn on the light (or uncover your eyes). How many balls do you see now? What are the colors of the balls? Do you still see the same number of balls, or have they changed in any way?"

E. Remarks: This is a gross test for second degree fusion, and it should be passed with ease by the patient. The interpretation of the various patient responses are:

   a. Report is two balls - suppression of appropriate eye.

   b. Two balls alternating - alternating suppression.

   c. Three balls - normal fusional response.

   d. Three balls becoming four balls - immediate response is normal but cannot maintain fusion.

   e. Three balls becoming two balls - immediate response is normal but quickly suppresses one eye under the impact of the binocular demand.

   f. Four balls - presence of 1st degree fusion (simultaneous perception).

   The patient may report a normal response of three balls, but even in this case it is well to question further whether they are all lined up in the same vertical plane, or if we have one of the balls displayed to the left or the right. This lateral displacement of one of the balls indicates the presence of so-called retinal slip.

   The second degree fusional test may be failed by patients because of the presence of a high lateral or vertical phoria. It is of interest in these cases to determine the amount of prism either laterally or vertically positioned to enable the subject to recapture normal second degree fusion.

F. Precautions:
   (1) Adjust stereoscope for maximum inhibition to psychic convergence.
   (2) Record all responses of the patient.
   (3) Set the stereoscope for infinity.
   (4) Since we have a nearpoint target, which is very similar to this target, be certain that you have the farpoint target.

G. Record:
   (1) The initial response of the patient.
   (2) The intermediate response (after five seconds of observation).
   (3) The final response (after an additional five seconds of observation).

6. *Stereopsis (third degree fusion) farpoint*

A. Target: stereogram DB-6D (Figure 21): stereoscope adjusted for infinity.

B. Procedure: Since we are testing stereo acuity of the patient at far, every precaution must be taken regarding the posture of the patient to minimize or inhibit psychic convergence. The stereogram contains 12 rows of symbols arranged within a black picture frame. Each row of symbols contains five simple forms: heart, ball, cross, box and star. One of the symbols in each row seems to stand out from the remaining symbols in the row. The patient may report that the target is doubled. In this case, move the slide holder toward the patient slowly, until he obtains single vision. The slide holder is now moved slowly back toward the normal infinity position. The patient is directed to report which symbol in each row is closer to him.

C. Normal: To report at least ten lines of the stereogram correctly. Each line correctly reported represents about four percent stereopsis.

D. Instructions to patient: "This card contains 12 rows of symbols within a black picture frame. You will note that each row contains five different symbols. In the first row- the one at the top - you will see a star, box, cross, heart, and ball. Do you notice that one symbol in this top row seems closer to you than the rest of the symbols in that line?"

Figure 21. Stereopsis (farpoint). DB 6D Keystone View Company.

(pause) "Does one of the symbols in the top row seem to float out towards you?" (pause) "Does one of the symbols in the top row seem to have air behind it?"

As soon as a correct response is obtained for the first row, the same questions are repeated for each row in turn, until the response on all 12 rows has been obtained. If the patient cannot give the correct response for the first line, question about the appearance of tiny symbols in the lower left and lower right of the black frame. These are suppression controls, and if they are absent the subject is using one eye.

E. Remarks: this is a gross test for stereopsis. A correct response on all 12 rows of the stereogram is equivalent to 48% stereopsis. Since this test becomes progressively difficult as you proceed from the first row towards the last row, it is important to encourage your patient in order to obtain his maximum response. Some patients will pass this test even though they have failed the second degree fusion test. The large, heavy black frame surrounding the stereopsis targets enables the subject with considerable lateral phoria to fuse this target; thus, he exhibits a stereopsis response.

F. Precautions:

(1) Adjust instrument and patient posture for maximum inhibition to psychic convergence.

(2) Encourage the patient to try all of the 12 rows of symbols.

(3) If patient fails on first row, ascertain whether failure is due to presence of diplopia, suppression or low steropsis.

(4) Be certain that patient understands what stereopsis means.

G. Record: That number of: rows correctly done.

If patient fails completely, designate cause of failure.

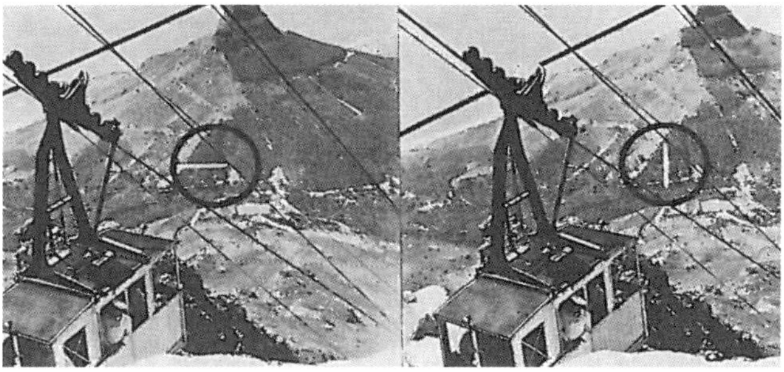

Figure 22. Macular suppression (far). BU21 Keystone View Company.

7. *Macular Suppression, Farpoint*

   A. Target: stereograph BU-21 (See Figure 22): stereoscope adjusted for infinity.

   B. Procedure: The patient must be able to fuse the target and report a single, clear picture. The patient is then interrogated regarding the appearance of the control marks. Have the patient draw how the marks appcar to him/her.

   C. Normal; The patient reports the presence of the perfect cross.

   D. Instructions to the patient; "Do you see one picture? Is the picture sharp and clear? Do you see any lines in the picture? (pause) Do you see a horizontal and vertical line in the picture? (For a young child draw a horizontal line on his back and a vertical line the same way) "Do you see both of these lines at the same time? What do these two lines look like?" (If the patient by this time has not described a cross), "are these two lines near each other? Do they look like a cross or a "T" lying on its side? Are both lines of the cross equally distant from you, or is one line closer to you than the other? Are both lines solid or is some portion of the lines fading or missing?"

   E. Remarks: Ask young children if they see the line running up-and-down. At the same time emphasize the direction by taking their finger and moving it in the same direction. Repeat this for the line going across, moving their finger in the horizontal direction this time. To verify the young patient response, have him draw on paper the way the lines look to him.

      The correct response is to see a perfect cross. However, a patient with the presence of a high lateral phoria may report that the lines cross each other, but that it looks more like a "T" lying on its side. In extreme cases of retinal slip, both lines may be displaced to such

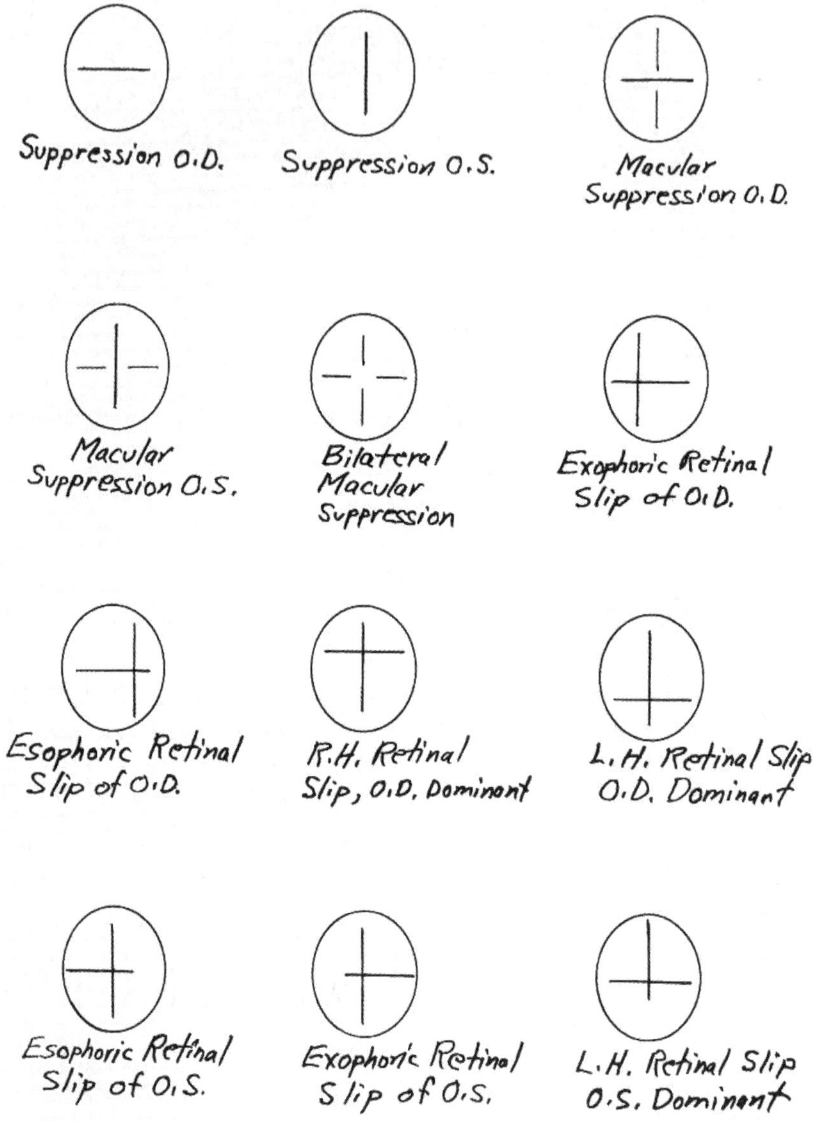

Figure 23.

a degree that they are both present but do not touch each other. The relationship of the vertical line to the center of the horizontal line will indicate whether the projection is crossed or uncrossed diplopia; therefore, the type of phoria which is causing the retinal slip may be determined (see Figure 23 for details).

If the patient reports the presence of only one control mark, it indicates a macular suppression of the eye corresponding to the side of the missing line. The control marks may alternate, the patient seeing only one control mark at a time, i.e., first the horizontal then the vertical line will appear. This indicates alternating suppression.

Even when the patient reports the presence of a perfect cross, it is important to question him further regarding the appearance of the control marks at the point of intersection. A small portion of the line at this point may be suppressed.

F. Precautions:

(1) Adjust the instrument and the posture of the patient so that you obtain maximum inhibition to psychic convergence.

(2) Question your patient carefully regarding the appearance of the two control marks.

G. Record: Record the exact appearance of the control marks upon immediate observation. Also note any changes as patient continues to observe the stereogram for ten seconds.

8. *Retinal Rivalry (Cortical Alternation)* Editors note: While these terms are not necessarily correct terminology today they were left unchanged for this discussion.

A. Target: black lines at 45° on one side and black lines at 135° on the other side of the stereogram (See Figure 24). The stereoscope is adjusted for infinity. A watch with a sweep second hand.

B. Procedure: The patient is adjusted to the instrument so that both feet are flat on the floor, and he is leaning slightly forward against the head of the instrument. The patient is asked to take his forefinger and to tap on the instrument table each time he sees a shift in

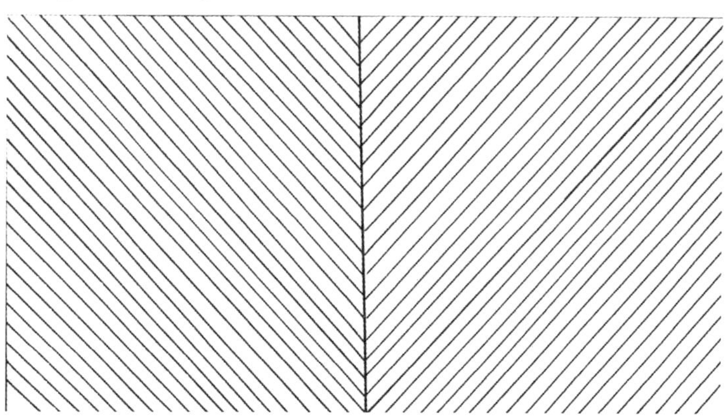

Figure 24.

the line, i.e., when he sees a preponderance of lines at 45° and they shift to 135°. Allow the patient a few seconds to make certain that he has understood your instructions before you start timing. Now time the number of taps made by the patient for a 30-second interval. This now becomes the rate per minute since two taps measure one complete cycle.

C. Normal: The normal rate for cortical alternation depends upon the age of the child:

(1) Seven years of age or less the expected rate is 20 cycles.

(2) From eight through 13 years of age, expected rate 25 cycles.

(3) 14 years or over, expected rate 30 cycles.

One standard deviation for this test is 5 changes per minute. Therefore, any patient exhibiting five changes less than the means cited would be considered as failing the test.

D. Instructions to patient: Look in the center of the picture at all times. You will note that you see a sort of basket weaving of crisscross lines. As you continue to watch in the center of the target you will see that the lines begin to shift and that you see one set of lines and then the other lines begin to come into view. I want you to tap on the instrument table with your forefinger each time that the lines shift as you watch the center of the target.

E. Remarks: Encourage the patient to observe the center of the target field at all times. You merely time the number of taps for a 30 second time interval. The original name for this visual skill test was retinal rivalry. It soon became evident that the retina could not rival that the phenomenon was cortical in nature. Therefore, the name cortical alternation is also used for this test. In addition, some authorities use the name "reciprocal replacement. The important fact is that you cannot have binocular vision without some alternation; only a complete monocular visual problem would give you a zero rate. Also, when we have a very fast rate (we have no norms for this) binocular vision as measured by stereopsis tends to break down.

F. Precautions:

(1) Instruct the patient carefully regarding the portion of the visual field that he is to observe and how he is to tap each time the lines shift at this fixation position.

(2) The number of taps per 30 seconds becomes the complete cycle rate per minute.

(3) Time your patient accurately.

(4) Patient must have both feet flat on the floor, looking slightly downward with his head placed firmly against the head rest.

G. Record:

(1) The cycle rate per minute.

(2) Which eye is used the most (clue to eye dominancy).

9. *Perimacular suppression (farpoint)*

A. Target: Split stereograms PG-16 and PG-19. These split targets consist of a small white fixation star on a black background and a heavy white ring on a black background. Stereoscope is adjusted for infinity.

B. Procedure: No fusion is possible in this test since we present a fixation target to one eye and a peripheral target before the other. The lateral position of the split targets is adjusted until the patient describes the star in the center of the ring. The patient is to observe both the white star and the white ring. We are testing for perimacular suppression of the eye which is located before the white ring. This test is therefore performed twice: first, with the circle before the right eye and the star before the left eye; second with the circle before the left eye and the star before the right eye. Have the patient describe the appearance of the circle as he maintains fixation upon the star.

C. Normal: The patient should be able to maintain the star inside of the ring. This indicates simultaneous visual ability. Fading of any portion of the white ring, or the disappearance of the ring, indicates perimacular suppression of the eye that corresponds to the eye which has the white circle before it. Each eye is tested in turn by reversing the position of the split stereograms.

D. Instructions to patient: "Tell me when the star is in the center of the white ring. Do you see the white star and the white ring all of the time? While looking at the star does any portion of the white ring disappear?"

E. Remarks: Some patients may have difficulty describing the appearance of the white ring. In this case have them draw what they see. Tell the patient to keep watching the star all of the time, but also tell him to be aware of the appearance of the white ring at the same time.

F. Precautions:

(1) Adjust instrument and posture of the patient in order to minimize psychic convergence.

(2) Be certain that fixation is always on the star.

(3) Encourage patient to describe completely the appearance of the ring.

G. Record:

(1) If patient can maintain simultaneous vision.

(2) The appearance of the circle as macular attention is directed at the star for each eye in turn. Have patient draw or record area of suppression using the clock dial designation.

10. *Hand and eye coordination (farpoint)*

A. Target: stereograms AN-1 and AN-9. AN-1 presents a gross number configuration on a simple background without any stereopsis demand. AN-9 presents a fine number configuration against a figural background which demands stereoscopic interpretation. The stereoscope is adjusted for infinity (see Figure 25).

B. Procedure: The height of the instrument must be adjusted so that the patient can rest his elbows on the instrument table and still maintain normal body posture. The patient is given two pointers of different colors. He is to hold one pointer in each hand in the same manner as if they were pencils. The patient orients the position of the pointers by using the eyepiece of the instrument as a starting position. The patient is to align the pointers before the eyepiece of the instrument so that they look like they are pointing toward the first number on the stereogram. The patient is to slowly advance both pointers from the eyepiece of the instrument toward the first number on the stereogram. Both pointers should land on this number simultaneously. The patient is to report any difficulty he experiences while he is pointing towards and touching the number on the stereogram. As soon as he has achieved a successful landing on the number, both pointers are moved back to the eyepiece of the instrument. The patient is now ready to advance to the next number on the target. This is repeated until the patient has made a complete circuit of all of the numbers on the target.

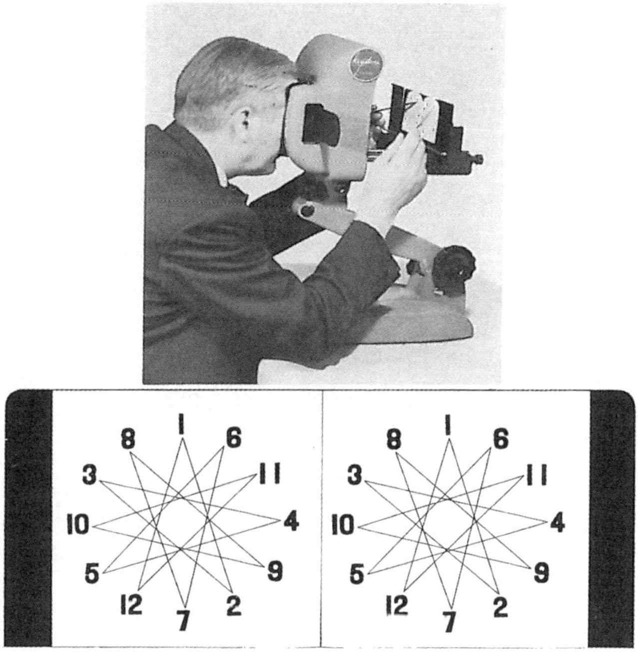

Figure 25. Hand-eye coordination (farpoint).

C. Normal: The patient should be able to point accurately to all of the numbers on both stereograms without reporting any doubling of the numbers, fading of one or both of the pointers, or not landing properly on the number with both pointers.

D. Instructions to the patient: "Take the two pointers and hold them as if they were pencils. Place both pointers in front of the eyepieces of the instrument. Now line the pointer tips so that they look as if they were pointing directly at number one on the card. Are both pointers aimed at the first number? Advance both pointers simultaneously and slowly toward number one until they both land on the target. If the numbers double or blur, or if the pointers fade or disappear, report this information immediately. If you see a single number one and both pointer tips touch the number, you can remove the pointers and place them back on the eyepieces of the instrument. Repeat this procedure for the next number, and etc."

E. Remarks: There is no other skills test which presents to the patient, in as vivid a form, his anomalous responses. There are few patients who can understand a verbal explanation of their visual deficiencies. But when a patient advances two pointers toward a number, and he can feel the front end of the pointer disappear every time he touches a number, he has had a self evident demonstration of his need for visual rehabilitation. The anomalous responses which the patient may report are:

1. Numbers are blurred. This indicates excessive stimulation of convergence by the use of the hands.
2. Numbers are doubled. This indicates poor fusion when precise binocular fixation is required.
3. One pointer present. This indicates suppression of the eye corresponding to the missing pointer.
4. Pointer tips are alternating. This indicates an alternating suppression.
5. Patient reports presence of both pointers, but you can observe that one pointer is inside of the number. This indicates a retinal slip associated with an esophoric tendency.
6. Same as case 5, but pointer tip is now on the outward side of the number. This indicates a retinal slip associated with an exophoric tendency.
7. Same as case 5, but pointer tip is now above the number. This indicates a retinal slip, associated with a hyperphoric tendency of the eye, associated with the high pointer.
8. The patient may ignore its one perceptual field and invade the target belonging to the other eye with a pointer. This indicates a more complex and deep-seated suppression of the eye corresponding to this hand.
9. The patient may report the presence of both pointers, but the tip of one pointer may be missing. This indicates a macular suppression of the eye corresponding to the pointer with the missing tip.

F. Precautions:

(1) Patient posture and instrument adjusted for maximum inhibition to psychic convergence.

(2) When the patient grasps the pointers make sure that he is not holding them so close to the front of the pointer that the hand comes in contact with the stereogram. The only physical contact between patient and stereogram should be the isolated pointer tips.

(3) Be certain that the patient understands your instructions. Repeat several times if necessary.

(4) If patient exhibits anomalous responses be sure and call these to his attention. You may do this by having him hold the pointers still. Remove his head from the instrument so that he can be certain that there are really two complete pointers present all of the time.

(5) Indoctrinate your patient to report what is happening all of the time.

G. Record:

(1) The numbers which double when he touches them.

(2) Any fading of pointers.

(3) Any invasion of the wrong perceptual field.

(4) Placement positioning of the pointers.

11. *Accommodative rock* (*accommodative facility*) *farpoint*

A. Target: reduced Snellen stereogram. Stereoscope adjusted for infinity position.

B. Procedure: Present two occluder paddles to the patient. He is to hold one paddle or occluder in each hand. Have him cover his right eye by covering the right side of the stereoscope, and determine if he can read the 20/20 reduced Snellen type with his left eye. Now have the patient occlude the other side, and see if he can now read the 20/20 reduced Snellen type with his right eye. The patient, by placing his elbows on the instrument table, will find it very easy to alternately occlude each eve. Have the patient "rock" back and forth three or four times so that you can note the facility of his response. While the left eve is occluded insert a minus 2.50 diopter lens in the left lens well, and have patient continue the alternate shift in the occluder paddles. With the right eye occluded, the patient must read the 20/20 reduced Snellen with his left eye through the minus 2.50 diopter lens. If he reports these letters clearly he must have accommodated two and one-half diopters. Now have the patient shift the occluder to his left eye. The patient must now inhibit two and one-half diopters of accommodation in order to see the 20/20 reduced Snellen letters clearly. Have the patient "rock" three or four times to be certain that he has good facility of accommodative change. Now shift the minus 2.50D lens to the right lens well and repeat the "rock."

C. Normal: ability to stimulate or inhibit two and one-half diopters of accommodation with facility.

D. Instructions to patient: "Place your elbows on the instrument table and hold one of these paddles in each hand. When I call 'right' I want you to cover the right eye of the instrument with the paddle and uncover the left eye. When I call 'left' I want you to cover the left eye with the paddle and uncover the right eye. I will always tell you which eye is to be covered by the occluder paddle. You will note that the target is a small group of letters. I want you to read aloud the smallest letters you can read as the occluder shifts from one side to the other."

E. Remarks: If patient fails this test, note whether he fails on the stimulative (minus lens side) or on the inhibitive side (plano side) of the stereoscope. The patient should be able to perform this test with ease, since an accommodative shift of only two and one-half diopters is demanded. Any failure (blurring) on the part of the patient indicates a poor facility of change in accommodation, regardless of the magnitude of his amplitude of accommodation. If the patient is able to perform this test, but only at a much slower pace, this should be noted. This test measures accommodative performance ability and not magnitude of accommodation. This is not an amplitude test; it is a facility test.

F. Precautions:

(1) Allow the patient to "rock" several times before you add the -2.50D. lens.

(2) Have children read the 20/20 reduced Snellen line in reverse, or call out for certain letters to be given at command. For example call out, "Third letter from the left, the last letter on the right and etc."

(3) Do not allow the patient more than three seconds to clear the print.

(4) Stimulative side: Side of the instrument in which the minus 2.50 diopter lens is located. Inhibitive side: Side of the instrument in which we have no lens inserted.

G. Record:

(1) Does the patient fail the test on the inhibitive or stimulative side?

(2) Did the patient clear the print quickly or slowly?

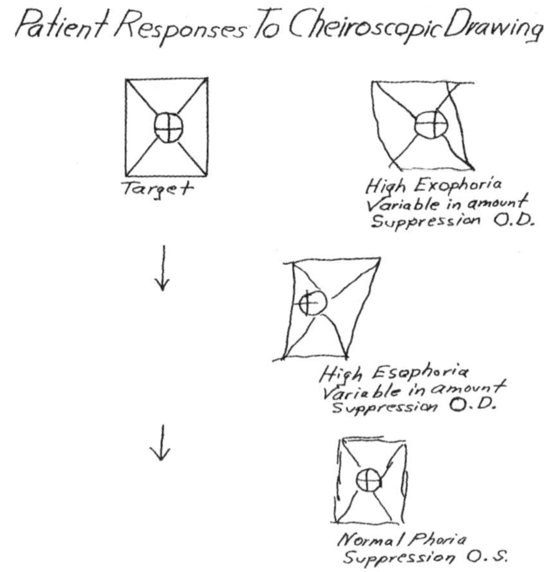

Figure 26. Patient Responses To Cheiroscopic Drawing

Patient Responses To Cheiroscopic Drawing

12. *Cheiroscopic Tracing*

A. Target: A simple line drawing of simple forms may be used. For suggested target see Figure 26: stereoscope is adjusted for infinity setting.

B. Procedure: The target is placed before the eye corresponding to the non-dominant hand, while the drawing paper is before the eye corresponding to the dominant hand. The target is placed close to the septum. The angle of the instrument is adjusted for normal writing angle. The patient is given a pencil. The pencil is held in the dominant hand at about three inches from the point of the pencil. The patient places his head in the stereoscope, and he places his pencil on the corner of the picture. If he has difficulty doing this, help the patient to orient his hand properly. The patient is now asked to trace over the picture. To him it seems that he is actually tracing over the picture. To the doctor, the patient is making a reproduction of the picture, on the paper, on the dominant hand side.

C. Normal: the ability to reproduce the target quickly and easily. Similar points of the picture and tracing should be 80mm for orthophoria. More than 80mm separation indicates exophoria; less than 80mm separation indicates esophoria.

D. Instructions to the patient: "Place your pencil on the upper right corner of the picture. Do you see the picture? Do you see the pencil tip? Now trace the picture with your pencil. Trace carefully and try to stay on top of the lines."

E. Remarks: Orthophoria for the correct-eye-scope is 87mm, but due to the psychic convergence involved, orthophoria separation of picture and tracing is 80mm. Unless precautions are taken to minimize psychic convergence even this figure may be too great. There should be no contact between the hand of the patient and the drawing platform of the instrument. The optical setting of the instrument is for optical infinity. The contact of the hand with the drawing platform of the instrument informs the patient that the target is close. Therefore, if the practitioner desires to estimate the amount of lateral phoria present, he must make certain that every effort is made to minimize psychic convergence.

The distance between the platform and the optical system of the cheiroscope is 200mm. At that distance, one prism diopter is equal to 2mm. Thus, when the distance between similar points of the target and the tracing is 85mm, we have 5mm. of exophoria (85 - 80 = 5), or if we convert into prism diopters, we have 2.5 diopters of exophoria (5/2 = 2.5). Any separation greater than the approximate orthophoria is indicative of exophoria, while any separation less than the orthophoric distance equals esophoria. For example, the distance between similar points of the target and the tracing is 70mm. We now have 10mm. of esophoria (80 – 70 = 10mm.), or if we convert into prism diopters, we have 5 diopters of esophoria (10/2 = 5).

If the patient's tracing is higher than the picture, it indicates the presence of hyperphoria associated with the eye corresponding to the dominant hand of the subject. This may be converted into prism diopters by dividing the amount of the vertical displacement of the tracing by two. If the tracing is lower than the picture, we have hyperphoria associated with the eye on the picture side of the instrument.

If the tracing is not complete, or if it is tilted to one side, it indicates a variable phoria. If the patient seems to be having difficulty making his tracing and has to stop and start several times, it usually indicates suppression. If the hand of the patient invades the picture side of the instrument, it indicates a more complete suppression of the eye corresponding to the dominant hand.

F. Precautions:

(1) Instruct your patient carefully as to the expected technique of performing this test.

(2) If your patient has difficulty in making his tracing, carefully check the placement of the picture. Usually, in these cases, the picture should be moved closer to the septum of the instrument.

(3) Have the patient inform you if the picture or pencil disappears. Instruct him to tap his pencil against the paper if the pencil disappears. Increase the illumination or use a very gross picture if the patient states that the picture tends to disappear.

(4) Don't allow the hand of the patient to rest on the drawing platform of the cheiroscope; only the pencil tip is to be in contact with the paper.

G. Record: The tracing itself should be part of your record. A comparison of this record with that obtained after the patient has received visual care provides a graphical record of progress.

13. Van Orden Star

A. Target: A Van Orden Target (see Figure 27) is placed on the drawing platform of the Cheiroscope. The instrument is set for optical infinity.

B. Procedure: the target is centered on the drawing platform of the Cheiroscope. The patient is given two pencils and told to hold one in each hand in the normal manner. The young child may need some help in holding the pencil with his left hand. The angle of the instrument is adjusted for normal writing posture. The patient is asked if he can see the two rows of dots. He then places one pencil at the right upper dot and the other pencil at the lower left dot. He moves both pencils toward each other diagonally scribing a path on the paper until they look like they meet at the center of the target. He now lifts his pencils free from the paper, and he moves the pencils back to the next lower dot on the right side and the next upper dot on the left side. He is again instructed to move his pencils toward each other diagonally until they look like they meet in the center and touch the other lines. The pencils are again lifted from the paper and moved back to the next dot down on the left and the next dot up on the right. To the patient, it appears that he is drawing a series of intersecting lines that meet in the center

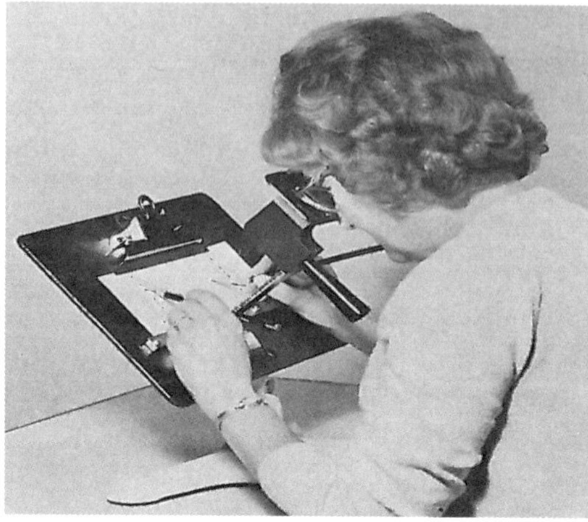

Figure 27. Van Orden Star

of the paper. The patient must be instructed to move both hands at the same time and not to move one hand and then the other.

C. Normal: A normal Van Orden Star pattern is reproduced in Figure 28.

D. Instructions to the patient: "Take one of these pencils in each hand. Now look through the eyepieces of the instrument. What do you see?" (pause) "Do you see two rows of black dots, one on the right side and one on the left side? Do you see both rows of dots at the same time? Now place your right pencil point on the top dot to the right, and place your left pencil point on the lower dot on the left. Now look at the center of the papers as if you are looking through white clouds far away. While looking straight ahead, move the pencils towards each other until they look like they touch in the center of the paper. Both pencils are to be moved at the same time. Now move your pencils back to the black dots, the right pencil on the next dot down on the right side and the left pencil on the next dot up on the left side. Again, draw the pencils toward each other until they look like they touch right in the center of the paper. This is repeated until all of the dots have been connected by pencil lines. It should appear to you as if you are constructing a star pattern."

E. Remarks: The patient starts the test with simultaneous perception and constructs a second degree fusional field. This is a dynamic measure of convergence response. The following are some typical responses: (1) All of the lines on one side come to a neat point, and the lines on the other side come to a neat point. The separation

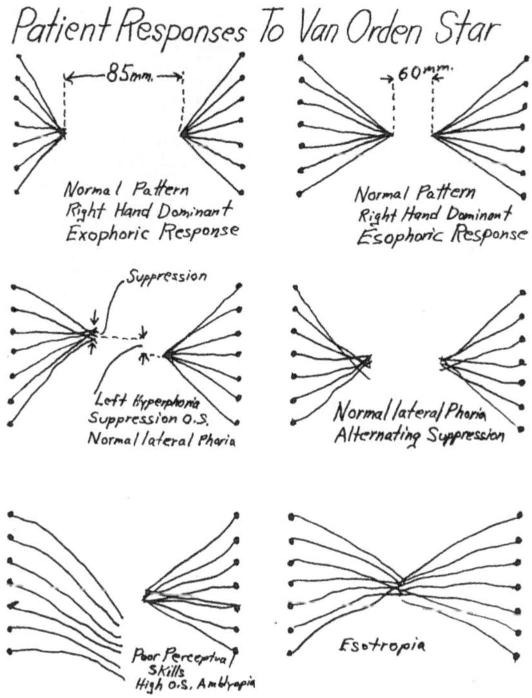

Figure 28. Patient responses to Van Orden Star

between the points is 65mm. This indicates a normal phoria and the presence of good binocular vision. (2) Both sets of lines come to a neat point, but the separation between the two points is less than 65mm. This indicates good binocularity but with an esophoric phoria. (3) Both sets of lines come to a neat point, but the separation between the two points is more than 65mm. This indicates good binocularity but an exophoric phoria. (4) Both sets of lines come to a neat point, but one set of lines comes to a common focus above the other set. A hyperphoria is indicated for the eye corresponding to the higher focus of lines. (5) Whenever the lines from a common side do not come to a single center but are somewhat divergent, this indicates suppression of the corresponding eye. (6) Because of the presence of a suppression, amblyopia, or lowered acuity, the patient with poor hand-and-eye coordination will produce a very poor star pattern with wide divergence of lines which usually do not have a common meeting center. The lines will be wavy and poorly constructed.

This type of record, taken before the patient has received his visual care and after he has finished his remedial work, presents in graphic form, the visual improvement obtained.

F. Precautions:

(1) Be sure that the patient understands your instructions. Before the patient starts his pattern, have him face you while you take two pencils and move them diagonally until they touch. Tell him this is what they will appear to be doing in the instrument, except that they will not actually touch but they will look like they touch. As soon as they seem to touch he is to discontinue his line and move the pencils back to the next dots.

(2) The pencils should seem to meet in the center of the paper.

(3) Only the pencil tips are to touch the paper. Do not let the patient rest his hands on the paper as he makes his lines.

(4) Normal nearpoint body posture is to be maintained.

G. Record: the drawing becomes part of the patient file.
The diagnosis should be written on the side of the drawing.

14. *Color Perception*

A. Target: stereogram DB-12 (instruction only) and DB-14 (Figure 29) (testing only) are used. Stereoscope is adjusted for optical infinity.

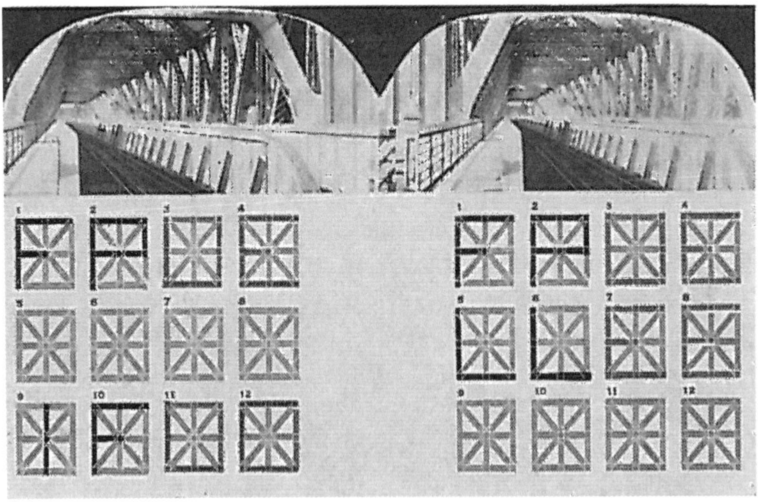

Figure 29. Color Perception. DB Keystone View Company.

B. Procedure: In order to familiarize the patient with the testing procedure the instruction card, DB-13, is inserted into the stereoscope. The patient's posture is adjusted for maximum inhibition to psychic convergence. The hues used in this stereogram are of such a nature that even a color blind individual can read the block letters in each row. The first row of the stereogram measures binocular color perception; the middle row measures right eye color perception; and the bottom row measures the left eye color perception ability. As soon as the patient is familiar with the testing stereogram it is removed from the stereoscope, and the testing stereogram DB-14 is inserted.

   We again ask the patient to identify the reddish block letters in each row of the stereogram. The letters that are not identified correctly are recorded.

C. Normal: Patient should read all twelve letters on stereogram DB-14 easily and rapidly.

D. Instructions to patient: (on instruction stereogram DB-13) "Do you see three rows of letters? Please look at the top row and read the four letters you see there. Now read the letters on the middle row; now the letters on the bottom row."

E. Remarks: If the patient reports diplopia by stating that the letters are doubled, repeat the test using monocular occlusion. This is not a color blindness test but a color perception test. A more suitable test for investigating color blindness would be the Ishihara or AO Co. Pseudo-Isochromatic plates.

F. Precautions:
   (1) Make certain that the patient understands your instructions.
   (2) Do not tell the patient that he is color blind if he fails this test. If the patient exhibits poor color perception, repeat the test with the Ishihara Plates to determine if color blindness is present.
   (3) Use the preliminary test card before using the diagnostic card.

G. Record: The letters which are incorrectly read should be recorded. If the patient is hesitant in reading some of the letters, this should be noted on the record form.

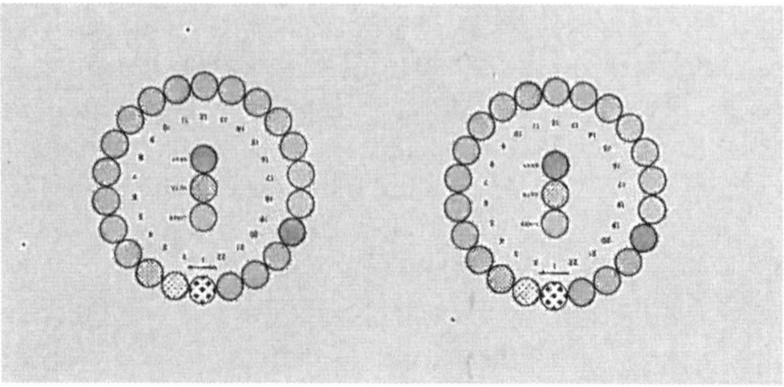

Figure 30. Visual Discrimination (near). DB 15 Keystone View Company.

If the patient is unable to read the letters on the monocular portions of the test, repeat the test using occlusion and see if elimination of binocular field conditions improves color perception.

15. Visual discrimination (near)

A. Target: stereograms DB-15, 16 and 17 (Figure 30). Stereoscope is adjusted for nearpoint.

B. Procedure: DB-16 is inserted into the slide holder. The Stereoscope should have a slight downward slope. The body posture of the subject should simulate normal nearpoint activity. Stereogram DB-16 measures right eye visual efficiency. In the center of the target we have three named circles containing lines, dots and a neutral gray. This is for patient indoctrination. Surrounding this is a circular pattern of small circles containing one of the three patterns lines, dots and gray. The lines and dots become smaller as we go from the first circle at the top and continue in a clockwise direction. The patient is to differentiate as to whether each circle contains lines, dots or gray. The patient continues around the circle pattern until he can no longer correctly identify the intent of the circle.

   The test is repeated for left eye acuity (DB-17) and binocular acuity (DB-15) at near.

C. Normal: The patient is to correctly identify the pattern present in each circle through numbers 15 or 16. This is equivalent to 20/20 visual acuity at near.

D. Instructions to patient: "In the center of this picture you will observe three circles. They are labeled lines, dots and neutral gray. All of the circles around the outside contain either lines, dots or neutral gray. Start with circle number 1 at the top of the picture, and going in a clockwise direction, tell me what is present in each circle - dots, lines, or neutral gray."

E. Remarks: This is an excellent nearpoint acuity test since it not only measures the ability of the subject to discriminate pattern differences, but it measures monocular ability under the conditions of binocular ground. Thus, this test can be used to determine the degree of nearpoint suppression. If on stereogram DB-16 (right eye acuity) the patient responds correctly through circle number 12, this is equivalent to 20/25. Now, when you occlude the patient's left eye, a correct response is obtained all the way through circle number 16 (equivalent to 20/20). Thus, this patient is exhibiting a small suppression of his right eye when the stress of binocular stimulus is imposed. It is therefore essential that we check the patient's response to the visual discrimination target under conditions of monocular occlusion, if he fails to attain standard acuity under the normal binocular conditions.

   Some success in identifying the visual discrimination targets can be obtained by guessing since you have one chance out of three of being correct. Therefore, some precaution must be taken in determining the acuity by these stereograms. For example, if the patient correctly identifies the pattern present in all of the circles through number 10, misses on 11, but calls 12 correctly – his score would be recorded as 10.

F. Precautions:
   (1) Patient must assume normal nearpoint posture.
   (2) Indoctrinate the patient as to the type of patterns he is to identify.
   (3) If patient has poor fusion, and complains of diplopia repeat test using monocular occlusion.
   (4) Whenever a patient does not attain standard discrimination ability, repeat the test under conditions of monocular occlusion so that we may identify the cause of the decreased acuity - suppression or amblyopia.

G. Record:
   (1) The O.D., O.S., and O.U. acuity.
   (2) Improvement in acuity upon occlusion.

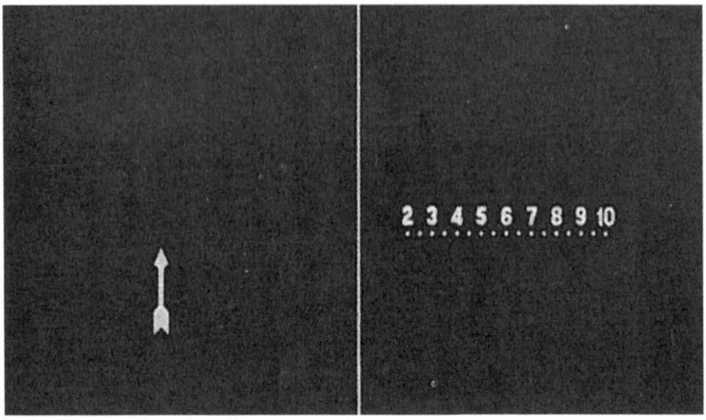

Figure 31. Lateral phoria (near). DB 9B Keystone View Company.

16. *Lateral phoria (near)*

    A. Target: stereogram DB-9B: (Figure 31). Stereoscope adjusted for near.

    B. Procedure: same as test B-3.

    C. Normal: arrow positioned between. 4.5 and 5.5.

    D. Instructions to patient: same as test B-3.

    E. Remarks: This test measures nearpoint visual posture. The arrow positioned below 4.5 esophoria; arrow above 5.5 indicates exophoria. For additional remarks see test B-3.

    F. Precautions:

       (1) Patient assumes normal nearpoint posture. See test B-3 for additional precautions.

    G. Record:

       (1) The number at which the arrow is pointing.

       (2) The extent of lateral movement of the arrow.

       (3) Note any tendency of the arrow to fade, blur or disappear.

17. *Fusion (second degree fusion) near*

    A. Target stereogram DB-5K: (Figure 32) Stereoscope adjusted for near.

    B. Procedure: same as for test B-5.

    C. Normal: The patient should see three balls or four balls quickly becoming three.

    D. Instructions to patient: same as test B-5.

Figure 32. Fusion (second degree-near). DB 5K Keystone View Company.

E. Remarks: Same as test B-5 except stereoscope is adjusted for nearpoint. Patient posture should be for near performance.

F. Precautions: (1) Patient assumes normal nearpoint posture. For additional precautions see B-5.

G. Record: The number of balls seen initially and the stability of this response. (See B-5.)

18. Macular Suppression at Near

A. Target: AN-71 or any nearpoint stereogram for the Telebinocular having horizontal and vertical control marks.

B. Procedure: Place the stereogram (AN-71) (see Figure 33) at the nearpoint setting of the instrument. The patient must experience stereoscopic vision. Procedure the same as B-7.

C. Normal: The patient reports the presence of a cross.

D. Instructions to patient: same as for B-7.

E. Remarks: same as for B-7.

F. Precautions:

(1) Patient assumes normal nearpoint posture for this test.

(2) Stereoscope is adjusted for nearpoint.

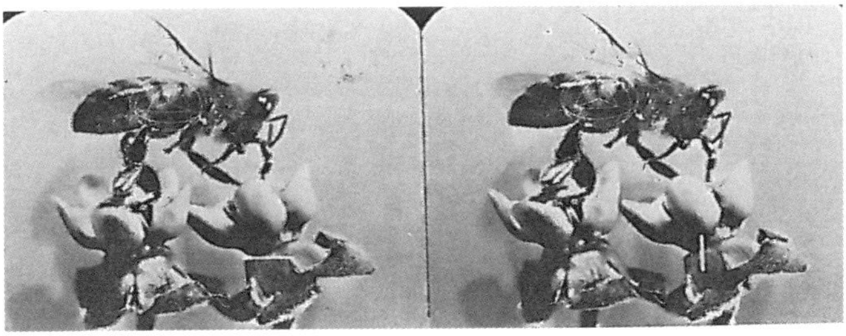

Figure 33. Stereogram (AN-71) Keystone View Company.

(3) Stereogram must have a separation of between 62 to 63 mm. between the center of the control marks (see B-7 for additional precautions).

G. Record: Have the patient describe or reproduce the appearance of the control marks. See B-7 for additional comments.

Special Tests

These are tests which require other types of instrumentation.

1. *Perceptual span*

A. Target: The targets consist of a series of digit groups from one to eight digits in size. Either a farpoint or a nearpoint tachistoscope may be used.

B. Procedure: The patient must be seated and with both feet flat on the floor. He should be leaning slightly forward. The patient assumes an attitude of relaxed alertness. He has a small pad and pencil for recording his observations. He is shown where the digit material will be located. He must be told not to stare at that point but to try and look beyond it. The patient must now be indoctrinated into the timing sequence of digit presentation. The operator will announce "ready," one second pause, now, one second pause, trip the shutter of the tachistoscope. The speed of flash will be 1/25th of a second. The patient records what ever he sees. The instrument is set for time exposure, and the patient is shown the digit group for a second time. If the patient has recorded the digit group correctly, the exposure is repeated using the next larger digit group. If the patient has made an error in reproducing the digit group, he is given another chance at a digit group of the same size. If he misses this size digit group for a second time, we consider that the material exceeds his perceptual ability. The digit groups are presented in ascending order, starting with one digit and going upward so that we can instill confidence in the patient's ability to perform at this exacting task.

C. Normal: The expected normal increases with the age of the patient, at six about two digits, at eight about three digits, at ten about four digits, at 13 or older five digits at 1/25th second exposure.

D. Instructions to patient: "I am going to flash some digits on the screen, and I want you to write down on this pad of paper what you see. You will be ready for the flash of the digits when I say 'ready', 'now' and then I will trip the shutter. I want you to be alert but not tense. Place both feet on the floor and lean slightly forward. I have shown you where the numbers will be located, but I don't want you to stare at that place. Try to look through the screen at that point as if it were further away. Now let's try it."

E. Remarks: There is considerable controversy as to the direct relationship between perceptual span and reading rate. This is understandable when we see the small range in perceptual span with age in comparison with the change in reading rate with age. Also, reading is a complex skill which involves a number of factors of which perceptual span is only one variable. The child with a poor perceptual span is handicapped in our modern complex environment.

   Always start perceptual span testing with one digit. This allows the subject to become thoroughly indoctrinated into the procedure followed and maintains proper motivation.

   Exposure time should be kept at 1/25th of a second since this is fast enough to prevent a second look and still is of sufficient time to allow an adequate stimulus.

F. Precautions:
   (1) Indoctrinate your patient thoroughly.
   (2) Do not vary your counting rate of 'ready', 'now' and flash.
   (3) Be certain that the patient has adopted the proper posture.
   (4) Encourage the subject to wait a second after the exposure before trying to record the digit combination. Muscular movement immediately after the exposure tends to erase the perception.

G. Record: the perceptual span of the subject.

2. *Reading rate and comprehension*

A. Target: reading test for grade level.

B. Procedure: It is desirable to use a reading test which investigates reading skills at a particular grade level. For this survey purpose the following tests are suitable:

   (1) Gates Reading Survey for Grades 3 to 10 (Bureau of Publications, Teachers College, Columbia University, New York, N.Y.) for adults; (2) Diagnostic Reading Tests, Survey Section, Forms A and B (Science Research Associates, Inc., 57 W. Grand Ave., Chicago 10, Ill.). *(Editor's note: Gates Oral Reading Survey from the Handbook of Diagnostic Tests*

by Lowry, available from OEP) In administering these tests the directions enclosed with the test must be followed.

C. Normal: as per test.

D. Instructions to patient: Read the directions as given in the test and have patient follow these instructions.

E. Remarks: The purpose of all training is to build speed and accuracy of response in the visual system. Our modern civilization places a tremendous premium on having an adequate ability in this skill. Fortunately it is not an innate ability, but one which is highly susceptible and responsive to training. The survey tests which have been suggested for reading rate and comprehension investigation serve the remedial reading teacher in the same manner as the usual visual skills tests serve the optometrists. These tests merely indicate whether or not the patient is up to or beyond his class level in this important ability of gaining information speedily from symbol groups on the printed page.

F. Precautions: Follow the printed instructions with the test and under no conditions deviate from them.

G. Record: Record your information in the units provided for in the test.

3. *Spontaneous Drawing*

A. Target: a sheet of white bond paper 8.5 x 11, #2 pencil without eraser.

B. Procedure: The patient is comfortably seated. The paper is centered before him with the 11-inch side parallel to him. The patient is given the pencil and told to make a drawing of a house. If he seems reluctant to start, make every effort to obtain a response. Don't offer any suggestions as to what details to add to the drawing. When the child pauses in his drawing merely ask in a normal tone of voice, "Are you finished?" Don't rush the patient.

C. Normal: This test should be performed on five year old children or older. We do not evaluate the drawing on the basis of artistic ability. From a visual standpoint we consider the following factors:

Approach to the task -

(1) Did a parent have to be present?

(2) Did the child turn to the doctor or parent for aid?

(3) Did the child start the drawing easily or was it necessary to coax him to start?

(4) Did the child start apologizing about his poor drawing ability before or during the drawing task?

(5) Once the child started the drawing task did he continue until he finished or was it necessary to urge him to finish?

Dependence upon the parent, needing suggestions in order to start his drawing, apologetic viewpoint, frequent starts and stops and wandering of attention all indicate the strong possibility of introverted tendencies or perceptual immaturity.

Motor Overflow -

(1) The observations of motor overflow give us clues as to his visual inadequacies and perceptual motor difficulties. The following factors should be considered:

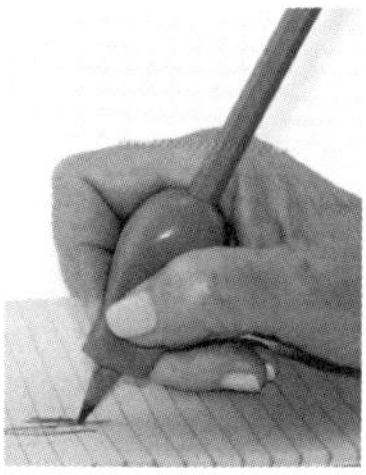

(2) Does the child hold the pencil in a normal finger method, or does he use the immature Palmer grasp?

(3) Observe for excessive effort used while making his drawing. How hard is he holding the pencil? Does he keep breaking pencil points? Does he have to wipe his hand as he makes his drawing?

(4) Observe for variations in working distance and estimate these variations to the nearest inch. Does he move excessively close as he continues the drawing?

(5) Head Tilt - A maintained head tilt gives us clues as to the possibilities of hyperphoria and/or anisometropia.

(6) Tension overflow - Does the child wiggle in his chair as he draws? Does he chew on his tongue or pencil? Does he sit on one leg? Does he swing his leg as he draws?

The greater the variations in motor overflow the greater the chance that we have visual distortions present.

Drawing -

In evaluating the drawing for visual factors consider the following:

(1) Positioning - Is the drawing free of the edges of the paper, or is it attached to the sides or the bottom of the paper for

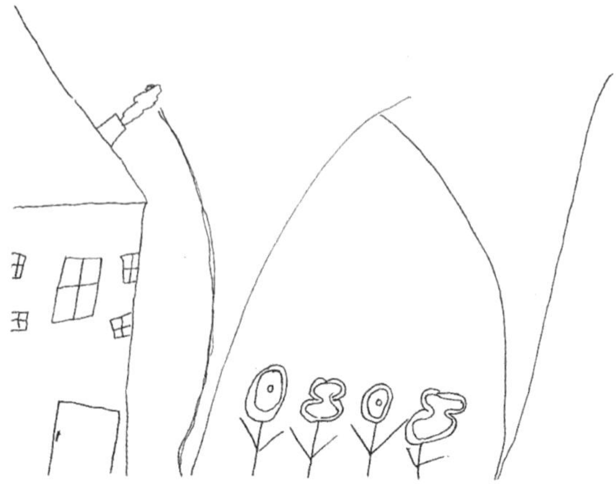

Figure 34.

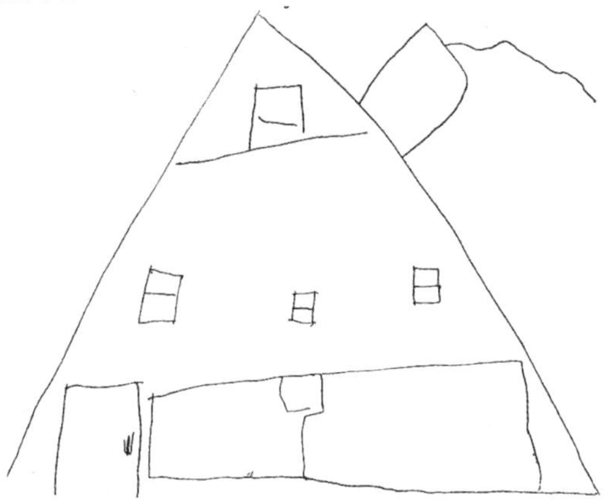

Figure 35.

support. Whenever the child finds it necessary to anchor his drawing it indicates that he needs this support to maintain his visualization. This lack of ability to draw free of the edge of the paper is normal for the five year old but indicates a lack of visualization ability in older children. Figure 34 is a spontaneous drawing made by Ezell, in second grade, 7 years old, reading level at the first grade. The size of the drawing indicates the possibility of the presence of hyperopia, but its immaturity of construction is obvious.

In addition observe the child if he changes the position of the paper as he makes his drawing. Often these rotations are done in order to avoid the use of oblique lines. This type of youngster is unable to follow a moving target and often has difficulty with reading. Figure 35 illustrates such a case and

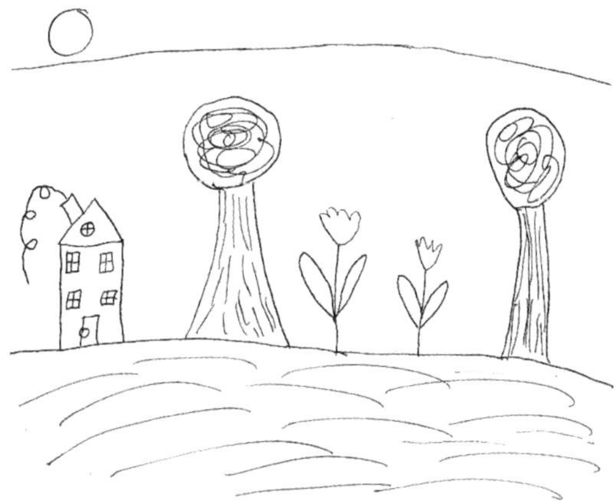

Figure 36.

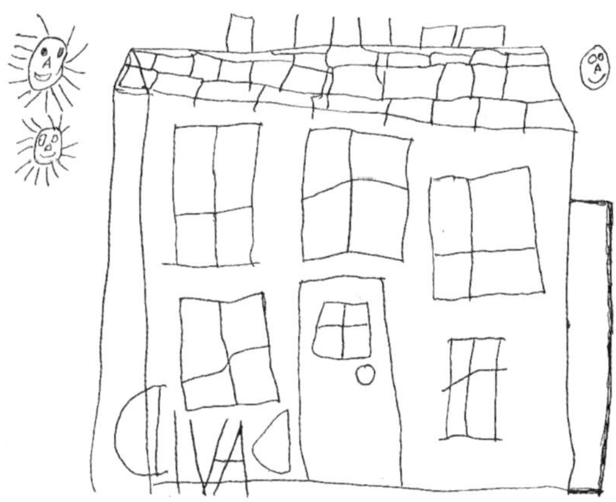

Figure 37.

the presence of the chimney at such an angle illustrates the positional difficulty experienced by the patient.

(2) Proportion - Does the drawing show that the child had an appreciation of the relative sizes of the various objects used in the picture? For example, if he has drawn a house, are the doors and windows in proper proportion to the total size of the house? If flowers are included in the picture, are they in proper size to the total size of the house? Note the large size of the flowers in relationship to the size of the house in Figure 36 as drawn by Jean age 6.

The total size of the drawing in relationship to the size of the paper gives us a clue to the type of refractive condition present. Figure 37 is a drawing made by David, age 6, who had a medium amount of hyperopia which was uncorrected

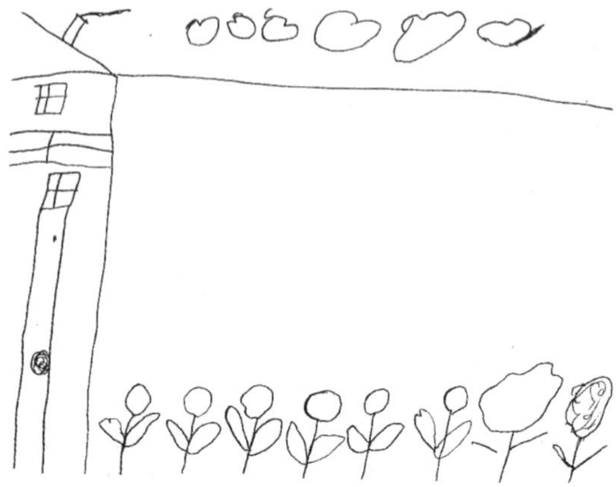

Figure 38.

(note reversals in the letters of his name). This youngster had a reading problem. His visual problem was evident not only from the refractive condition present but, in addition, the motor-visual skills of rotations, fixations, accommodative rock and nearpoint of convergence tests were failed.

(3) Line construction - The type of lines used in constructing their drawing of a house provide excellent clues as to their perceptual-motor development. The following age norms are based on children from a metropolitan area of above average socio-economic advantages:

Vertical lines - 4 to 4,1/2 years

Horizontal lines - 5 to 5,1/2 years

Oblique lines - 6 to 6 1/2 years.

Figure 38 is a drawing made by M.T., female, age 7, failing first grade for the second time. She made the oblique roof line by rotating the paper so that it was drawn as a vertical line. While the child had the paper in a rotated position she drew the chimney as perpendicular to the roof. The same low order performance was evident in her visual tests.

(4) The number of objects - A drawing consisting of a single object is a lower order performance than a drawing containing several objects. The number of objects present in the drawing must be balanced against the detail in these objects. Thus, a child drawing a house having several details shown would be graded higher than a mere outline of a house with a couple of stick trees. The highly oral child will often draw a simple

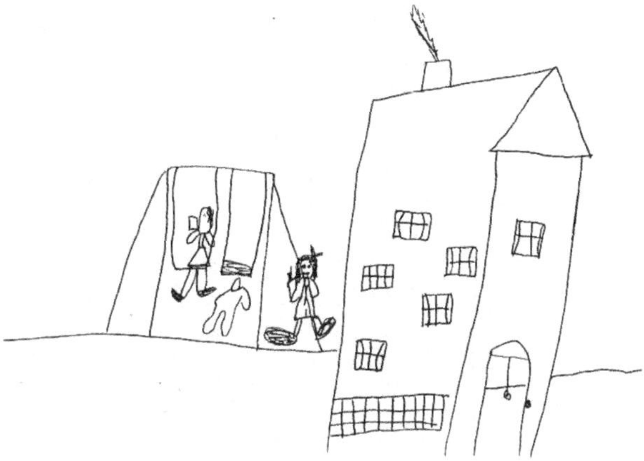

Figure 39.

figure and present a very detailed account regarding the drawing. These children often do well in the lower grades but start having scholastic difficulties when silent reading starts in the third grade

(5) Perspective - The appearance of perspective in the drawing is a good indication that some stereopsis is present. N.M., female, age 6 1/2, had excellent stereopsis for her age and made Figure 39. Note the effort to show the depth of the house. However, it must be understood that this type of observation cannot be used with older children who develop a more sophisticated knowledge of perspective.

6) Directionality - The reading requirements of our civilization require a left-to-right directionality. The child not having this directionality will reverse words, have poor fixations, and be retarded in his reading ability. Directionality can be appraised from a patient's spontaneous drawing by observing where he starts on the paper and the direction in which he makes his lines. Inspection of the finished picture will often reveal additional clues, i.e., the direction of the smoke arising from the chimney; the direction that a car, bicycle, train or other objects are facing; the direction that the people in the drawing are facing; the direction that a bird is flying; and the direction that trees and flowers are bending in the wind. Michael, 6 1/2, failing first grade, drew the house on the far right of the paper. He had difficulty with oblique lines and rotated his paper; he made the smoke from the chimney go to the left, and he finally added the tree on the left of the

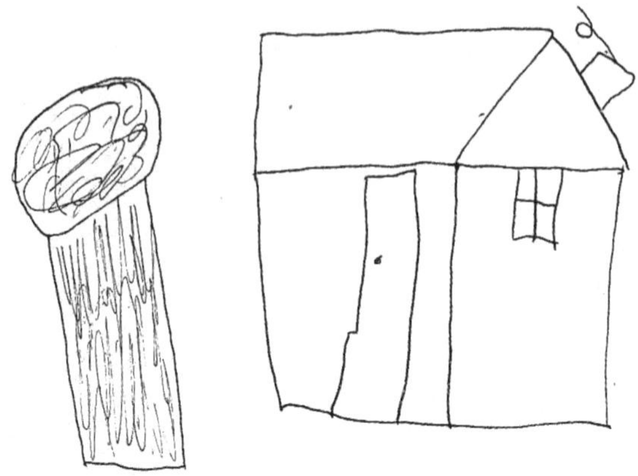

Figure 40.

house. Note that the tree is slanted toward his left. In his cheiroscopic drawing he made the same right-to-left lines. His drawing is Figure 40.

D. Instructions to patient: "Take this pencil and make me a picture of a house." Don't pay any further attention to the child unless he stops his drawing activity. At this time merely ask if he is finished or would he like to continue.

E. Remarks: Spontaneous drawings have been used by psychologists to determine personality disorders, and they have been used by educators to estimate intelligence and to predict reading readiness. From a visual standpoint we are interested in spontaneous drawing for clues as to: (1) the organization of the child's visual space world; (2) the quality of the child's hand and eye coordination; (3) his visual directionality; (4) the age level of his visual development and its direction; (5) the postural misalignments and variation in working distance that may predict future visual changes. A series of spontaneous drawings while the child is under visual care provide a graphic illustration of his progress.

F. Record: the spontaneous drawing.

Visual Efficiency Score

The present method of informing the patient of his visual performance on the visual skills battery has been to merely list each test that he failed. This presents a complex picture to the patient which has little meaning to him. This type of presentation does not inform the patient how his visual skill performance would compare with a normal population. Similarly, the practitioner has often found it confusing to evaluate a visual skills battery as to whether the deviations noted are significant or of minor importance.

In order to simplify visual skills data presentation, a visual efficiency score was devised (see Figure 41). Twenty primary visual skills tests are rated on a five-point scale. Perfection in performance on all 20 skills would result in a score of 100%, whereas; failure in all of the tests would result in a score of 20%. Utilizing this procedure on a general population of kindergarten children and of college students, and assuming a straight line relationship between visual efficiency score and age has resulted in the following average score values:

Age	Minimum Visual Score
5	66
10	75
15	80
20	85

It is to be expected, since maturational factors are present in some of the visual skills tests, that the norm value obtained for kindergarten children would be lower than for older students.

The use of the visual efficiency score has simplified the presentation of visual skills performance to the patient. This has several advantages, particularly from a professional sales viewpoint, for it presents to the patient his performance ability in terms of a number. The patient can understand that the seriousness of his visual decrements increases with the lowness of the score below the average value, Thus, a college student that scores 70 when his norm value is 85 can appreciate the difference between these values. Another college student that scores 83 when his norm value is 85 would perhaps not be able to appreciate the difference or lowering of his visual performance tests. The visual efficiency score can be utilized to inform the patient as to the effectiveness of the lenses prescribed or the visual training program undertaken. To illustrate this use of the visual efficiency score let us suppose that initially the patient had a score of 70 (age 10); lenses were prescribed and a progress examination performed in four weeks. The progress examination revealed a visual performance score of 80. It was obvious to the patient as well as the parents, how much better the child was performing visually. A home visual training program was initiated to see if further change could be obtained. The next progress report revealed a score of 92. The parents were extremely satisfied in the visual improvement obtained by their child. In order to use the visual performance score as described, the testing procedure and scoring method to be presented must be carefully followed.

Instructions For Evaluating Visual Skills Profile

Instructions for evaluating visual skills profile

1. *Binocular rotations*

Score 1: At least one eye cannot make a rotational movement.

Score 2: Both eyes follow target but extremely irregular movements.

Score 3: Both eyes follow target with irregular movements in one sector.

Score 4: Both eyes follow target with good movements but with slight irregularities.

Score 5: Perfect binocular rotational ability.

2. *Monocular rotations*

Method of grading eye movements same as binocular test. Performance graded on the poorer eye.

3. *Saccadic fixations*

Score 1: Patient can only change fixation with extreme effort and use of head movements.

Score 2: Several gross errors are made in over-shooting.

Score 3: Patient makes only one gross error in over-shooting or under-shooting.

Score 4: Only a slight inaccuracy in making fixation changes.

Score 5: Fixation changes are perfect.

4. *Near-to-far fixations*

Method of scoring same as for saccadic fixation test.

5. *Nearpoint convergence*

Score based on objective measurement recorded to the nearest inch and check in the appropriate column of form.

6. *Donders amplitude of accommodation*

Measurement performed on 20/20 nearpoint Snellen and converted into diopters. This value compared to the following expected values.

Age	Amp	Age	Amp
10	14	40	4.5
15	12	45	3.5
20	10	50	2.5
25	8.5	55	1.5
30	7.5	60	1.0
35	6.5	65	0.5

7. *Simultaneous perception*

Score 1: Patient sees only the dog or the pig.

Score 2: Dog and pig both present, widely separated.

Score 3: Dog and pig both present, head of dog above pig.

Score 4: Dog and pig both present, dog not directly above pig.

Score 5: Dog and pig both present with perfect vertical alignment.

8. *Fusion at far*

Score 1: Patient reports two balls.

Score 2: Patient reports four balls with movement.

Score 3: Patient reports four balls with stable position.

Score 4: Patient reports four balls going into three, or three balls going into four balls.

Score 5: Patient reports three balls.

9. *Stereopsis*

Score as indicated on visual skills profile form.

10. *Accommodative facility*

Any farpoint line stereogram can be used as a target. The stereogram is set at infinity in the stereoscope. Insert a minus 2.50 diopter sphere before one eye. Use alternate occlusion and inquire if the picture is sharp and clear before each eye. Shift position of lens and repeat. Score as indicated on visual skills profile form.

11. *Lateral phoria*

Check patient response in the column on the visual skills profile form that is closest to the response. If the patient response falls in between values given on the form, check the higher number (i.e.-patient response 6; score 2).

12. *Vertical phoria*

Score the patient as given on the visual skills profile form.

13. *Visual efficiency at far, O.D.*

Score as per the percentage scale on the stereogram and check the appropriate column on the form.

14. *Visual efficiency at far, O.S.*

Score as per the percentage scale on the stereogram and check the appropriate column on the form.

15. *Hand and eye coordination*

Score 1: Patient reports the presence of one pointer.

Score 2: Both pointers are present but numbers are doubled.

Score 3: Normal response, but one pointer tip is missing.

Score 4: Normal response, but pointer exhibits exo or eso landing response.

Score 5: Perfect response.

16. *Fusion at near*

Score same as the farpoint fusion test.

17. *Macular suppression at near*

Any split stereogram containing horizontal and vertical control marks may be used. Test is performed at nearpoint stereoscope setting.

Score 1: One control mark is reported

Score 2: Alternate suppression is reported.

Score 3: The central portion of one of the control marks is missing.

Score 4: Both control marks are present but they do not form a perfect cross.

Score 5: Perfect response.

18. *Lateral phoria at near*

Check the patient response in the proper column. Round off numbers to the highest value.

19. *Visual Efficiency at near, O.D.*

Record the patient response on the percentage scale and check this value in the proper column of the form.

20. *Visual efficiency at near, O.S.*

Score in the same manner as for test number 19.

Conclusion

In no other way can such a wealth of information regarding the visual performance of the patient be obtained as in these visual skills tests. In no other way can the patient's binocular skill at both farpoint and nearpoint be appraised. These tests demonstrate to the patient his visual difficulties and the improvement in his visual efficiency after he has had his visual rehabilitation. These tests demonstrate to the vision specialist the type of visual problem present and what adaptations the patient has made because of the environmental stress to which he has been exposed.

Name:________________________Case No:______Date:_______Sex (m) (f)

Wearing (No Rx) (Old Rx) (   ) Visual Efficiency Score:_____

	Test name	1	2	3	4	5	Doctor notes
	Binocular Rottions	No ability to follow	Poor movements	Fair movements	Good, very slight defect	Excellent	
	Monocular Rotations	No ability to follow	Poor movements	Fair movements	Good, very slight defect	Excellent	
	Saccadic Fixations	Extremely poor	Poor fixations	Fair fixation	Good, very slight defect	Excellent	
	Near-to-far fixations	Extremely poor	Poor fixations	Fair fixation	Good, very slight defect	Excellent	
	Nearpoint convergence	8"	6"	4"	3"	To nose	
	Donders amplitude	1.50D Below normal	1.00D Below normal	0.50D Below normal	Expected for age	Above expected for age	
Far	Simultaneous perception	Monocular vision	Sim. per. but far apart	Sim. per. but overlap	Sim. per. Slightly far apart	Sim. per. Directly above	
Far	Fusion	Two balls	Four balls move	Four balls stable	4 > 3 3 > 4	Three balls	
Far	Stereopsis	Misses four lines	Misses three lines	Misses two lines	Misses one line	All correct	
Far	Accommodative facility (-2.50)	Complete blur on both sides	Complete blur on one side	Partial blur on one side	Very short blur on one side	No blur on either side	
Far	Lateral phoria	5.5 or 13.5	6.5 or 12.5	7.5 or 11.5	8.5 or 10.5	9.0 or 10.0	
Far	Vertical phoria	□ or ✸	+ or ♥	Ō	ϴ	ϴ	
Far	Vis. Eff. O.D.	60%	70%	80%	90%	100%	
Far	Vis. Eff. O.S.	60%	70%	80%	90%	100%	
Far	Hand and eye coordination	Monocular vision	Doubling of numbers	Pointer tips missing	Normal, slight errors	Perfect coordination	
Near	Fusion	Two balls	Four balls move	Four balls stable	~~4 > 3~~ ~~3 > 4~~	Three balls	
Near	Macular suppression	Monocular vision	Alternate suppression	Macular suppression	Displaced cross	Perfect cross	
Near	Lateral phoria	2.5 or 7.5	3.0 or 7.0	3.5 or 6.5	4.0 or 6.0	4.5 or 5.5	
Near	Vis. Eff. O.D.	60%	70%	80%	90%	100%	
Near	Vis. Eff. O.S.	60%	70%	80%	90%	100%	

Figure 41. Visual skills profile.

The usual question asked is, "How many of these tests should be taken on a particular patient?" The obvious answer is to take as many of these tests as you possibly can. The case history information will usually give you some clue as to the problem present, and professional judgment will dictate how many of these skills tests should be performed on a particular patient. As an absolute minimum the following should be taken on every patient: (1) rotations and fixations (2) nearpoint of convergence (3) Brock string (4) visual efficiency at near and far (5) hand and eye coordination. Since patients are constantly being referred to our offices who have failed a battery of skills at a screening program at school, industry or application for driver's license, it is extremely important that more skill testing be performed on patients if we are to determine the reason for such referral and what remedial measures to institute.

CHAPTER VI
Visual Tests

There are many different procedures for performing all of the regular optometric tests. One of the many contributions of Dr A. M. Skeffington is his program of standard procedures for performing various optometric tests. This establishment of a "standard practice" does not mean that other methods are not as good as or perhaps even better than the testing routine presented. But if a common technique is followed, we will all obtain comparable results for the same patient.

Since we all admit that optometric tests are primarily of a psychological nature and since the visual system is complex, the testing situation must be controlled if reliable results are to be obtained. Not only must the testing procedure remain constant, but questions and rapport with the patient also must remain constant. To minimize these effects, Dr A. M. Skeffington developed a method of visual analysis in which similar tests, i.e., performed by the same testing procedure, but differing in spatial direction, are compared with each other. For example, convergence at far is compared to abduction at far; positive fusional reserve is compared to negative fusional reserve, etc.

Standard procedures, once learned, make it possible to concentrate upon patient response rather than upon some variation in technique. The magnitude of the patient response and the quality of his response are both very important. Two patients may have the same statistical test magnitude, but one patient may perform the test easily and rapidly, while the second patient may complain of difficulty (pain, nausea, etc.). The difference in performance ability of these two patients is diagnostic.

It is also important that the testing proceed rapidly and smoothly from one test to another. A smooth, machine-like performance establishes patient confidence and improves the reliability of the test results. A clumsy, slow, inadequate, irregular performance reduces test reliability. The visual examination should be a smooth-flowing, routine experience for the patient in order to instill proper patient-doctor relationship.

Editors Note: This text was first published in 1958. The Optometric capability for the examination of ocular integrity has changed. Please keep that in mind as you read certain parts of this section on Ophthalmology. It is being republished with almost no change from the original.

1. Ophthalmoscopy

Optometrically, we are concerned with the visual problems of the non-pathological case. The first procedure must be to determine the presence or absence of pathology. If evidence of pathology is found, the patient must be referred to the proper practitioner who is fully qualified to make a more exhaustive physical examination, diagnosis and institute treatment.

Optometric office experience indicates that approximately one percent of all patients seeking optometric services have a pathological condition requiring other attention and referral. Good visual achievement cannot be expected until the pathological condition has been eliminated. The presence of a pathological condition does not necessarily preclude continuation of the analytical examination because many of these cases may need immediate lens application or visual training. For example, a diabetic, under insulin control, will still need lens application, even though typical fundus changes are present. Professional judgment must be exercised to determine the proper procedure for any particular case.

To examine the right eye of the patient, the direct ophthalmoscope is held in the right hand with the index finger in the proper position to turn the lens wheel attached to the eyepiece of the instrument. The patient is directed to observe a target directly ahead and about six feet above the floor. The optometrist holds the instrument firmly to his brow and in such alignment so he can see through the peep-hole. The instrument is placed as closely as possible to the eye of the patient. When examining the patient's right eye, the doctor holds the instrument in his right hand and uses his right eye. Similarly in checking the patient's left eye the instrument is held in the left hand and the left eye is used for observation.

To reduce patient discomfort, it is best to always use the minimum intensity of illumination necessary in order to clearly observe any defects that may be present. The light should never be thrown upon the macular area until the doctor is ready to observe this portion of the fundus. Many patients experience discomfort from the light source when the macula is checked.

The observation should be started with the maximum plus in the instrument and a careful check made of the cornea, lids, cilia and conjunctiva for any abnormalities. By reducing the plus power in the instrument, the anterior surface of the lens and the iris can now be observed. As the plus power is reduced progressively in the instrument, the movement gradually is from the anterior surface of the lens, to the posterior surface of the lens and through the vitreous filled space between the lens and retina. Of primary interest to the doctor is the presence of infiltrations or foreign elements.

As the reduced amount of plus in the instrument is reached, allowing observation of the fundus, it is well to withdraw the instrument to a distance of about 20" from the eye of the patient and to note any opacities. This new position of the instrument reveals a red background and any opacities will be visible as black objects. If any opacities are observed, their location may be judged by having the patient look up. If the object moves rapidly in the same direction as the eye, the object is located on the cornea. If the object moves slowly in the same direction as the eye movement, it is located at the anterior surface of the lens. If the particle does not move with the movement of the eye, the object is near the center of the lens. If the particle moves in the opposite direction of the eye movement it is located at the posterior surface of the lens. Opacities located in the vitreous will seem to move in a direction opposite to the eye movement, but they will slowly float back to the original position.

In examining the fundus, the optometrist is primarily interested in four features: disc, vessels, fundus field and macular area.

The disc should be observed for: (a) size and shape; (b) margin of disc sharp and clear; (c) normal physiological cupping; (d) pigmentation or any other irregularities.

The vessels should be observed for: (a) diameter of veins to arteries should be 2:1; (b) axial streaking on arteries; (c) vessels should course uninterrupted over the fundus; (4) no pulsation of arteries.

The fundus field should be observed for: (a) free of exudations, hemorrhages or pigmentation; (b) uniform color.

The macular area should be observed for: (a) sharp macular reflex; (b) area free of blood vessels, exudates or deposits.

The examination described is now repeated for the left eye of the patient.

2. Ophthalmometry

The ophthalmometer is an instrument which enables determination of the power of the cornea in its principal meridians. The difference in the refracting power of the principal meridians gives the gross cylinder and axis. To estimate the net cylinder necessary to correct the astigmatic condition of the eye, two factors must be considered. The first modifying factor is the influence of physiologic astigmia which averages -0.50 X 90°. The second modifying factor is that the cylinder is measured at the corneal surface and the correcting cylinder is worn at 15 mm. to 19 mm. from the cornea. The modifying factor for this is that it increases the minus cylinder by one-fourth. Javal combined these into a rule which bears his name. The method of calculation is illustrated in these examples:

Example 1:

43.00 X 5°
44.00 X 95°
-1.00 X 5° gross cylinder
-0.25 X 5° correction factor for distance
________(1/4 X 1.00 = 0.25)
-1.25 X 5°
0.50 X 90° physiological astigmia
-0.75 X 5° net cylinder

Example 2:

40.25 X 15°
44.00 X 105°
-3.75 X 15° gross cylinder
-1.00 X 15° correcting factor for distance
________(1/4 X 3.75= 1.00)
-4.75 X 15°
-0.50 X 90° physiological astigmia
-4.25 X 15° net cylinder

3. Habitual phoria at far

All habitual tests are performed through the lenses used by the patient for that particular test distance. If the patient is not wearing glasses, the test is performed with the patient fixating through plano. If possible, the patient's old correction should be used since improper placement of optical centers may be a contributory cause of the patient's complaint.

The patient is directed to observe the distant fixation target. The usual target for this test is the 20/20 Snellen letters. If the patient cannot see these letters, the size of the target should be increased until they can be identified by the patient. The patient is told to close his eyes and the dissociating device and measuring prism are positioned before his eyes. The patient is dissociated by six prism diopters base-up before the left eye. The measuring prism is placed before the patient's right eye and it is turned to 12D base-in.

The six diopters base-up before the left eye will cause the patient to see the lower image with his left eye and the upper image with his right eye. The prism base-in positioned before his right eye will create uncrossed diplopia so that the doctor will be able to tell the patient what he will see when he opens his eyes. The patient now is asked to open his eyes and the doctor states, "You now see two rows of letters, with the upper target to the right of the lower target." On confirmation from the patient, the doctor states, "I am going to move the targets so that one group of letters will be directly above the other group of letters. As soon as you see this alignment tell me to *stop*." Now begin the reduction of the amount of base-in prism before the right eye and the doctor again states to the patient, "Do you notice the targets moving closer? Have they lined up one directly above the other yet?" As reduction of the amount of base-in prism continues, the doctor should continue urging the patient to watch the targets and report as soon as vertical alignment has been obtained.

As soon as vertical alignment of the targets is obtained either one eye of the patient should be occluded, or he should be instructed to close his eyes. If any base-in prism still remains in the measuring prism, it is recorded as prism diopters of exophoria; if the measuring prism contains prism base out, it is recorded as prism diopters of esophoria. It is important to eliminate the dissociated condition as soon as the end point of the test is reached, otherwise the patient may feel uncertain in his response as the target starts to swing out or in again because of unstable convergence condition.

If the patient is a very high exophore, the initial amount of base-in prism placed in the measuring device may not be sufficient to create a condition of uncrossed diplopia. In these cases, base-in prism should be added until the patient reports the upper target to the right of the lower target.

In some cases the patient may insist that he can see only one target. You have several possibilities for this response. First, the patient may have a high hyperphoria and the six base-up is not sufficient to induce diplopia.

This can be corrected by increasing the amount of base-up prism until diplopia is elicited. Second, the patient may suppress one eye and, therefore, report the presence of only one target. This may be eliminated by increasing the amount of dissociation or by placing a red glass before the suppressed eye.

Habitual Phoria at Far

Test distance: 20'
Target: 20/20 Snellen (or smallest readable).
Lenses in place: habitual distant correction.
Dissociating device: 6 base-up O.S.; 12 base-in O.D.
Illumination: target well-illuminated 20 foot candles of illumination (f.c.).
Phoroptor adjustment: far pupillary distance.

13A. Habitual phoria at near

This test is a repetition of the preceding test with the fixation distance changed from 20' to the nearpoint testing distance of 16". This test is performed through the patient's near-point glasses. If no correction has been worn at near, this test is performed through plano.

The target is the reduced Snellen 20/20 letters placed at 16" from the patient. The patient is again dissociated by 6D base-up before the left eye and sufficient base-in prism turned before the right eye to create uncrossed diplopia (15-20PD). The patient will again report the upper target to the right and the amount of base- in is slowly reduced until vertical alignment of the targets is obtained. Base-in prism remaining in the rotary is recorded as diopters of exophoria; base-out prism as diopters of esophoria.

Habitual Phoria at Near

Test distance: 16".
Target: 20/20 reduced Snellen (or smallest).
Lenses in place: Habitual near-point correction.
Dissociating device: 6 base-up O.S.; 15 base-in O.D.
Illumination: target well-illuminated 20 f.c.
Phoroptor adjustment: near pupillary distance.

4. Static retinoscopy

The retinoscope is an instrument for observing the focal point of a beam of light which has passed through all of the refracting surfaces of the eye. We can adjust the amount of lenses before the patient's eye so that this emerging beam will come to a focus at any desired distance from the patient. To minimize experimental error and because of anatomical factors, it is customary to perform this test at either a 20- or 26-inch working distance. The working distance, once selected by the practitioner, must remain constant throughout the test.

The patient, throughout this test, must maintain fixation upon a target at 20'. Since the patient is observing a distant target and we have added sufficient lenses to bring the emerging beam of light to a focus at the working distance, we must correct our finding by the lens equivalent of this working distance. The correction factor, which is subtracted from the total lenses, is two diopters for a 20-inch working distance and one and a half diopters for a 26-inch working distance.

The phoropter is adjusted for the distant pupillary distance of the patient. The patient is instructed to observe the distant fixation chart and to ignore the flashing light. The practitioner uses his right eye to examine the right eye of the patient. A constant working distance must be maintained. Sufficient plus lenses are added before the right eye of the patient so that a definite "against" motion is seen in all meridians. Now the amount of plus is reduced by 0.25 diopter steps until the reflex is neutral in all meridians (spherical finding), or until neutral in one meridian is obtained and against motion in the other principal meridian (astigmatic finding). If a neutral motion is obtained in all meridians, the dioptric equivalent of the working distance is subtracted from the total lenses in the phoroptor, and the remainder recorded as the static retinoscopy test value for that eye.

If a neutral motion is obtained in one meridian, but there is an against motion in the other principal meridian, minus cylinder lenses are added in quarter diopter steps with the axis parallel to the neutral motion meridian. When sufficient minus cylinder has been added to change the original against motion to a neutral condition, the patient's astigmatic status has been neutralized. There should now be a neutral motion in all meridians. This should be checked by moving in a little closer to the patient, which should change the motion from neutral to *with*; by moving away from the patient, the motion should change from neutral to *against*. Now, the dioptric equivalent of the working distance is subtracted from the spherical portion of the test and the remainder recorded as the test result. For example:

O.D. +1.00 (total lenses
O.S. +1.00 -1.00X90° in phoroptor)
Working distance = 26" (1.50 D.)
We would record as No.4:
O.D. -0.50
O.S. -0.50 -1.00X90°

In examining the patient's right eye, the refractionist manipulates the retinoscope with his right hand and uses his right eye. In examining the patient's left eye, the refractionist manipulates the retinoscope with his left hand and uses his left eye. This is necessary so that the patient at all times will be able to fixate upon the distant target.

Summary Static Retinoscopy

Test distance: Patient fixation distance 20' Working distance 20"or 26".
Target: Snellen chart.
Lenses in place: start test from plano.
Illumination: medium illumination.
Phoroptor adjustment: far p.d.

5. Dynamic retinoscopy at 20"

The phoroptor now contains the gross lenses used in the static retinoscopy finding. The refractionist positions himself at 20" from the patient, and the patient is cautioned to observe a fixation target near the retinoscope. The refractionist's working distance and the patient's fixation distance are the same. Sufficient plus is now added in 0.25D steps before each eye so that an against motion is obtained. The refractionist now reduces the plus before each eye in 0.25 steps until a neutral motion is obtained in each eye. This is *high* neutral. The total lenses in the phoroptor before each eye are recorded as the dynamic retinoscopy at 20 inches. No correction is made for working distance since the patient's fixation distance and the refractionist's working distance are in conjugation.

Summary Dynamic Retinoscopy 20 Inches

Test distance: Patient fixation distance 20" Working distance 20".
Target: reduced Snellen letters (or equivalent).
Lenses in place: gross No.4.
Illumination: normal.
Phoroptor adjustment: near p.d.

6. Dynamic retinoscopy at 40"

The phoroptor now contains the lenses used in the dynamic retinoscopy at 20". This test is performed at 40" from the patient and the patient is to observe a fixation target in the plane of the retinoscope. It should be noted that the fixative distance of the patient and the refractionist's working distance are the same. Usually we will see an against motion when this test is started with the lenses in place from the dynamic retinoscopy at 20". If either a neutral or a with motion is observed, sufficient plus sphere should be added to obtain a definite against motion in both eyes. The plus sphere power is now reduced in 0.25D steps until a neutral motion is observed in each eye. The total lenses in place before the patient's eyes is recorded as the dynamic retinoscopy finding at 40".

Summary Dynamic Retinoscopy at 40"

Test distance: Patient fixation distance 40". Working distance 40".
Target: reduced Snellen letters (or equivalent).
Lenses in place: dynamic retinoscopy at 20".
Illumination: normal.
Phoroptor adjustment: near p.d.

7. Distant subjective test (basic finding)

Any adequate subjective technique requires that the following factors be considered:

(a) Sufficient plus sphere initially to obtain maximum inhibition to accommodation.

(b) Verification of the amount of cylinder by at least two subjective techniques.

(c) Verification of the astigmatic axis by two subjective techniques.

(d) The vision in each eye balanced under binocular conditions and under a slight blur.

(e) The subjective test is concluded under single binocular conditions and starting with a "fog" of 0.75D.

(f) The binocular fog is reduced in 0.25 steps until patient obtains a visual acuity of 20/20. This means that the patient can correctly identify the letters of the 20/20 line and one or two letters on the 20/15ths.

Sufficient initial inhibition to accommodation will be obtained if the subjective test is started with the total lenses in place from the dynamic retinoscopy finding. If for any reason a dynamic retinoscopy test cannot be performed, the patient should be blurred with plus sphere until he can just identify the 20/200 Snellen letter.

The astigmatic axis may be determined by any of the following methods: (1) clock-dial - the patient selects the darkest line and by the use of the rule of 30, the minus cylinder axis is determined; (2) cross-cylinder check test - the handle of the cross-cylinder is aligned with the tentative cylinder axis and as the patient observes a Snellen target the cross-cylinder is flipped. If the axis is correct, the patient will detect no difference in the visibility of the target in either position. If the patient reports that the letters are clearer in one position than the other, the axis of the minus trail cylinder should be moved in the direction of the red dot of the cross-cylinder when it is in the preferred position. This is repeated until the Snellen target is equally clear in either position of the cross-cylinder.

Any of the following procedures may be used to determine the amount of the cylindrical correction: (1) clock-dial - sufficient minus cylinder added to make all the lines equally dark and black; (2) T-chart - sufficient minus cylinder added to obtain equality of the two groups of lines which are at right angles to each other; (3) cross-cylinder check test - the cross-cylinder is flipped from the position where the minus cylinder axis corresponds with the minus cylinder axis of the tentative cylindrical correction, to the second position where the plus cylinder axis of the cross-cylinder corresponds to the minus cylindrical axis of the tentative cylinder. The patient, thus, has the choice between the appearance of the Snellen target through more or less minus cylinder. By this rapid change in the amount of cylinder, the patient can decide which situation improves his visual acuity.

After determining the monocular refraction for each eye, the patient should be blurred with an additional 0.50D of plus sphere. Now the Risley prisms are adjusted before each eye, 3 base-up before the O.S. and 3 base-down before the O.D. The patient will now experience diplopia and will see the upper target with the right eye and the lower target with the left eye. The target is the 20/30 Snellen line of letters. At this point, the patient should be asked to report whether the two targets are equally clear, or if one is clearer than the other. If the patient reports that both targets are equally clear or blurred we have binocular balance of acuity. If the patient declares that one target is clearer than the other, additional plus is added in 0.25 diopter steps to the eye which has the better acuity, until the patient reports equality of visibility. If equality of vision is impossible to obtain, the patient is left with the dominant eye having the best acuity.

The dissociating prisms are then removed and the remainder of the test is finished under single binocular conditions. The plus sphere is reduced in 0.25 steps until the patient obtains 20/20 vision. If for any reason the patient does not obtain 20/20 vision, the lens combination which gave the maximum visual acuity is recorded as the finding. The greatest plus power through which the patient attains standard acuity is recorded as the *basic finding* or the *subjective finding.*

8. Induced phoria at distance

The procedure for this test is identical with the habitual phoria test at far (No.3) with the only exception that the test is performed through the subjective finding.

Summary Induced Phoria at Far

Test distance: 20' (6 meters).
Target: 20/20 Snellen letters (or smallest visible).
Lenses in place: subjective finding.
Dissociating device: 6 base-up O.S.; 15 base-in O.D.
Illumination: good illumination, 20 f.c.
Phoroptor adjustment: far p.d.

9. True adduction at distance

This is the first fused prism test which is performed. The patient is observing the distant Snellen chart and is reading silently the 20/20 line or the smallest letters visible. The subjective finding is in place and the Risley prisms are positioned so that they can be turned into a base-out direction. While the patient is viewing the smallest Snellen letters visible (usually the 20/20 line) through the subjective finding and the prisms (at zero position), an additional plus 0.25D sphere is added to each eye. The patient is asked if he noticed the blur produced by this simultaneous addition of the plus sphere. The plus 0.25D spheres are removed and the patient instructed that this same blur will be produced again. As soon as he notices this condition, he is to report "blur." Now both rotary prisms should be turned in the base-out direction, simultaneously and slowly. As soon as the patient reports "blur," the total amount of base-out prism in both rotary prisms is recorded. The amount of base-out prism needed to cause a blur equivalent to an 0.25D plus sphere above the subjective finding is recorded as the true adduction finding.

Summary True Adduction at Far

Test distance: 20' (6 meters).
Target: 20/20 Snellen or smallest visible.
Lenses in place: subjective finding.
Prisms in place: both Risley prisms in position to turn base-out.
Auxiliary lenses: plus 0.25D spheres O.U. to demonstrate blur.
Illumination: normal 20 f.c.
Phoroptor adjustment: far p.d.

10. Convergence at distance

When the patient has reported that the target is blurred and the data for test No. 9 has been recorded, we continue turning more base-out prism binocularly and the patient is asked to report when the target doubles. When diplopia has been reported, the amount of base-out is recorded as the break point for the test. The refractionist now requests the patient to report when the targets become one (reversion to single binocular vision). The amount of base-out prism in the Risley rotaries is slowly decreased, binocularly, and the amount of prism in place when the patient reports single vision is recorded as the recovery portion of the test. Two results are recorded for this test and expressed as a fraction - *break/recovery*. For example: patient reports double vision with a total of 19D base-out; and reports recovery of fusion with 10 base-out still in the rotaries. This would be recorded as 19/10.

Occasionally, the patient will not be able to regain fusion until base-in prism has been introduced. In this case, the recovery is recorded as a minus value. For example, patient reports diplopia with 15 base-out; regains fusion with 3 base-in. This would be recorded as 15/-3.

At times the patient may report that the target is not doubling, but that it seems to move to one side. The direction of movement detected by the patient should be determined. It now can be determined which eye is suppressing. If the patient suppresses his right eye, he will report the target moving to his right; if he suppresses his left eye, he will report the target moving toward his left.

Summary Convergence at Distance

Test distance: 20' (6 meters).
Target: 20/20 Snellen or smallest visible.
Lenses in place: subjective finding.
Prisms in place: Both Risley prisms in position to turn base-out.
Illumination: normal 20 f. c.
Phoroptor adjustment: far p.d.

11. Abduction at distance

This finding has the same procedure as the previous test. It differs in that the stimulus is applied in the base-in direction. This test also has a break point and a recovery value, and the data is recorded in the same manner as for No. 10. Example: diplopia reported at 10 base-in; recovered fusion with 6 base-in. This would be recorded as: 10/6.

As in the preceding test, the patient may report that the target is moving to one side rather than giving the expected response of diplopia. In this case, the direction of movement should be ascertained, and then it can be determined which of the patient's eyes is suppressing. For example, the patient reports the target moving toward his right. This is due to suppression of his left eye. When the patient reports the target moving toward his left, this is due to suppression of his right eye.

Summary Abduction at Distance

Test distance: 20' (6 meters).
Target: 20/20 Snellen or smallest visible.
Lenses in place: subjective finding.
Prisms in place: both Risley prisms in position to turn base-in.
Illumination: normal 20 f. c.
Phoroptor adjustment: far p.d.

12. Vertical phoria and ductions at distance

This test consists of two parts: first, the vertical phoria test and, second, the vertical duction test. The general procedure for the phoria test is the same as No. 3 test. The phoria is taken through the subjective finding with the patient observing the Snellen target. The patient is dissociated with 10 to 15D base- in before the right eye. About 6 to 8 prism diopters base-up is placed before the left eye. The patient will have uncrossed diplopia. He will see the upper target with his right eye and the lower target with his left eye. The patient is asked to report when the targets are aligned horizontally (directly across from each other) and the amount of base-up is slowly reduced before the left eye. Any base-up remaining in the prism before the left eye when the patient has reported horizontal alignment would be recorded as diopters of right hyperphoria, and any prism base-down remaining in the prism before the left eye would be recorded as diopters of left hyperphoria.

Upon completion of the vertical phoria portion of the test, both Risley prisms are turned so that they can operate in a base-down or a base-up direction. Both rotaries should now read zero. The patient is again observing the Snellen target through the subjective finding and prism base-down is introduced before the right eye. The patient is cautioned to report as soon as the target doubles. The amount of prism base-down is noted as soon as the patient reports diplopia. Now, the amount of prism base-down is slowly reduced until the patient reports single vision. This would be recorded as right supraduction. Then prism base-up is turned in before the right eye and the patient again asked to report when the target doubles. This is recorded as the break finding.

The amount of base-up before the right eye is gradually reduced and the patient is asked to report when he regains single vision This is recorded as the recovery value. This duction is known as right infraduction. For example, the following duction values are obtained with prism applied before the right eye of the patient, 4 base-down to break, 2 base-down to recovery; 5 base-up to break and 3 base-up to recovery. This would be noted on the case study analysis sheet as: right supraduction 4/2; right infraduction 5/3.

If it is necessary to reduce the amount of prism before the right eye to such a degree that the opposite prism direction is entered, the recovery value is recorded as a minus value. For example, 5 base-up before right eye for diplopia regains single vision with 1 base-down before the right eye. This would be recorded as: right infraduction 5/-1.

Summary Vertical Phoria	**Vertical Ductions**
Test distance:	
20 feet (6 meters).	20 feet (6 meters)
Target:	
20/20 Snellen.	20/20 Snellen.
Lenses in place:	
subjective finding.	subjective finding.
Prisms in place:	
6 base-up O.S.; 10-15 base-in O.D.	Risley prisms positioned to turn base-up or base-down.
Illumination:	
normal 20 f. c.	normal 20 f. c.
Phoroptor adjustment	
far p.d.	far p.d.

13B. Induced phoria at near

This test is performed in the same manner as the No. 13A test. It differs in that this phoria test is taken through the subjective finding. This is a near-point test. The reduced Snellen target is placed at 16" and well illuminated. The phoroptor is adjusted for the near pupillary distance. The patient is dissociated by means of 6 diopters base-up prism before the left eye and 15 diopters prism base-in before the right eye. The patient will now have uncrossed diplopia and will see the upper target with his right eye and the lower target with his left eye. The amount of prism base-in now is reduced before the right eye until the patient reports vertical alignment of the targets. Any prism base-in remaining in the rotary prism is recorded as prism diopters of exophoria and any prism base-out in the rotary would be recorded as diopters of esophoria.

Summary Induced at Near

Test distance: 16".
Target: 20/20 reduced Snellen (or smallest visible).
Lenses in place: subjective finding.
Prisms in place: 6 base-up O.S.; 15 base-in O.D.
Illumination: normal 20 f.c.
Phoroptor adjustment: near p.d.

14A. Dissociated cross-cylinder.

The cross-grid target (three horizontal lines and three vertical lines) is placed at 16" from the patient. Dissociation is performed by placing three base-up before the left eye and three base-down before the right eye. He will now report the presence of two cross grid targets, one higher than the other. Because of the positioning of the prisms, the higher image will be before the right eye and the lower image before the left eye. The patient is asked if the lines are equally clear and black in the upper target and in the lower target. If the astigmatic correction is correct, the patient should report that the vertical lines of the cross grid and the horizontal lines of the target are equally clear and black.

If the patient reports inequality in the lines of either target, additional plus sphere should be added and the patient again questioned as to the appearance of the lines. If they are still unequal, additional minus cylinder is added with axis at 90° to the darkest lines, until the patient reports equality of the horizontal and vertical lines of the target.

The cross-cylinders are introduced before each eye with minus cylinder axis (red dot) at 90°. The illumination is dimmed (about two foot-candles). Plus sphere is added in 0.25D steps before each eye until the patient reports the vertical lines darker and blacker in both the upper and lower target. The plus sphere is now slowly reduced in 0.25D steps until equality of the lines is obtained for each target. If equality of the lines is impossible because the patient reverses from vertical lines, the darkest, to horizontal lines, the darkest, with a reduction of an 0.25D in plus sphere, record the total lenses in place that leave the vertical lines the darker. When equality of the lines in both targets is obtained, the total lenses in place are recorded as the dissociated cross-cylinder finding. For example:

O.D. +1.00 -.50 X 90° vertical lines darker
O.D. +0.75 -.50 X 90° lines equal

Recorded would be:
No. 14A O.D. +0.75 -.50 X 90°

Summary Dissociated Cross-Cylinder

Test distance: 16".
Target: cross-grid.
Lenses in place: subjective finding.
Prisms in place: 3 base-up O.S.; 3 base-down O.D.
Auxiliary device: cross-cylinders (0.50D) with red dot at 90° before each eye.
Illumination: dim.2 f. c.
Phoroptor adjustment: near p.d.

15A. Induced phoria through the unfused cross-cylinder

This is a nearpoint phoria test taken through the lenses in place at the completion of the dissociated cross-cylinder test. The illumination is increased to normal intensity. The prism before the left eye is increased to 6 base-up; the prism before the right eye is adjusted to 15D base-in. The target remains the cross-grid, and the cross-cylinders remain in place. The patient will have uncrossed diplopia, with the upper target to the right of the lower target. The amount of base-in is slowly reduced until the patient reports vertical alignment of the targets. Any base-in prism remaining in the measuring prism is recorded as exophoria; if base-out is in the measuring prism, it is recorded as diopters of esophoria.

Summary Induced Phoria Through Unfused Cross-Cylinder

Test distance: 16".
Target: cross-grid.
Lenses in place: dissociated cross-cylinder finding.
Prisms in place: 6 base-up O.S.; 15 base-in O.D.
Auxiliary device: cross-cylinders remain in position as in No. 14A.
Illumination: normal 20 f.c..
Phoroptor adjustment: near p.d.

14B. Binocular cross-cylinder

The dissociating and measuring prisms used in the previous test (No. 15A) are removed. The cross-grid target remains in the same position. The illumination is dimmed to two foot-candles. The cross-cylinders remain as before. The patient will now report a single cross-grid target. We again question the patient to compare the horizontal and vertical lines and to report which lines are the darkest or blackest. Since the lenses in place are those from the dissociated cross-cylinder test, we usually obtain the response that the vertical lines are the darkest. If the patient reports that the lines are equal or that the horizontal lines are the darkest, sufficient plus sphere should be added in 0.25 steps O.U. until the patient reports the vertical lines the darkest. We now reduce the plus in 0.25 D. steps O.U. until the patient reports equality of the lines. If equality of the lines cannot be obtained, we leave the patient with the lenses which leave the horizontal lines the darkest. The total lenses in place are recorded as the fused cross-cylinder test.

Summary Binocular Cross-Cylinder

Test distance: 16".
Target: cross-grid.
Lenses in place: dissociated cross-cylinder finding.
Auxiliary device: cross-cylinders (0.50 D.) in place O.U. red dot at 90°.
Illumination: dim 2 f.c.
Phoroptor adjustment: near p.d.

15B. Induced phoria through fused cross-cylinder

This is another near-point phoria test which is performed through the lenses in place at the completion of the fused cross-cylinder test. A reduced Snellen 20/20 target is placed at 16". The patient is dissociated by means of six diopters base-up prism before the O.S. and uncrossed diplopia is established by placing 15D base-in before the O.D. The illumination is increased to normal. The cross-cylinders are removed. The patient should report seeing two groups of letters, with the upper group to the right. The patient now is asked to report when the targets are aligned vertically and then reduction is started of the amount of base-in before the right eye. As soon as the patient reports alignment of the targets, any base-in remaining in the Risley prism is recorded as diopters of exophoria. If the measuring prism contains base-out, it is recorded as diopters of esophoria. This test is the final phoria test in the examination.

Summary Induced Phoria Through Fused Cross-Cylinder

Test distance: 16".
Target: 20/20 reduced Snellen.
Lenses in place: fused cross-cylinder finding.
Prisms in place: 6 base-up before O.S.; 15 base-in before O.D.
Illumination: normal 20 f. c.
Phoroptor adjustment: near p.d.

16A. Positive relative convergence

This is a nearpoint base-out-to-blur-out prism test. The lenses through which this test will be taken depend upon the refractive condition of the patient. The lenses used must always be noted upon the examination form. If the patient is a non-presbyope, hyperope or emmetrope, the test is taken through the subjective finding. If the patient is a presbyope, the test is taken through the net fused cross-cylinder test lenses. If the patient is a myope, the test is taken through the habitual near-point lens correction.

With the correct lenses in place, the patient's attention is fixed upon the target and he is told to report when he is no longer able to read a single letter of the 20/20 lines. Both Risley prisms are positioned before the patient so that they can be turned in the base-out direction. Normal illumination is used in this test. As the patient continues to observe the target, the amount of base-out is gradually increased (binocularly at same rate of speed) until the blur-out point is reached. The total amount of base-out before both eyes is recorded as the positive relative convergence test.

Summary Positive Relative Convergence

Test distance: 16".
Target: 20/20 reduced Snellen.
Lenses in place: (a) non-presbyope, hyperope or emmetrope-No. 7.
(b) presbyopic hyperope or emmetrope; 14B net.
(c) myope: habitual minus at near.
Prisms in place: Risley prisms positioned to turn base-out.
Illumination: normal 20 f. c.
Phoroptor adjustment: near p.d.

16B. Positive fusional reserve

This is a continuation of the previous test. As soon as the total amount of prism base-out necessary to blur-out the 20/20 reduced Snellen target has been recorded, we continue turning more base-out prism binocularly until the patient reports that the target has doubled, is starting to move to one side, or that the target has become clear. As soon as one of these responses is obtained, the total amount of base-out prism in both Risley prisms is recorded as the break.

Now reduction is started of the amount of base-out and the patient is instructed to report as soon as the targets go together and become one. As soon as binocular single vision has been regained, the total amount of base-out in both prisms is recorded as the recovery.

These two results are recorded as break/recovery. For example, the patient reports diplopia with 26 base-out; he reports single vision with 10 base-out. This would be recorded as 26/10. In some cases, the patient may not regain single vision until base-in prism has been introduced. In this instance, the amount of base-in would be recorded as the recovery, but must have a minus sign to indicate its opposite nature. For example, the patient reports diplopia with 16 base-out; regains fusion with 4 base-in. This would be recorded as 16/-4.

The normal response under increasing amounts of base-out is for the patient to report diplopia. In some cases, the patient will report the target moving to one side. This indicates that the patient is suppressing. If the patient suppresses his right eye, he will report the target moving to the right. If the patient suppresses his left eye, he will report the target moving to his left. When this occurs, the total amount of base-out prism in the rotaries is recorded and a notation is made on the examination form as to the eye that is suppressing. For example, 10 base-out, target moving toward the right. Recorded as: 10 O.D. supp.

Summary Positive Fusional Reserve

Test distance: 16".
Target: 20/20 reduced Snellen.
Lenses in place: same as for No. 16A.
Prisms in place: Risley prisms to turn base-out.
Illumination: normal 20 f. c.
Phoroptor adjustment: near p.d.

17A. Negative relative convergence

This test is the complete blur-out of 20/20 reduced Snellen target by prism base-in. It is, therefore, similar to positive relative convergence, except that the binocularly applied prism is in the base-in direction. The total amount of base-in present in both Risley prisms when the target is blurred out is recorded as the negative relative convergence.

Summary Negative Relative Convergence

Test distance: 16".
Target: 20/20 reduced Snellen.
Lenses in place: same as for No. 16A.
Prisms in place: Risley prisms in position to turn base-in.
Illumination: normal 20 f. c.
Phoroptor adjustment: near p.d.

17B. Negative fusional reserve

This test is a continuation of the negative relative convergence test. As soon as the patient reports the target blurred out, we continue adding prism base-in binocularly until the patient reports the target doubled, cleared, or moved to one side. The moment the patient reports any of these responses, a total is made of the amount of base-in in both Risley prisms and recorded as the negative fusional reserve test.

The next step is reduction of the amount of base-in prism, which is done slowly and equally before each eye. When the patient reports that the diplopia is gone and he has recovered fusion, the total amount of base-in prism in both rotaries is recorded as the negative fusional reserve test. This test has two parts, just as the positive fusional reserve test and its value is recorded in the same way. For example, patient reports diplopia with 24 base-in, regains fusion at 17 base-in. This would be recorded as 24/17.

If instead of reporting diplopia, the patient states that the target is moving to the right, it indicates his left eye is suppressing. If the patient states that the target is moving to his left, it indicates suppression of his right eye.

Summary Negative Fusional Reserve

Test distance: 16".
Target: 20/20 reduced Snellen.
Lenses in place: same as for No. 16A.
Prisms in place: Risley prisms in position to turn base-in until diplopia; reduce amount of base-in until regains fusion.
Illumination: normal.
Phoroptor adjustment: near p.d.

18. Vertical phoria and duction at near

This test is performed in the same manner as the vertical phoria and duction at far, except that it is taken at near. The first portion of this test is the vertical phoria. The target is the 20/20 reduced Snellen line. The target is at 16 inches from the patient. The patient is dissociated by means of a 15D base-in prism before his right eye, and a 6D base-up prism is placed before his left eye so that he will report the presence of two targets, with the right target higher than the left target.

The patient is instructed to read the letters of the target and to report as soon as the two targets are horizontally aligned. When horizontal alignment (directly across from each other) is reported, any base-up remaining in the measuring prism before the left eye is recorded as diopters of right hyperphoria. If base-down prism is found in the measuring prism before the left eye, the phoria is recorded as diopters of left hyperphoria.

The rotary prisms are now rotated so that they can introduce prism base-up or prism base-down. The patient is observing the 20/20 reduced Snellen line at 16". At this point, prism base-up is gradually introduced before the left eye, and the patient is asked to report as soon as the target doubles (break point). The total prism base-up before the left eye is recorded as break portion of right supraduction. The amount of base-up before the left eye is slowly decreased and the patient is asked to report when the targets become one. The amount of base-up before the left eye at this point is recorded as the recovery portion of right supraduction.

The next step in the procedure is in the base-down direction before the left eye and again the patient is asked to report when the target doubles. We also determine through this procedure the amount of base-down before the left eye when the patient regains single vision. This would be the recovery portion of right infraduction. The test results are recorded in the same manner as for test No.12.

Summary Vertical Phoria and Vertical Duction at Near

Test distance: 16".	16".
Target: 20/20 reduced Snellen.	20/20 reduced Snellen.
Lenses in place: subjective finding.	subjective finding
Prisms in place: 6 base-up O.S.; 15 base-in O.D.	Risley prisms positioned so that they can turn prism base-down or -up.
Illumination: normal 20 f. c.	normal 20 f. c.
Phoroptor adjustment: near p.d.	near p.d.

19. *Amplitude of accommodation.* The rotary prisms are removed. The reduced Snellen target is replaced with a paragraph of 0.62 em type. The target is placed at 13 inches from the patient. The illumination is bright. The subjective finding is in place.

The patient is asked to read the print at the 13-inch distance. If the patient can read the target, minus sphere is added in 0.25 diopter steps binocularly until the patient reports that the target is definitely blurred. The amount of minus added above the subjective finding is added to 2.50 diopters to give the binocular amplitude. For example, subjective +1.00: The total lenses in place upon completion of test is -3.00. What is the amplitude of accommodation? +4.00 + 2.50 = 6.50 diopters of amplitude.

If the patient is presbyopic, difficulty in reading the target will be found. In these instances, plus sphere is added binocularly in 0.25 diopter steps until the patient reads the print with difficulty. The additional plus above the subjective is subtracted from 2.50 to obtain the amplitude. For example, subjective finding: +1.00; total lenses in phoroptor upon completion of test is +2.00. What is the amplitude? +1.00 has been added above the subjective; therefore, amplitude = 2.50 - 1.00 or 1.50 diopters of amplitude of accommodation.

Because of the necessity for computing the amount of lag for the cross-cylinder tests, this test is performed immediately after the induced phoria test at near (No. 13B).

The test described is repeated monocularly to determine the right eye and left eye amplitude of accommodation.

Summary Amplitude of Accommodation

Test distance: 13".
Target: 0.62 em type.
Lenses in place: subjective finding.
(a) presbyope - plus sphere added until print is readable.
(b) non-presbyope - minus sphere added until print becomes difficult to read.
Illumination: normal 20 f. c.
Phoroptor adjustment: near p.d.

20. Positive relative accommodation

A row of 20/20 reduced Snellen letters is placed at 16" from the patient. The lenses in place represent the subjective finding, except as noted in the positive relative convergence test. As the patient continues to read the letters on the target, minus sphere is added binocularly in 0.25 steps until the patient states that *all* of the letters are blurred out. The total minus sphere added above the control lenses in place is recorded as positive relative accommodation. For example, subjective finding is a +1.00 O.U.; total lenses in place -2.00. What is the amount of positive relative accommodation? The total minus sphere added is a -3.00 diopters. This amount, therefore, is recorded as the P.R.A.

Summary Positive Relative Accommodation

Test distance: 16".
Target: 20/20 reduced Snellen.
Lenses in place: (a) non-presbyopic hyperopes and emmetropes-test is taken through No.7 (subjective).
(b) presbyopes-test is taken through 14B net.
(c) myopes-test is taken through the habitual minus at near.
Illumination: normal 20 f. c.
Phoroptor adjustment: near p.d.

21. Negative relative accommodation.

The same fixation target and test distance is used for this test as in the positive relative accommodation test. This test differs from the preceding test in that we are going to determine to what extent we can inhibit accommodation while fixation is maintained at 16". We therefore add plus sphere in 0.25D steps to the control lenses in place, until the patient states that all of the letters are completely blurred out. The amount of plus above the control lenses in place is recorded as the N.R.A. For example, control lenses in place: -1.00; total lenses in place after completion of test +2.00. What is the amount of the N.R.A.? The total plus added is +3.00. Therefore, this is the N.R.A.

Summary Negative Relative Accommodation

Test distance: 16".

Target: 20/20 reduced Snellen.

Lenses in place: (a) non-presbyopic hyperopes and emmetropes: taken through subjective finding.

(b) presbyopes: taken through 14B net.

(c) myopes: taken through the habitual minus at near.

Illumination: normal 20 f. c.

Phoroptor adjustment: near p.d.

CHAPTER VII
Significance of the Visual Tests

A. Introduction

The probe bodies used in our investigation of the visual pattern of the patient are *lenses and prisms*. Lenses are used for their specific effect upon the accommodative pattern; prisms are used for their specific effect upon the convergence pattern.

There are four basic changes that can be performed with prisms and lenses. They are:

1. *Convex sphere*-Inhibit accommodation-The induced change is as *if* the object moved away from the plane of regard. The size change observed is that the target appears larger.

2. *Concave sphere*-Stimulate accommodation-The induced change is as *if* the object is moved closer to the observer. The size change observed is that the target appears smaller.

3. *Base-in prism*-Inhibit convergence-The induced change is as *if* the object is moved away from the plane of regard. The size change observed is that the target appears to become larger.

4. *Base-out prism*-Stimulate convergence-The induced change is as *if* the object is moving closer to the observer. The size change observed is that the target becomes smaller as it comes closer. These four basic changes of spatial projection are schematically shown in Figure 42. Thus, each of our optometric tests can be classified according to the spatial direction and type of pattern probing occurring. This has been done in Table 6. You will note that three of our optometric tests, namely, convergence at far, positive fusional reserve and negative fusional reserve have been listed as tests which influence the accommodation pattern as well as the convergence pattern. This reflex activity of the accommodation pattern occurs when we stimulate or inhibit convergence past a certain value; the pattern is completely utilized and the overflow stimulus begins to activate its sister pattern. We must remember that the subject reacts as an entity to the testing situation. The stimulation or inhibition of one segment of the visual pattern can be continued for some time without affecting another portion of the visual pattern because of the buffer area present in the central nervous system. Thus, if we were to stimulate the

> convergence pattern by means of base-out prism, we could continue this stimulation without an overt action of the accommodation pattern as long as the buffer area has not been completely utilized. When the buffer area (or latitude of performance) is completely utilized, continuing stimulation of the convergence pattern will result in an overt action of the accommodative pattern, and the patient will experience a blur. The extent and integration of these buffer areas in the central nervous system determines the limit of stimulation or inhibition of one segment of the visual pattern without affecting the other portion. The amount of this latitude or relationship in the central nervous system necessary to maintain a functional flexibility between the pattern of accommodation and the pattern of convergence depends upon the learned relationship existing at the moment; the interest of the organism in the visual situation; the size, color, contrast, and complexity of the peripheral field of the stimulus object; the quantity and quality of the illumination; the physical posture of the subject; the mental and emotional level of the organism; and many other variables. This emphasizes the importance of standardizing our testing procedures, equipment, targets, and illumination, if we are to have statistical reliability, to our measures of organismic visual responses.

There are those who state that the analytical examination has been ritualized, that it regimented the optometrist, and that it does not allow for freedom of action so that we may utilize professional judgment. If these same individuals would examine neighboring fields of science, they would see the same rigid formulations. The field of chemistry comes to mind. If we are to test the boiling point of water, it makes no difference what quantity of water may be present. If we proceed to a salt mixture, the amounts of each of the ingredients become important in determining the physical properties of the system. If we proceed to a colloidal mixture, we find that we must now regulate not only the amounts of each of the ingredients but also the order in which they are added, the speed with which they are added, and the length of time at which the mixture has been heated (past history of the gel). The good organic chemist learns from bitter experience the importance of following the cookbook recipes, if he is to end up with a beautiful dyestuff rather than a tarry mess. Deviations from the cookbook recipe are done only after prolonged experimentation. Let us consider the educational psychologist who is interested in the action of the organism to his external environment. He has long understood the importance of standard testing procedures. In many of the psychological tests, the exact instructions to be given to the subject are recorded. Even the tone of the examiner's voice can change the validity of a test.

CONVEX SPHERES

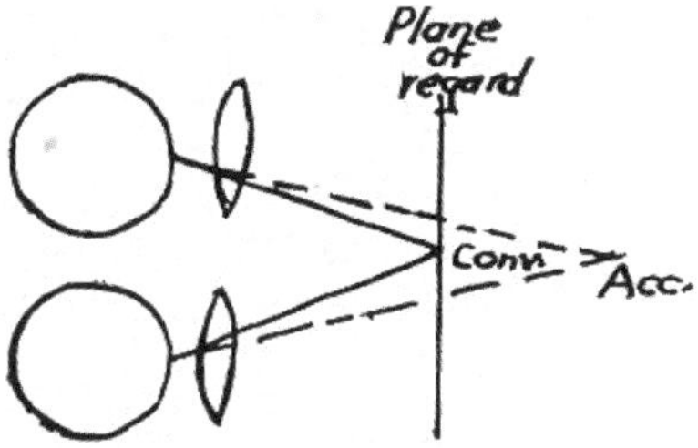

Convergence at the plane of regard
Accommodation is away from the plane of regard

CONVEX SPHERES

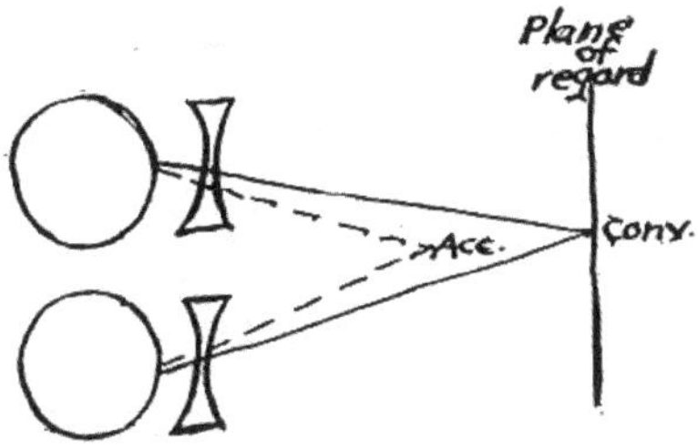

Convergence at the plane of regard
Accommodation has moved toward the observer

BASE-IN PRISM

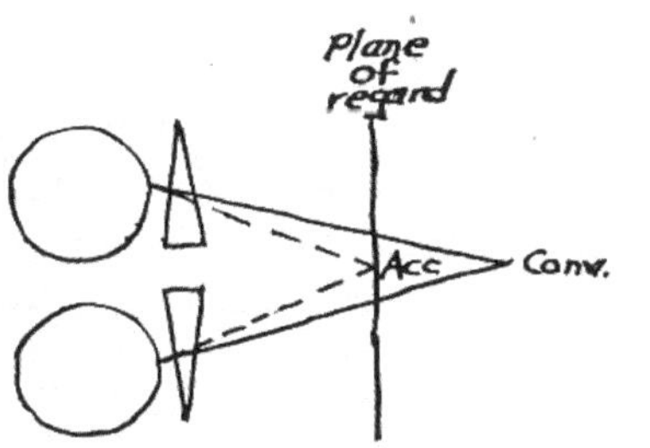

Accommodation at the plane of regard
Convergence is away from the plane of regard

BASE-OUT PRISM

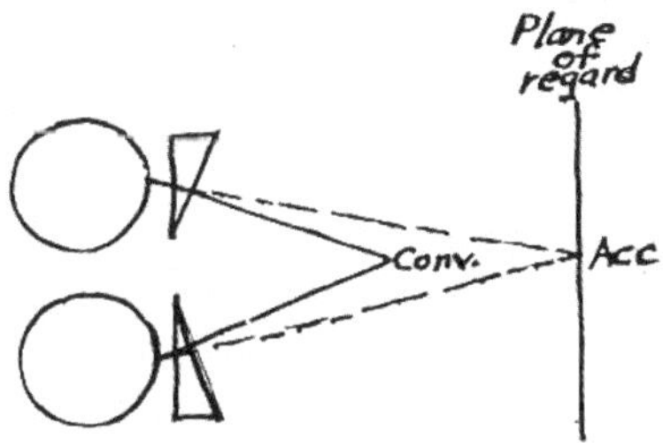

Accommodation at the plane of regard
Convergence has moved toward the observer

Figure 42. Effect of lenses and prisms on accommodation and convergence.

We must remember that the human organism is an exceedingly complex structure of infinite abilities in equilibrium with a complex external environment, internal environment (physiological) and a mental environment. In order to test this complexity with any validity, all variations as to testing procedure, order of testing, targets, illumination, and patient posture must be rigidly controlled. It is for this reason that the analytical procedure has been routinized. When answers which seem incredulous are obtained from patients, it is well to remember the phrase which originated from our biological laboratories: "The test animal does not lie. It is better to question ourselves as to procedure, target, illumination and environmental surroundings than to use the hackneyed expression; "The Patient is Neurotic."

B. The development of a diagnostic syndrome.

In the beginning, when our concept of a visual problem was merely acuity, it was sufficient to consider only the magnitude of a visual test. As our concept of what constituted a visual problem broadened to include visual performance and visual achievement, it became evident that the magnitude of a test value was not sufficient identification for a visual problem. A series of norms or expected values for the key optometric tests were determined by A.M. Skeffington and his associates. By comparing our test values for a particular patient against these norms, we could readily determine whether our values were lower or higher than these norm values. Thus, a pattern or syndrome began to develop. This was an important contribution to visual analysis since it recognized that these experimental values for a particular patient will fluctuate from time to time, depending upon the demands of the external environment, physiological state of the subject, and his emotional level. Thus, while the magnitude of these various visual tests may fluctuate, their relationship to the norm value is much more stable. That is, a phoria test, which tends to be in eso, will continue so rather than vary haphazardly. This fluctuation in amount is evident from the visual data presented in Table 7 which concerned two observers who were given a complete visual examination at weekly intervals for a period of ten weeks. The next advance in stabilizing the syndrome was the comparison of tests to each other; i.e., static retinoscopy compared against the subjective at far; base-in tests compared to base-out tests; and nearpoint accommodative tests compared to farpoint accommodative tests. Therefore, for the purpose of diagnosis we are interested in the magnitude of the static retinoscopy test; but we are also interested in the comparison of this test to the distant subjective test.

We have three types of visual problems. They are: the poor reader, accommodative interference (fatigue) or a convergence interference (fatigue) pattern. As has been shown in Table 6 (I and II) all of our optometric tests investigate either the accommodative pattern or the convergence pattern.

The accommodative mechanism that functions through a smooth muscle mechanism is slow acting; the convergence mechanism which functions through a striated muscle mechanism is fast acting. It is obvious that whenever we have two mechanisms which must coordinate their activity, where one is fast acting and the other mechanism is slow acting, the slower functioning mechanism becomes the pace setter. It is thus that the great majority of all visual problems are accommodative interference cases (B-Type). The remainder of the visual problems are convergence interference

Table 6. (Part I)

Test No.	Name	Operational Name
3	Habitual Phoria at Far	Base-In prism needed for vertical alignment of dissociated images.
13A	Habitual Phoria at Near	Same as above.
4	Static Retinoscopy	Plus sphere needed for flicker neutralization of motion while patient is fixating at far.
5	Dynamic Retinoscopy at 20 inches	Same as above with patient fixating at 20 inches.
6	Dynamic Retinoscopy at 40 inches	Same as above with patient fixating target at 40 inches.
7	Subjective (Basic Finding)	Maximum plus to standard acuity while patient fixates target at 20 feet.
8	Induced Phoria at Far	Same as Test No.3, performed thru No.7.
9	True Adduction at Far	Base-Out prism to 0.25 D. blur at far.
10	Convergence at Far	Base-Out to Break and Recovery at far.
11	Abduction at Far	Base-In to Break and Recovery at far.
13B	Induced Phoria at Near	Same as Test No. 13A, performed thru No.7
14A	Dissociated Cross Cylinder Test at Near	Maximum plus to equality of line target under dissociation thru cross-cylinder.
15A	Phoria Thru 14A	Base-In prism to vertical alignment of dissociated line target thru 14A.
14B	Fused Cross Cylinder Test at Near	Maximum plus to equality of line target under fused conditions thru cross cylinders.
15B	Phoria Thru 14B	Same as 15A, Control lenses 14B.
16A	Positive Relative Convergence	Base-Out to blur out at near on reduced 20/20 Snellen.
16B	Positive Fusional Reserve	Base-Out to Break and Recovery at Near.
17A	Negative Relative Convergence	Base-In prism to blur out at near on reduced 20/20 Snellen.
17B	Negative Fusional Reserve	Base-In to Break and recovery at Near.
19	Amplitude of Accommodation	Minus sphere to blur on 0.62em type at 13 inches.
20	Positive Relative Accommodation	Minus sphere to blur out at near on reduced 20/20 Snellen.
21	Negative Relative Accommodation	Plus sphere to blur out at near on reduced 20/20 Snellen.

cases (C-Type). Proportionately 95% of all cases are accommodative or B-Type, and the remaining 5% are convergence or C-Type cases.

If an interference exists in the accommodative pattern (see Fig. 43), this interference acts as an inhibition to the stimulus arriving at the pattern from the higher neurological levels. Therefore, the visual pattern is forwarding equal stimulation to both the accommodative and convergence patterns. We, therefore, would have the stimulus to the converging pattern

Table 6. (Part II)

Test No.	Portion of Visual Pattern Tested	Type of Probing Used	Spatial Direction
3	Convergence	Inhibition	Away from plane of regard
13A	Convergence	Inhibition	Away from plane of regard
4	Accommodation	Inhibition	Away from plane of regard
5	Accommodation	Inhibition	Away from plane of regard
6	Accommodation	Inhibition	Away from plane of regard
7	Accommodation	Inhibition	Away from plane of regard
8	Convergence	Inhibition	Away from plane of regard
9	Convergence	Stimulation	Toward organism
10	Convergence (Accommodation)	Stimulation	Toward organism
11	Convergence	Inhibition	Away from plane of regard
13B	Convergence	Inhibition	Away form plane of regard
14A	Accommodation	Inhibition	Away from plane of regard
15A	Convergence	Inhibition	Away from plane of regard
14B	Accommodation	Inhibition	Away from plane of regard
15B	Convergence	Inhibition	Away from plane of regard
16A	Convergence	Stimulation	Toward organism
16B	Convergence (Accommodation)	Stimulation	Toward organism
17A	Convergence	Inhibition	Away form plane of regard
17B	Convergence (Accommodation)	Inhibition	Away from plane of regard
19	Accommodation	Stimulation	Toward organism
20	Accommodation	Stimulation	Toward organism
21	Accommodation	Inhibition	Away from plane of regard

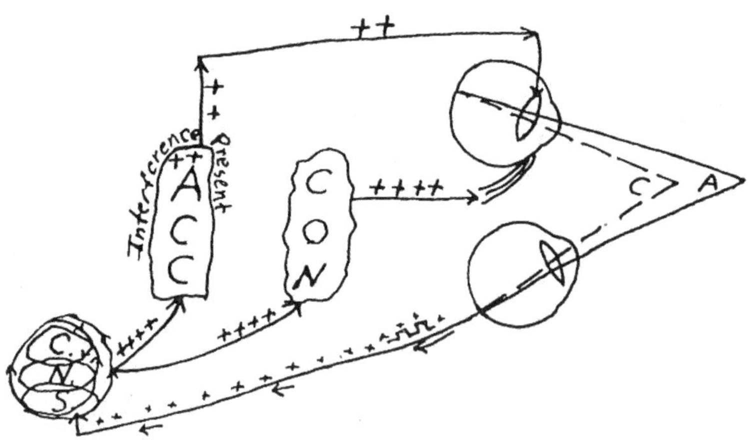

Figure 43. Development of a B-type case.

forwarded practically unchanged to the convergence mechanism, while this same amount of stimulus entering the accommodative pattern would be partially absorbed because of the existing interference, and only a portion would be forwarded to the accommodative mechanism. Because of

Table 7.

Phoria Tests					Duction Tests		
#3	#8	#13A	#13B	#10	#11	#16B	#17B
1/2 S	1 S	4 X	2 X	22/8	8/2	22/11	19/8
11/2 S	11/2 S	3 X	2 X	20/5	6/1	12/4	25/17
1/2	1 S	3 X	2 X	28/8	9/4	16/8	18/4
1 S	1 S	3 X	3 X	23/9	8/3	14/8	25/6
1 S	1 S	2 X	1 X	24/8	10/3	14/7	23/9
1 S	1 S	1 X	1 X	23/11	9/3	23/11	21/3
1 S	1 S	2 X	2 X	24/8	8/2	16/7	22/10
1/2S	1 S	1/2 X	1/2 X	20/9	10/4	21/12	19/6
2 S	2 S	1 X	Ortho	22/7	11/4	24/12	21/6
1 S	1 S	3 X	3 X	27/9	10/4	22/12	21/7

Accommodative Tests

#4	#7	#5	#14A	#14B
+.50	+.25	+2.00	+1.00	+1.25
+.75	+.50	+2.25	+1.50	+1.75
+.50-.25x.75°	P1.-.25x25°	+2.25	+1.50	+1.25
+.75	+.25	+2.00	+1.50	+1.25
+.50	+.25	+2.00	+0.75	+0.50
+1.00	+.50	+2.75	+1.00	+0.75
+.75	+.25-.50x20°	+1.75	+1.00	+0.75
+.75	+.50	+1.75	+1.00	+0.75
+.50-.25x115°	+.50-.25x15°	+2.25	+1.00	+1.00
+1.00-.25x55°	+.75-.25x55°	+2.75	+1.50	+1.50
+.75-.25x110°	+.25	+2.00	+0.25	+0.25
+1.00	+.25	+2.25	+0.50	+0.50
+.75-.25x125°	+.25-.50x15°	+2.50	+0.75	+0.50
+.75	+.50-.25x160°	+2.50	+0.75	+0.50
+.50-.25x180°	+.50-.25x20°	+2.00	+1.25	+0.75
+.75-.25x180°	+.50	+2.00	+1.25	+0.75
+.75-.25x180°	+.25	+2.25	+0.75	+1.25
+1.00-.25X180°	+.50	+2.25	+1.00	+1.50
+.75	+.25	+2.50	+1.25	+0.75
+1.00	+.50	+2.75	+1.25	+0.75

this accommodative interference, we have a spatial warping with accommodation away from the organism and convergence projected toward the organism. Therefore, in performing any of our optometric tests which create this spatial configuration typical of the accommodative interference case, we can expect that test value to be relatively high. If the optometric test creates the opposite spatial configuration, we would expect that test to be relatively low in value. Thus, for the accommodative interference case (B-Type), we can expect minus lens tests to be low, plus lens tests to be high, base-out tests to be high, and base-in tests to be low. Whenever the probe body causes a reversal in the habitual spatial projection, that test value will be low; if the probe body creates a spatial configuration similar to that of the habitual pattern, that test value will be high.

Table 8.

	Accommodative		Convergence	
	Stimulation	Inhibition	Stimulation	Inhibition
Tests No.	(10) (16B) 20	5, 6, 14A, (17B), 21	9, 10, 16A, 16B	11, 15A, 17A, 17B
B-Type	Low	High	High	Low
C-Type	High	Low	Low	High

Figure 44 presents the schematic diagram of the convergence interference (C-Type) case. We note that it is the opposite of the B-Type case. We thus can state that any test which creates the spatial configuration of accommodation towards the organism and convergence away from the organism will be high in amount. Those optometric tests which create the reverse of this configuration will be low in amount. Thus, minus lens tests will be high; plus lens tests will be low; base-out tests will be low; and base-in tests will be high.

You will note that convergence at far (No. 10) is a direct stimulation to convergence at far, but simultaneously, because of the close relationship between accommodation and convergence, we will have the indirect stimulation of accommodation also. Therefore, this test has been entered as a convergence as well as an accommodative test. For the same reason, positive fusional reserve and negative fusional reserve have been included as both convergence and accommodative tests, Thus, the informative sequence for a B-Type case will be:

5-9   6   14A   16A-21
10-11-16B-17B   15A   17A-20

The typing, as you can observe, is complex. The duction pattern for a particular B-Type case depends upon whether it is a B1 or a B2 and its deteriorated status. Thus, we have:

B-Type Case

Time ↓   B1 ↓   B2 ↓

11 – 16B   11 -17B

10 – 16B   10 – 17B

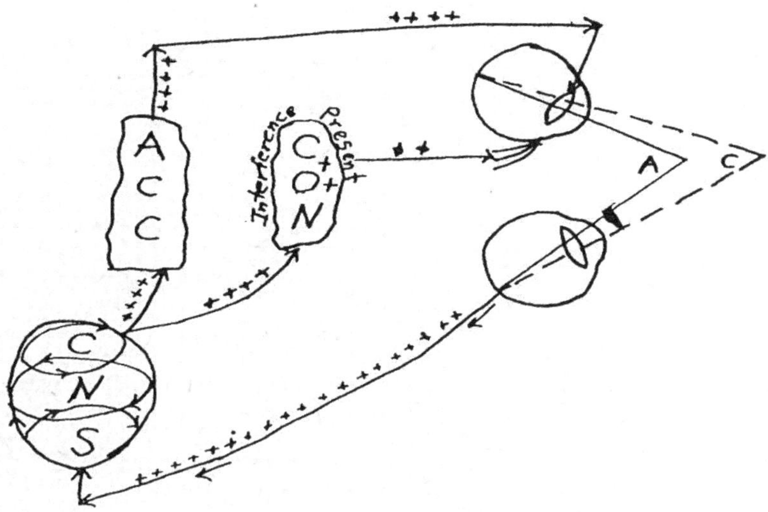

Figure 44. Development of a C-type case.

Although true adduction test (No.9) is high in the initial stages of myopia, for the typical hyperopic B-Type case true adduction is typically low, in comparison to its expected value. Thus, a typical B1 case would have the following informative sequence:

$$\frac{\text{5 \quad 6 \quad 14A \quad 16A-21 \quad 19}}{\text{9-11-16B \quad 15A \quad 17A-20}}$$

A typical B2 case would have the following informative sequence:

$$\frac{\text{5 \quad 6 \quad 14A \quad 16A-21 \quad 19}}{\text{9-11-17B \quad 15A \quad 17A-20}}$$

Thus, from Table 7 we can construct the informative sequence for the C Type case:

$$\frac{\text{15A \quad 15A \quad 17A -20}}{\text{(17B) – 5 – 9 – 10 - 16B \quad 14A \quad 16A -21}}$$

We find in the early stages of the C-Type ease that true adduction (No.9) is usually up to its expected value. Since convergence stimulation creates a reversal in the habitual spatial pattern for a C-Type case (see Fig. 44), we find that positive fusional reserve (No. 16B) will be lower in amount than the negative fusional reserve (No. 17B). Therefore the informative sequence for a typical C-Type case becomes:

$$\frac{\text{15A \quad 15A \quad 17A-20 \quad 19}}{\text{5 – 10 - 16B \quad 14A \quad 16A-21}}$$

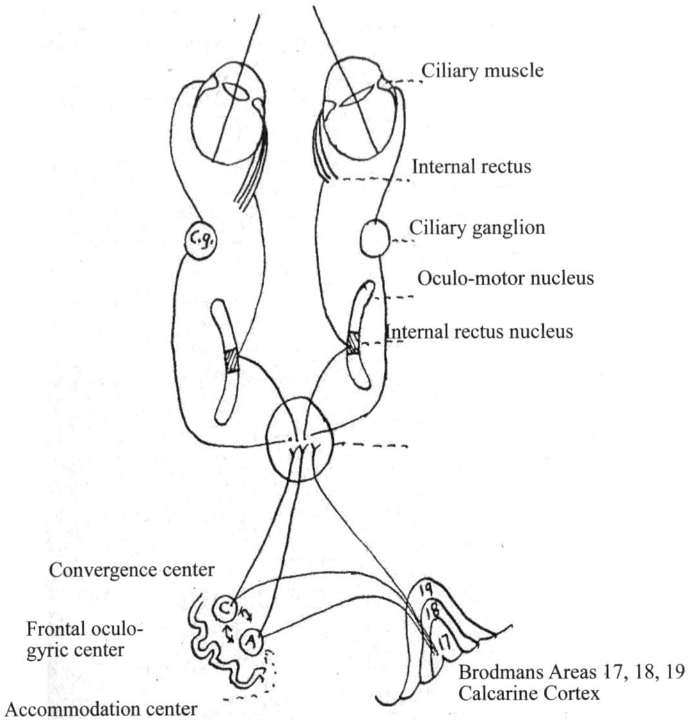

Figure 45. A schematic diagram of the functional relationship between accommodation and convergence.

If you will note the informative sequence for the B1-Type, you will observe that if the visual problem has existed for some time the duction pattern of the case will be as follows: No's. 10-16B low. The similarity of this deteriorated B-Type and C-Type case is obvious. Thus, the B-Type case assumes many guises as the degree of the deterioration increases. The statement has been made that a skilled physician is one who can differentiate and identify syphilis, because this disease can simulate and duplicate the pattern of almost any type of disease. The same statement is true for visual science, in that the skilled practitioner is one who can identify a true B-Type case, because it also can assume many disguises. Figure 45 presents the relationship between accommodation and convergence.

To illustrate the spatial configuration of the B-Type case, the following case data has been plotted on a skew chart (see Fig. 46).

The effect of visual stress is a restriction in spatial latitude, and in some of the test values we have had a spatial reversal. Man is a space binding animal. The protracted concentration within a restricted area results in a

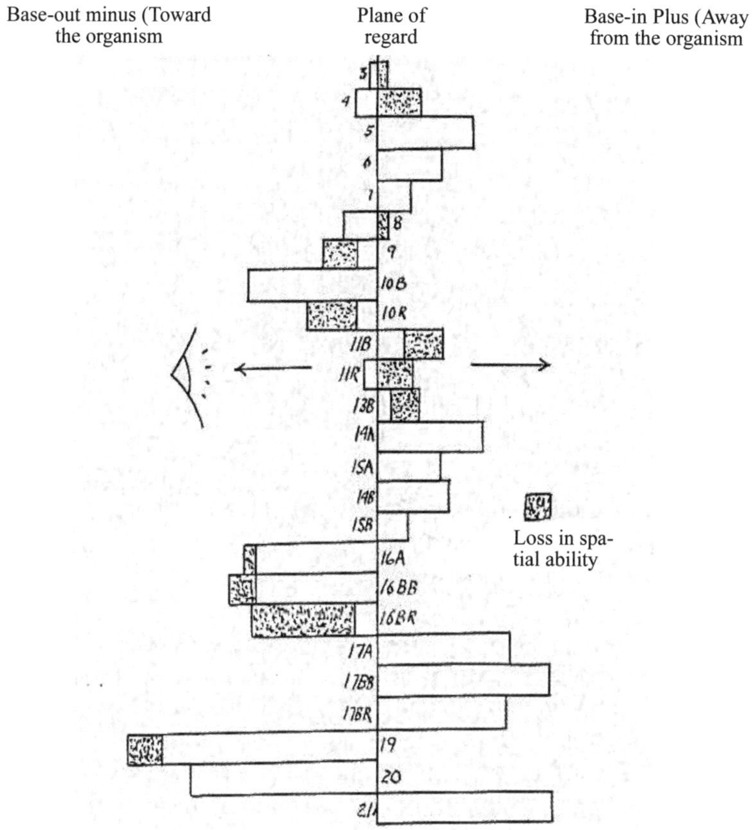

#3	1Eso	#10	19/3	#16A	X
#4	-0.50	#11	4/-2	#16B	18/3
#5	+2.25	#13B	2 Exo	#17A	19
#6	+1.50	#14A	+2.50	#17B	24/18
#7	++0.75	#15A	8 Exo	#19	5.00
#8	5Eso	#14B	+1.50	#20	-4.50
#9	3	#15B	6	#21	+3.25

Figure 46. Skew Chart

diminished ability to perform spatially. It is the purpose of visual care to restore this freedom of spatial movement.

The Case Typing

The case typing determines whether the patient can utilize full plus lens application or whether a minimum plus lens application must be used. The term "full plus" refers to the maximum lens values found in the subjective at far (No.7) and the M.S.D.A. at near. The analytical tests which make up the case typing are the fusional reserve tests at both far and at near. These are commonly called the duction tests and there are four of them - positive and negative fusional reserve at far (No.10 and No.11) and the positive and negative fusional reserve tests at near (No.16B and No.17B). Optometry recognized very early in its clinical development the importance of the duction tests in determining the lens prescription. Two rules of thumb emerged from this clinical experience:

1. All duction tests at far and near are high. It was found that whenever all of the duction test values exceeded their expected values that the patient did not have a binocular difficulty. In fact, these people very rarely sought visual care until presbyopia started to develop. Therefore, they needed very little in the nature of a lens correction.

2. Duction tests at far and at near are low. Similarly, it was found that when these same duction tests were low that subjective complaints started to multiply. In fact, the lower the magnitude of these findings, presuming that the patient has not developed suppression, the greater were the number and intensity of subjective complaints. Therefore, the lowering of these duction tests was a signal that a correction was needed. It was soon found that with certain duction patterns only a partial correction must be used.

Thirty years ago the various schools of optometry were teaching various rules regarding when to apply a partial lens correction, none of which were entirely satisfactory. It was Dr. A. M. Skeffington and his research associates that developed the importance of the time factor in visual analysis. They reasoned that the more recent the visual problem, the more conducive it would be to accept the full lens values as found subjectively and by means of the cross-cylinder tests at near. They further stated that the older the visual problem the more conservative we should be in prescribing plus lenses. These two statements are based on the psychological observation that recent learning patterns are easy to erase but learning patterns which have existed for a long time are very difficult to change. Lenses tended to change visual learning patterns since they created new relations between accommodation and convergence. Therefore, if these changes were recent, we could utilize full plus lens attack. However, if the visual problem was of long standing the patient would tend to reject visual changes created by the lens application.

From the duction pattern evolved the concept of case typing which is merely a graphical statement of which ductions are lower than their expected value. The problem now is to determine which duction pattern indicates that the visual problem is of recent origin. We have the following possible low duction patterns:

11-16B

11-17B

10-16B

10-17B

Which of these duction patterns is the most recent? Let us consider the farpoint ductions. If the visual problem is of recent origin, it has not as yet spread to farpoint (See Fig. 47) and, therefore we would expect that both ductions at far would be high. However, when we turn base-out prism at far (No.10) we are stimulating convergence so that we have the spatial movement of both accommodation and convergence toward the patient (convergence is closer of course). This is a normal situation that the patient has done many times, i.e. the movement of convergence and accommodation toward himself. Therefore, this finding in a recent visual problem would tend to be *high.* If we consider the base-in duction at far (No.11) for a recent visual problem, we have a different set of circumstances. This movement of convergence beyond the plane of regard at

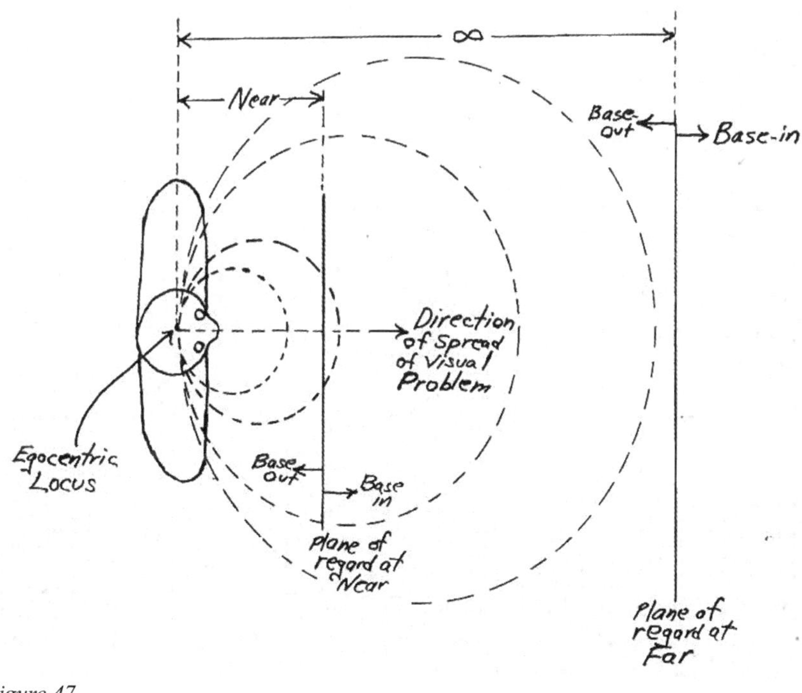

Figure 47.

infinity is a completely artificial skill that has never been organismically used. We would expect, therefore, that the magnitude of this test would be the first to collapse upon the beginning of a visual problem. As far as the farpoint ductions are concerned, we would expect in a *recent* visual problem to have, No.11 the low duction. This would indicate that full plus may be used. However, if the visual problem has lasted for a considerable period of time, we now have the movement of interference to reach the farpoint position (See Fig. 47). As the problem spreads from nearpoint toward farpoint we have the gradual erosion of the magnitude of the No.10 duction. Therefore, whenever the #10 duction becomes lower than the No.11 duction we know that the visual problem has either lasted for a long time or the patient has been exposed to very high environmental demands. This means that this type of visual pattern is going to be very difficult to change and so we must be conservative in the lens changes that we propose for the patient. Therefore,

_____ recent problem, will tolerate full lens values
11

_____ advanced visual problem, cut plus, be conservative.
10

Let us now consider the nearpoint ductions and their effect upon the lens application. The expected values for both the base-out duction at near (No.16B) and the base-in duction at near (No.17B) are approximately the same (21 p.d. compared to 22 p.d.). The visual problem starts at the patient's working distance which is usually closer than 16 inches, As we turn base-in prism at near for the beginning visual problem, the spread of the visual problem has not progressed to beyond the plane of regard and, therefore, we would expect (No.17B to be high. However, for the beginning visual problem, as we start to turn base-out prism at near, we very quickly enter the spatial area where the patient has visual distortions and, therefore, perceptual rapport with the plane of regard cannot be maintained and the patient will double under the base-out stimulus demand. If the visual problem is recent as far as the nearpoint ductions are concerned, we would expect to have (No.16B as the low duction. However, if we consider the advanced visual problem which has already spread to farpoint, we will find the reverse situation will be present. Under the stimulus demand of base-out prism the finding will be low and the base-in movement beyond the plane of regard will also be low. The base-in finding (No.17B), since it moves into the more recent spatial area in which the patient as yet has not organized it, will be the lower of the two test values. Therefore,

_____ recent problem, will tolerate full lens values
16B

_____ advanced visual problem, be conservative
17B

Let us now consider the total duction patterns and their significance in lens application.

11 - 16B
↓ ↓

RECENT FAR VISUAL PROBLEM — RECENT NEAR VISUAL PROBLEM

Thus, the No.11 and No.16B tests being low indicate a recent visual problem and will readily accept the maximum plus found in the subjective tests at far and at near.

When we have:

11 - 17B
↓ ↓

RECENT FAR VISUAL PROBLEM — ADVANCED NEAR VISUAL PROBLEM

the duction pattern of No. 11 and No.17B tests low, we are beginning to have a more advanced visual problem. We have the conflict of one duction indicating that full plus is acceptable and the other duction test indicating that we should be more conservative in our lens application. In this set of circumstances, since the patient will tolerate more lens power at near than at far, the wise procedure is to cut or reduce the magnitude of the lens application at far and prescribe full plus at near. This pattern indicates a more advanced visual problem but as yet has not reached the full spatial distance at farpoint. The reason we are more conservative at farpoint in reducing the lens values to be prescribed is that the patient has less tolerance for changes in visual habits at far which involves considerable spatial movement and depth perception. At nearpoint the patient is working from a seated posture involving limited depth perception factors. Therefore, at the nearpoint distance the patient will tolerate the full plus of the subjective at near (M.S.D.A.).

The duction pattern of:

$$\overline{10 - \quad 16B}$$

↓ ↓

ADVANCED FAR VISUAL PROBLEM — RECENT NEAR VISUAL PROBLEM

With the No.10 and No.16B duction tests low, we have the development of a visual problem which has now spread to farpoint. This indicates a more advanced visual problem. However, we have the seeming conflict that with the No.16B duction being the low finding at near a simpler problem is present. This is because both No.16B and No.17B are low, but No.16B is the lower of the two. Under these circumstances the more conservative approach is used and we cut plus at both far and at near. The final duction pattern is:

$$\overline{10 - 17B}$$

↓ ↓

ADVANCED FAR VISUAL PROBLEM — ADVANCED NEAR VISUAL PROBLEM

This is the most advanced stage of the visual problem, and it calls for the reduction of lens application for both far and at near.

Classification of the analytical tests. All of our optometric analytical tests can be placed in one of the following categories:

1. Those findings which measure the protection available for the pattern of convergence.
2. Those findings which measure the protection available for the pattern of accommodation.
3. The measurement of the extent of the potential of inhibition existing between the patterns of accommodation and convergence.
4. The measurement of the extent of the learned relationship existing between the patterns of accommodation and convergence.
5. The measurement of the extent of the degree of organization existing between the patterns of accommodation and convergence.
6. The measurement of a latitude of performance within the visual pattern to preserve single and clear vision in the face of changes in total behavior due to advancing age.

Table 9.

Duction Pattern	Time Factor	Lens Application
10-16B	Beginning Visual Problem	Full Plus Can be Prescribed
11-17B	Intermediate Visual Problem	Reduce Plus at Far Full Plus at Near
10-16B	Advanced Visual Problem	Reduce Plus at Far and Near
10-17B	Advanced Visual Problem	Reduce Plus at Far and Near

Table 10.
A Classification Of the Optometric Tests

Category Measures	Test No.	Type of Test
1. Protection to Convergence	3, 13A, 8, 13B, 15A, 15B	Phoria Tests
2. Protection to Accommodation	4, 5, 6, 14A, 14B	Retinoscopy and cross-cylinder tests
3. Potential of Inhibition	9, 16A, 17A, 20, 21	Blur Tests
4. Learned Relationships	10, 11, 16B, 17B	Duction Break Tests
5. Degree of Organization	10, 11, 16B, 17B	Duction Recovery Tests
6. Protection of Acc. Against Senility	19	Amplitude of Accommodation

The Optometric analytical tests have been classified into the six categories in Table 10. These various categories provide the optometrist with the adaptations which have been made by the Organism in order to adjust to the impact of our modern nearpoint visual environment.

C. Measurement of the protection available to the pattern of convergence

The latitude of protection in the central nervous system, for the protection of the convergence pattern, is measured by determining the phoria value. In order to perform a phoria test the following conditions must be present: (1) A dissociating device to fracture the normal figure-ground characteristics of the binocular visually observed terrain. (2) A target with sufficient identification demand to localize accommodation. (3) The target to be located at a particular test distance.

We normally define a phoria in terms of the overt movement of the eyeballs upon dissociation, i.e., exophoria is the movement of the eyeballs outward in relation to a line from the object to the center of rotation of the eye. Similarly, esophoria is an inward movement of the eyeballs in relation to a line from the object to the center of rotation of the eye. This movement of the eyeballs can only occur when the normal binocular space lattice has been ruptured by a dissociating device. Whenever single vision is impossible because of changes in size, color, intensity, or position of the stimuli reaching each eye we have this destruction of the fusional ability, and we obtain this overt action of the eyeballs. *Without the dissociating device we have no way of determining whether a patient has* 10 *esophoria or* 10 *exophoria.* The exophoria or esophoria must still be present whether or not we have a dissociating device in place. This poses three questions. (1) Where is the exophoria or esophoria located? (2) What does the dissociating device do? (3) What makes the eyes turn when the dissociating device is in place? Let us answer these questions in the reverse order. What makes the eyes turn when we place a dissociating device before one eye of the patient while he is fixating a target? The eye must turn because of the action of the muscles, in particular the activity of the lateral group. But what caused the muscles to become active? A neural impulse must have gone to the muscle group for them to become active. Where did this neural impulse pattern come from? It must have come from the central nervous system. Thus, the answer to the third question is a neural impulse pattern from the central nervous system.

The obvious answer to the second question is that the dissociating device makes single vision impossible. The dissociating device must do something more than this. Without the dissociating device in place, the eyes are in a normal position for the particular fixation distance. The presence of the dissociating device alters this situation, and we now have an outward positioning of the eyes if the patient has exophoria, or an inward positioning of the eyes if the patient has esophoria. Thus, the dissociating device removed a dam which had been preventing the flow of the neural impulse pattern from the central nervous system to the extrinsic musculature. Technically, this dam which was removed by the presence of the dissociating device was *the necessity for inhibition.* Thus, when the dissociating device is not present these impulses are *inhibited* from flowing to the extrinsic musculature.

We can now answer the first question. Exophoria or esophoria must be located in the central nervous system. Both exophoria and esophoria are innervational patterns of inhibition located in the central nervous system.

Table 11.

The Effect Of Sustained (30 minutes) and Dissociated Binocular Effort Upon Near Phoria, After Stenhouse (Brit. J. Ophthalmol 29, 37 [1945])

Near Phoria	Before	After
8 Exo	4	6
6 Exo	5	4
4 Exo	14	10
2 Exo	34	18
1 Exo	5	6
Ortho	5	7
2 Eso	5	12
4 Eso	1	8
6 Eso	0	2
MEAN	2.3 Exo	1.0 Exo

What, then, is the difference between these two phorias? We usually accept the answers. Exophoria is when the eyes turn out; esophoria is when the eves turn in. But again, this is merely the external appearance of the phenomena. Exophoria is present at birth, and it seems to be maturationally developed. Esophoria seems to develop when we have tensions.

Exophoria, from the functional viewpoint, is defined as a developmental or maturational relationship within the visual behavior pattern, between areas of that pattern (of inhibitory nature), operationally active to preserve the integrity of performance of the convergence pattern. The question arises, "How does exophoria preserve or protect the convergence mechanism?" The nervous system components are usually at different levels of activity which is the usual state of affairs. If we consider the enormous activity of the organism as he goes about in his environment, and if the skeletal nervous system is in ascendancy, the convergence pattern (center?) will receive a greater degree of stimulus than the accommodative pattern (center?). This will result in extra stimuli to the convergence pattern which must be absorbed or inhibited if the status quo of the organism is to be maintained. This is the function of exophoria. If the patient has 10 exophoria in the morning when he reports to his desk job we would expect, because of this absorption or inhibition, that the amount of exophoria will decrease. Stenhouse published the effect of sustained and dissociated binocular effort for a period of thirty minutes upon the near phoria. His data is tabulated in Table 11. You will note that initially only six out of the 73 observers exhibited esophoria at nearpoint. After completion of the visual task we see that 22 of the observers now have esophoria at near. Thus, the exophoria buffer area under continuous impact will gradually lessen in amount, and if the visual conditions are

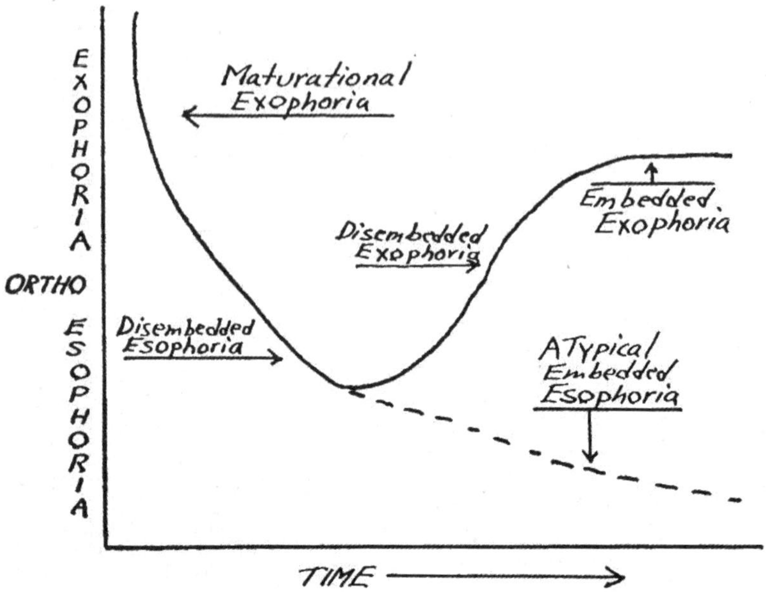

Figure 48. The effect of time upon the amount and type of phoria.

of such intense nature, we will have orthophoria and finally the organism will go into esophoria. Figure 48 depicts the typical change in the nearpoint phoria with time. You will note the rapid decrease of the exophoria and finally the dip into esophoria. We now have two possible organismic responses. The usual response is for the organism to start rebuilding the buffer area of exophoria. He will build sufficient exophoria so that regardless of the intensity of the task he will have sufficient ability to maintain an exophoric condition. We find that many students and accountants, because of the visual demands of their task, will build high exophoria. We also have the individual who cannot learn how to build sufficient latitude of performance (exophoria) on his own, and he will oscillate between exophoria, esophoria, exophoria, etc. and repeat this cycle over and over again. He seems never to be able to stabilize his visual pattern unless he can receive plus lens application and visual training. The atypical response to the nearpoint task is the individual who develops more esophoria and finally structures or stabilizes with a high degree of esophoria. Examples of these three types of responses are given in Table 12. They are based on experimental measurements on college students which were taken three times per week (every other day) for a period of seven weeks.

Thus, when we examine the patient and find esophoria which is an active state of inhibition and therefore undesirable, we are interested in the answers

Table 12.
The Variation In Nearpoint Phoria Values With Time For College Students Who Were Examined Three Times Per A Week For A Period Of Seven Weeks

	Typical Variation of Exophoria	Atypical Esophoria	Embedded Exophoria
1	1 Eso	5 Eso	18 Exo
2	Ortho	4 Eso	12 Exo
3	3 Exo	2 Eso	16 Exo
4	3 Exo	2 Eso	14 Exo
5	3 Exo	Ortho	10 Exo
6	3 Exo	2 Eso	14 Exo
7	5 Exo	3 Eso	14 Exo
8	3 Exo	Ortho	14 Exo
9	5 Exo	2 Eso	13 Exo
10	3 Exo	2 Eso	13 Exo
11	1 Exo	5 Eso	14 Exo
12	3 Exo	3 Eso	16 Exo
13	2 Exo	5 Eso	11 Exo
14	3 Exo	3 Eso	14 Exo
15	½ Eso	4 Eso	14 Exo
16	1 Eso	4 Eso	12 Exo
17	4 Exo	4 Eso	13 Exo
18	3 Exo	5 Eso	16 Exo
19	3 Exo	5 Eso	16 Exo
20	1 Exo	2 Eso	18 Exo

to two questions. (1) Is this the transient esophoria which is the typical organismic response upon the first impact of the visual task? (2) Is this esophoria the atypical type which has been of long duration and embedded in his visual pattern? Table 13 lists the diagnostic differences between these two types of esophoria.

Esophoria differs from exophoria in that it is an emergency condition and organismically undesirable. The patient characteristically will make every effort to eliminate it and re-establish the more desirable exophoria. The presence of esophoria is indicative of a visual problem. Esophoria is an inhibitory pattern in the central nervous system for the purpose of protecting the convergence pattern. It is an inhibitory pattern since the movement of the eyeballs inward does not occur unless some dissociating device is in place. We further classify esophoria as an active state of inhibition. We use the term active since the esophore is inefficient and, therefore, this type of inhibition must be on a higher neurological level than the state of inhibition of the exophore.

Although we normally think of our measurement of exophoria and esophoria as displacements laterally, since we use lateral prism for their measurement, it is obvious that we can consider these phoria values as overt movements in space; the esophore projecting closer to him than the plane

Table 13.

	Transient Esophoria.	**Embedded Esophoria**
Case History	Severe complaints. Difficulty performing nearpoint tasks.	"Dull" complaints. Performs satisfactory to himself but with consider able effort.
Amount	Between 1-7 Eso.	Between 5-22 Eso.
Type of Pattern	Disembedded.	Embedded.
Effect of Plus	Plus spheres reduce the amount of Eso.	Plus spheres have very little effect upon the amount of the phoria.
Age	Under 20 yrs.	20 yrs. or over.
Effect of Fatigue	The amount of the Eso fluctuates during the examination	Stays fairly constant.

of regard; the exophore projecting away from his plane of regard. These are illustrated in Figure 49. Table 14 compares exophoria and esophoria

EXOPHORIA = ORTHOPHORIA = ESOPHORIA

From this equation, we see that orthophoria is not a static condition of perfection of so-called muscle balance; but it is a dynamic state of balance in which all of the buffer area of exophoria has been used up because of a sustained environmental demand; or that the patient is beginning to rebuild an adequate buffer area in proceeding from esophoria toward exophoria. The orthophore is in a precarious position, and the sooner he can be brought over toward the exophoria side the better. Thus, one of the fundamental purposes of visual training or lens application must be to aid the patient obtain an adequate area of inhibition, the development of exophoria.

For the purpose of measuring the amount of protection available to the convergence pattern several phoria tests are taken. They are:

1. Habitual phoria at far (No.3)
2. Habitual phoria at near (No.13A)
3. Induced phoria at near (No.8)
4. Induced phoria at near (No.13B)
5. Induced phoria through the plus of the dissociated cross cylinder test at near (No.15A)
6. Induced phoria through the plus of the fused cross cylinder test at near (No.15B)

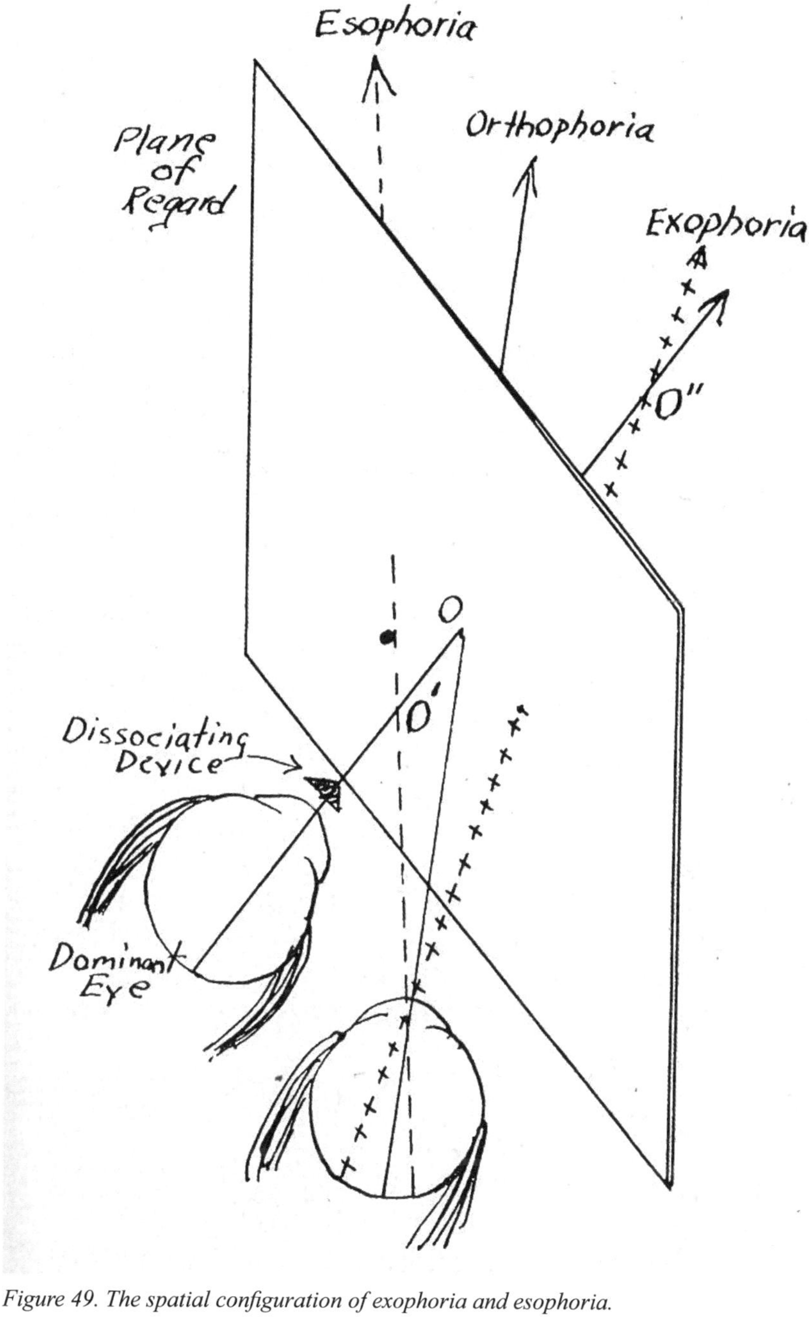

Figure 49. The spatial configuration of exophoria and esophoria.
Esophoria-Spatial projection is in front of the plane of regard as if object is at 0'.
Orthophoria-Spatial projection is at the plane of regard at 0.
Exophoria-Spatial projection is in back of the plane of regard, as if object is at 0".

Table 14.
A Comparison Of Exophoria And Esophoria

	Exophoria	Esophoria
Movement of the eyeball under dissociation	Outward	Inward
Measured by	Base-In prism	Base-Out prism
Type of Diplopia	Crossed	Uncrossed
Spatial Projection	Away from the plane of regard	Toward the organism
Purpose	Protection of Convergence (Maturationally normal)	Protection of Convergence (Emergency situation)
Efficiency	Highly Efficient	Inefficient
Type of Protection	Area of Inhibition (Sub Cortical?)	Active State of Inhibition (Higher Cortical Level?)
Present	In the visual efficient	In the inefficient producer and accident prone individuals

The interpretation of the phoria tests taken through our cross cylinder lenses will be discussed under the cross cylinder test. It is sufficient to state at this time that we use these phoria values for the purpose of obtaining a lag.

Thus we perform phoria tests in order to determine the following: 1) the extent of the visual problem; 2) the effect of a lens upon convergence; 3) to determine a lag; 4) type of visual problem (embedded or disembedded); 5) type of visual care needed (lenses, visual training, or a combination of both).

The normal value for the latitude essential for adequate achievement in the environment depends upon the test distance at which the measurement is performed. At the farpoint, we find that the mean value is ½ exophoria, and at the nearpoint the mean value is 6 exophoria. Therefore, it is desirable that the organism have slightly more than these values so that we can be assured that sufficient latitude of performance is present in the convergence pattern for efficient performance.

D. Measurements of the protection available to the pattern of accommodation.

The protection available to the organism against blurred vision is *hyperopia.* Hyperopia is the amount of this protection available in the accommodative pattern. By classical definition hyperopia is an eyeball which is too short for its refractive power. Thus, light rays entering such an eye with accommodation at rest come to a focus beyond the retinal plane, or the converging rays are intercepted by the retina before they can come to a focus. This is a definition of a hyperopic optical system, and it is merely an abstraction which has little relation to clinical experience.

A dimensional analysis of an object can be performed in one of two ways, i.e. (1) We can determine the physical dimensions of the object, or (2) we can determine the amount of a standard liquid which can be poured into the object. When we consider the visual mechanism, it is obvious that we can never clinically determine the location of the focus in the eyeball. Therefore, the classical definition is merely an interesting physical abstraction. It is impossible, in a living system, to ever have accommodation at rest, and it also is difficult to apply the term focus when we consider the visual mechanism. Focus is defined as that point on the luminous conoid which gives the maximum intensity of energy per unit area. When we refer to a corrected lens system on an optical bench this point can be found. If we consider the eyeball (with its high dioptric power. and its several asymmetric refractive surfaces of varying densities, its components not on the same axis and with all the inherent defects of such a complex refracting system) it can be readily shown that instead of a focus in one plane we have a considerable range over which the conditions of maximum flux density per unit area is present. Thus, there is *latitude of focus* rather than a *point focus.*

Since we cannot determine readily the physical dimensions of eyeballs we must use the second method for the measurement of hyperopia. We can define hyperopia as a condition in which the subject must use more than the normal amount of accommodation for the test distance in order to maintain standard acuity; or, a hyperope is the refractive condition of a subject who will maintain standard farpoint acuity through convex spheres. This is an operational or clinical definition of hyperopia since it tells us what we do in order to measure it.

Hyperopia has also been defined as the amount of accommodation free of convergence with fixation at far. This is based on the clinical procedure of placing plus spheres before the eyes of a hyperope, and he still maintains single vision at far and clear farpoint vision.

These clinical definitions of hyperopia aided us in understanding the measurement of hyperopia, but they still leave the questions unanswered: (1) What is the value of hyperopia? (2) Where is it located? (3) What is its function?

The act of accommodation, in order to maintain a retinal-intensity-gradient conducive to satisfactory interpretation by the subject, is hyperopia. The amount of this accommodation at any particular moment depends upon the following factors: (a) previous activity of the subject, (b) the intensity-demand of the particular activity, (c) the physical environmental factors of color, illumination, size, contrast, motion and distance, (d) intellectual demand of the target. From the abstract, theoretical definition, hyperopia is a dimension analysis of the eyeball. From the clinical viewpoint, hyperopia is measured by the amount of accommodation involved.

Up to this point, we have been considering merely the clinical measurement of hyperopia; but it is obvious that the accommodative mechanism does not function without an innervational pattern from the central nervous system. Thus, the hyperope, for any particular fixation distance, has a particular type of innervational pattern the amount of which depends upon the previously mentioned factors. This innervational pattern proceeding to the accommodative mechanism provides the hyperope with a balance or degree of compensation between environment and interpretation. If we change environmental factors, for example, size of target, the amount of accommodation in effect will diminish as the size of the target increases. Similarly, if we vary the interpretive demand, the amount of accommodation in effect will also vary. For example, five students, whose average age was 23, had an average dynamic retinoscopy test value at a test distance of 20 inches while reading 20/40 reduced Snellen of plus 1.50 diopters. These same students, at the same test distance, gave an average dynamic retinoscopy test value of plano when reading an advanced book on psychological optics. *Thus, hyperopia provides man with a latitude of performance in the central nervous system for the purpose of providing clear vision in spite of fluctuations in either external or internal environmental conditions.* Hyperopia is, therefore, a protective device and in man's primitive environment was of survival value.

We can understand why we may have a group of individuals of the same age who all have the same amount of hyperopia and who still need a variety of visual services depending upon the environmental demands and interpretive factors. It is obvious that when this latitude of performance is not adequate for the environmental demands placed upon the individual that some form of adaptation must occur. The usual change is a decrease in the amount of hyperopia, but when emmetropia is reached the patient may go into minus projection and finally into myopia. He may cancel certain visual skills; or he may retreat from the task or perform at a very inefficient level. The presence of emmetropia is thus a sign of trouble. The patient no longer has any latitude of performance and he is characteristically a poor performer.

It is only in the case of the absolute hyperope, where we have insufficient amplitude of accommodation for the existing dimensional hyperopia, that we have the physical conditions present of converging rays of light entering the eyeball. They do not give a retinal-intensity-gradient that is conducive to a satisfactory interpretation. It is this person who needs convex lenses for the restoration of acuity. This is the prosthetic application of plus lenses.

The accommodative mechanism is a slow acting device. Allen (Allen, M J. *The response of the intra-ocular muscles of the dog and cat to electrical stimulation.* Am J Optom. 1950;27:287) states, "The ability of an individual to grade the amount of his accommodation is evidence which seems to support the conclusion that the human ciliary body is also a multiunit smooth muscle. If this is true, then we can predict that the human accommodative reaction time should be relatively long; due in part to the latent period of the ciliary muscle. Furthermore, due to the relatively slow contraction and relaxation of this type of muscle, the rate of change of human accommodation should be low." The accommodative mechanism functions much more slowly than the convergence mechanism. Whenever we have a dual mechanism performing a common cooperative act, the slower moving portions of the mechanism become the pace setter. Thus, the accommodative pattern is the pace setter and clinically we find that the great majority of all visual problems are accommodative problems.

Five analytical tests are performed in order to determine the amount of latitude of performance in the accommodative pattern. The tests determine the amount of protection in the accommodative pattern at farpoint test distance, intermediate, and at nearpoint (see Table 15).

The testing conditions for the static retinoscopy (No.4) test are arranged for maximum inhibition to accommodation with farpoint fixation. These conditions are: (a) extra plus spheres before each eye; (b) gross fixation target; (c) dim light; and (d) flickering light in one eye which tends to create dissociation. Since expected distant phoria is an exophoria we would have some inhibition to accommodation. Therefore, we would expect for the unimpaired visual pattern to have more hyperopia found in the static retinoscopy test than in the subjective at far. Upon the impact of the nearpoint visual environment, with its protracted period of concentration, the stimulus pattern will not be inhibited under these testing conditions; and we would expect to find a static retinoscopy test value which is now lower than the subjective at far. The static retinoscopy test at far is an objective measurement of negative relative accommodation at far.

Table 15.

Test No.	Test Name	Test Distance	Type of Test
#4	Static Retinoscopy	20 ft.	Objective
#5	Dynamic Retinoscopy @ 20"	20"	Objective
#6	Dynamic Retinoscopy @ 40"	40"	Objective
#14A	Dissociated Cross Cylinder Test	16"	Subjective
#14B	Fused Cross Cylinder Test @ Near	16"	Subjective

Dynamic retinoscopy (No.5) performed at 20 inch fixation distance is an objective measurement of negative relative accommodation at 20 inches. In performing the static retinoscopy test, the fixation distance is at 20 feet, and the measurement is performed usually at 26 inches (See Fig. 50). Therefore, there must be a correction factor to convert the test value to a 20 foot distance. In the case of the dynamic retinoscopy at 20 inches (No.5), the fixation distance and the measuring distance are the same. Therefore, the gross value is recorded. In performing the dynamic retinoscopy test at 20 inches every effort is made to maintain patient's accommodation and convergence at the target. The target usually used for this test is the reduced Snellen letters 20/40-20/60. The target is usually gross; the illumination is dim; the light flicker from the retinoscope tends to inhibit convergence; and the working distance is outside the normal nearpoint attention distance of the average worker. We have certain conditions which are inhibitory in nature, and so we might expect more plus spheres to be accepted by the patient. These factors make it difficult to use the dynamic retinoscopy test at 20 inches without first correcting the value found for the influence of convergence upon accommodation at that test distance. This correction factor is called a lag. The maximum lag possible would be the equivalent of the fixation distance into lens diopters. Since this is 20 inches, the maximum lag is 2.00 D. In order to determine the amount of convergence in this particular test, a phoria should be performed at 20 inches upon completion of the dynamic retinoscopy test at 20 inches. The maximum convergence involved at 20 inches is two meter angles, or twelve prism diopters. That is, if we performed this test and obtained a value of plus 2.00 diopters, and we measured the associated phoria and found a value of 12 exophoria, this would give us a lag of 2.00 diopters. Therefore, the net dynamic retinoscopy is plano. This is emmetropia at a 20 inch fixation distance. Calculating the lag for the dynamic retinoscopy at 20 inches by this method would require extra phoria determination. The correlation between dynamic retinoscopy at 20 inches and the dissociated cross cylinder test at 16 inches is highly significant (r = 0.8 to 0.9).

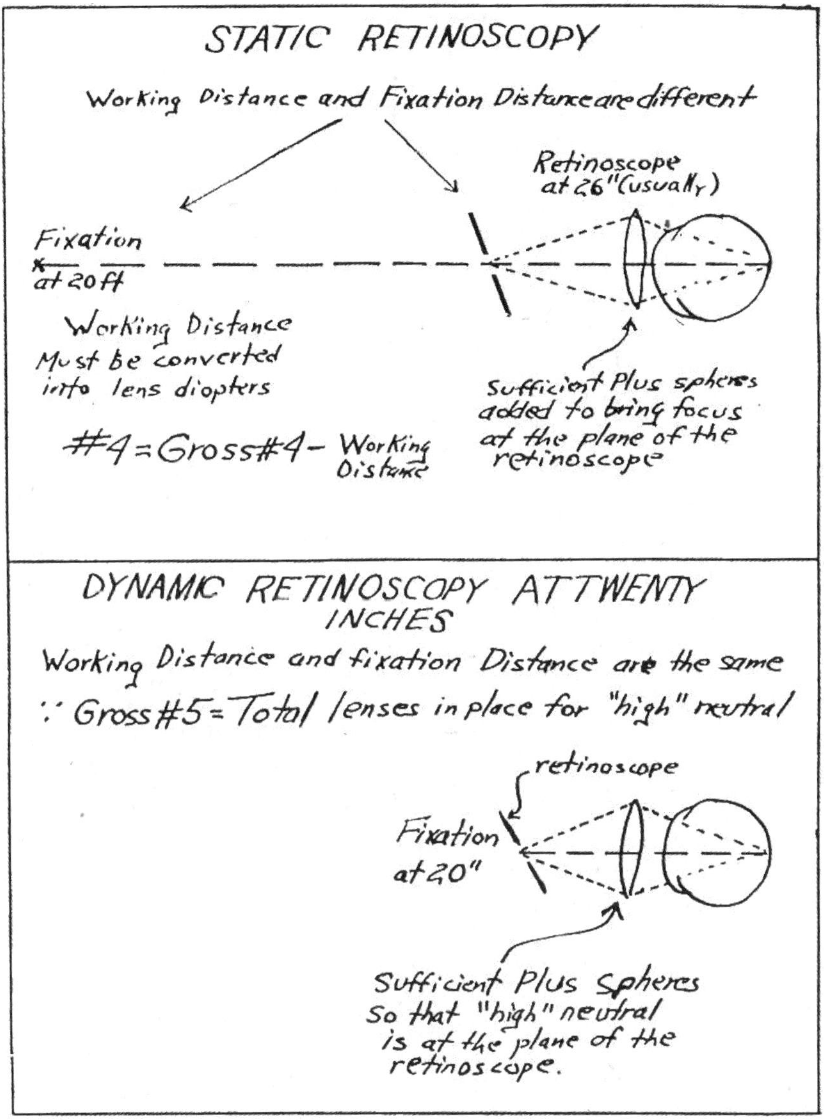

Figure 50. Comparison of static restinoscopy and dynamic retinoscopy at X-X 20".

Therefore, a weighted lag table for the dynamic retinoscopy test at 20 inches was constructed based upon the phoria taken through the lens values for the dissociated cross-cylinder test at 16 inches (No.15A). This weighted lag table based upon the phoria taken through the dissociated cross-cylinder test lenses is adequate for most purposes; but if the dynamic retinoscopy test (No.5) differs from the dissociated cross-cylinder test at

16 inches (No.14A) by 1.00 diopter or more, than a phoria should be taken through the lens values of the dynamic retinoscopy test at 20 inches, and the lag computed from this phoria. Regardless of the amount of exophoria present, we can never have a greater lag than the dioptric equivalent of the fixation distance.

When we have subtracted the lag from the gross dynamic retinoscopy test at 20 inches, we have obtained a net dynamic retinoscopy test value (net No.5). The net dynamic retinoscopy test at 20 inches is the negative relative accommodation at a 20 inch fixation distance which is free of the influence of convergence. This value, net dynamic retinoscopy test at 20 inches can now be compared with the static retinoscopy test at far. For the unimpaired individual we would expect to find the net dynamic retinoscopy test value to be higher in plus than the static retinoscopy test value. As impairment develops, the amount of the net dynamic retinoscopy test value in relation to the static retinoscopy decreases, and finally the net dynamic retinoscopy test value becomes equal to the static retinoscopy test value. If the intensity of the environmental impact continues, the dynamic retinoscopy test value will now become less in plus than the static retinoscopy test.

The dynamic retinoscopy test at 40 inches (No.6) is a measurement of the negative relative accommodation at an intermediate fixation distance. We would expect, for a fixation distance of one meter, that the maximum lag to be deducted from the gross dynamic retinoscopy test at 40 inches would be 1.00 D. We find that a phoria taken at 40 inches more closely approximates the farpoint phoria average of one-half exophoria than it does the nearpoint phoria average of 6 exophoria. As soon as we proceed outside of reaching distance there is a rapid drop to approximately farpoint test values. Therefore, an empirical lag of one-quarter diopter was established for this test. In order to convert the gross dynamic retinoscopy test at 40 inches we deduct a lag of one-quarter diopter, and we obtain a net dynamic retinoscopy test value.

This lag of 0.25 D. is deducted from the Gross No. 6 test regardless of the type or magnitude of the far or near phorias. This is the only dynamic accommodative test which is handled in this arbitrary manner. In the unimpaired individual, we find that the net dynamic retinoscopy test at 40 inches (Net No.6) is higher in plus than the static retinoscopy test lenses. As visual impairment develops at the intermediate distance the amount of the net dynamic retinoscopy test value at 40 inches decreases and becomes less in plus than the static retinoscopy test.

The cross cylinder tests at near (Nos. 14A & 14B) differ from the proceeding measures of negative relative accommodation in that the tests are subjective in nature, and the test is performed at 16 inches which duplicates closely the average nearpoint working distance of the patient. The dissociated cross-cylinder test at near (No.14A) is performed under test conditions conducive to the maximum inhibition of direct and conditioned accommodation. These experimental conditions are: the cross-cylinders, cross-grid target, dim illumination, dissociating device and the use of plus spherical lenses. Under these test conditions both accommodations and convergence are free to function in space according to the learned spatial relations of the individual. This test probes deeply into the elementary structure of the visual pattern at near. Under these conditions of maximum inhibition, we will have overt movements away from the plane of regard. The extent of these movements will depend upon the latitude of performance present in the accommodative pattern (hyperopia) and the latitude of performance present in the convergence pattern (exophoria). This test, since it allows overt movements to occur both in the accommodative and convergence pattern simultaneously, presents a deep probing into the warf and woof of the visual pattern. In the dissociated cross-cylinder test (No.14A) we have:

1. Cross cylinders, dim illumination, plus spheres inhibit direct accommodation.

2. Dissociating prisms inhibit conditioned accommodation.

Thus, the dissociated cross-cylinder test measures both the direct and conditioned inhibition to accommodation.

In the phoria test through the lenses of the dissociated cross-cylinder test (No.15A) we have:

1. Dissociating prisms inhibit direct convergence.

2. Plus spheres inhibit conditioned convergence.

Thus the phoria through the lenses of the dissociated cross-cylinder test at near measures both the direct and conditioned inhibition to convergence.

The relationship between direct and conditioned accommodation and direct and conditioned convergence at the normal 16 inch test distance is 2.50 diopters of accommodation and 15 diopters of convergence; or six diopters of convergence are associated with one diopter of accommodation. In order to convert the phoria in exophoria into its equivalent accommodative effect one merely divides the prism diopters by 6. This equivalent accom-

Table 16.
The Variation In ACA Ratio As Determined By The Morgan Method

Subject: Pollack	Parker	Gosnell
1. 2.75	1. 2.50	1. 3.62
2. 2.62	2. 1.25	2. 4.25
3. 4.87	3. 4.25	3. 4.00
4. 2.87	4. 4.50	4. 5.25
5. 3.75	5. 1.62	5. 2.00
6. 4.67	6. 4.37	6. 4.25
7. 1.75	7. 4.37	7. 4.37
	8. 1.87	8. 4.50
	9. 2.25	9. 4.12
	10. 3.50	

modative effect at 16 inches can never be greater than 2.50 diopters. This value is the maximum allowable lag.

Under the conditions for inhibition of accommodation present while performing this test, we would expect that the patient would accept the dioptic equivalent of the testing distance. That is, the dissociated cross-cylinder test value minus the subjective sphere should be equal to 2.50 diopters. Clinically, we find that the average value of this add is 0.75 diopters. Some of the accommodation which the cross-cylinder does not inhibit is due to the psychic accommodation. It becomes obvious that the mere presence of a stimulus target at 16 inches from the patient is no assurance that he is accommodating geometrically for that distance. The work with "book" retinoscopy has shown that when the organism is searching for meaning we have maximum accommodative response; when the organism is reading material within his grade level we have minimum accommodative response. Under cross-cylinder testing conditions the organism is telling us how much accommodation he is willing to give up at 16 inches with the conditions of maximum inhibition. When the patient exhibits a gross cross-cylinder test which is in less plus than the subjective finding, he is exhibiting, under conditions for maximum inhibition to accommodation, an excessive stimulus to accommodation. This is a complete rejection of plus lens application at nearpoint. These are the hyperopic patients who complain of their glasses being too strong and yet have better than standard acuity at far through them.

In order to determine the amount of inhibition to accommodation due to the cross-cylinder, dim illumination and the plus spheres, we must correct the inhibition to accommodation because of the presence of exophoria. This correction factor, for the influence of convergence upon accommodation, is termed a lag. A conversion factor of 6:1 is used. This is based

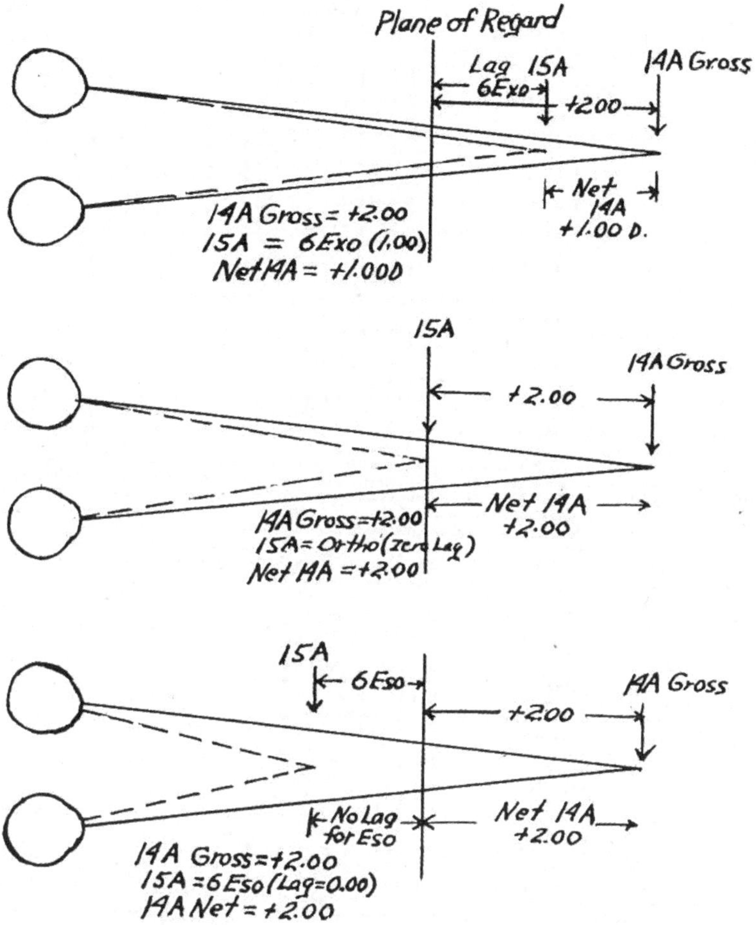

Figure 51. The spatial relationships between No. 14A and No. 15A (Accommodation free from Convergence).

upon the normal experience of the emmetrope of utilizing 2.50 diopters of accommodation and 15 prism diopters of convergence when he looks at 16 inches. The functional school is often asked, "Why do you use a six-to-one relationship when the average value for the ACA ratio is 4:1?" Experimental data has shown that the ACA ratio is highly variable. A true determination of the average ACA ratio for a particular subject could only be determined after several measurements over a period of several days. The high variability of ACA ratio measurement is shown in the data of Table 16. The ACA ratio was determined by direct measurement (Morgan method) for a two diopter change in accommodation. Each measurement was repeated four times. In spite of all these precautions, the considerable variation in ACA ratio is obvious.

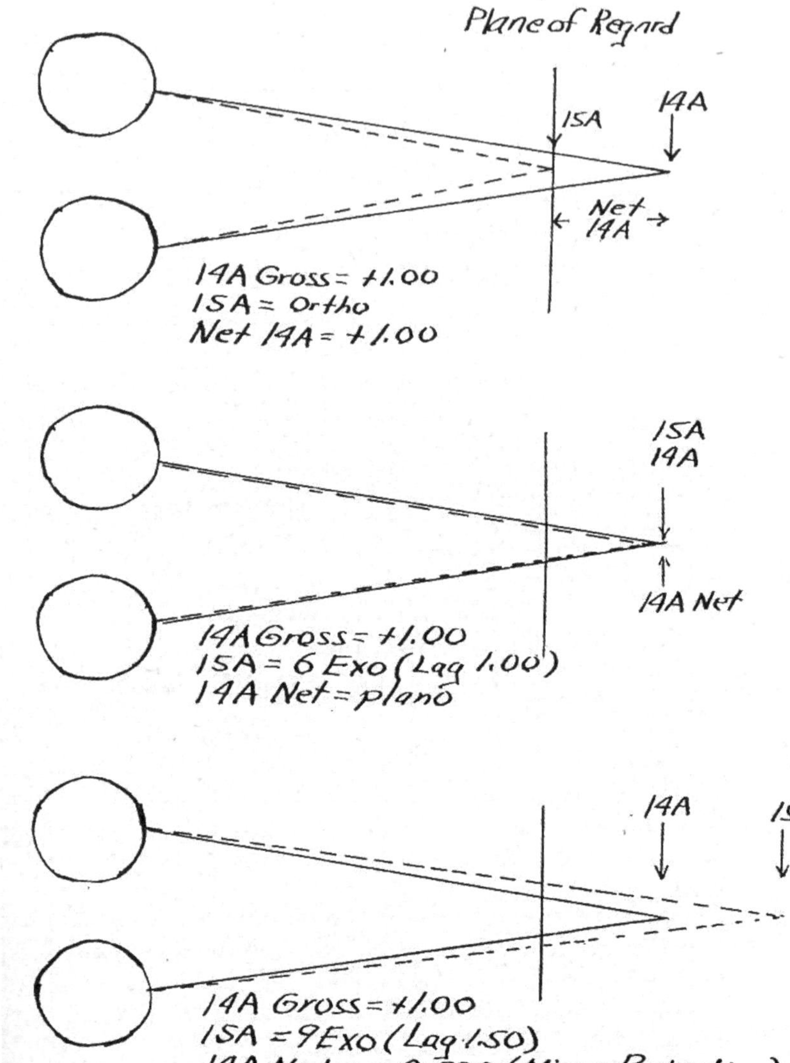

Figure 52. The spatial development of minus projection.

The average ACA ratio for the general population is 4.0 with a standard deviation of 2.0 units. On the basis of this data, the chances of an ACA ratio greater than 6:1 occuring is 15.87%; while the chances of an ACA ratio less than 6:1 occurring is 84.13%. Thus, the odds are 5:1 that our particular patient will not have an ACA ratio greater than six-to-one. The lag calculated from the exophoria found when taken through the lenses of the dissociated cross-cylinder test at near (No.15A) will be lower on the average than its actual value. The resultant net dissociated cross-cylinder test will, therefore, be higher than its actual value. When we consider that we have a zero lag for those cases having orthophoria or esophoria in the phoria test taken through the dissociated cross- cylinder test (No. 15A), the odds are better than 5:1 that the calculated net No.14A is higher in plus than its actual value. *This is why it has become axiomatic to never prescribe more plus than the net cross-cylinder lens values at near for constant wear.* The cross-cylinder values are the maximum plus at near-point. We must now have some counterchecks to verify the acceptance of this maximum plus. The first check is that the cross cylinder plus must not reverse the habitual equilibrium pattern. The second check point is that the cross-cylinder plus must be acceptable according to the duction pattern. Figure 51 presents the spatial relationship between the dissociated cross-cylinder test (No. 14A) and the phoria through the lenses of the dissociated cross-cylinder test (No. 15A). The net dissociated cross-cylinder test value (No. 14A) represents the spatial distance away from the plane of regard when the distance of No. 14A is greater than the No. 15A. The net cross-cylinder test value represents the amount of accommodation free of convergence at the nearpoint testing distance.

Figure 52 illustrates the development of minus projection. We have minus projection at near when the cross-cylinder test value is in plus (or at least plano), and the amount of exophoria present in the associated phoria test (No.15A) creates a lag of such an amount that the net cross-cylinder amount is in minus. This is not myopia at near but rather the development of minus overtones. When the direct inhibition to accommodation by plus spheres produces a conditioned change in convergence of such magnitude that the movement of the convergence change is greater than that of the accommodative change, we speak of the resultant effect as being minus projection. In the development of myopia at near, it is believed that the following sequential changes occur:

1. Hyperopia at near of greater magnitude than the hyperopia at far
2. Hyperopia at near of equal magnitude to that found at far.
3. Less hyperopia found at near than at far.
4. Minus projection at near of low amount.
5. Minus projection at near of high amount.
6. Minus at near.
7. Myopia at near.

The organism can explore any portion of the cited sequence. The extent of the adaptation at near and the type of adaptation followed will depend upon many factors. Some of these factors are:

Factors	No. 14A Net	No. 14B Net
Efrfect upon Acc. 1. Cross-cylinders Plus lenses Dim illumination 2. Dissociating device	1. Direct inhibition to accommodation 2. Conditioned inhibition to accommodation	1. Direct inhibition to accommodation 2. Not present
Effect upon Conv. 1. Dissociating device 2. Plus lenses	1. Direct inhibition to convergence 2. Conditioned inhibition to convergence	1. Direct inhibition to convergence 2. Conditioned inhibition to convergence
Comment	We have tried both direct and conditioned factors present ∵ full lag is deducted Since we have at near 15Δ ≎ 2.50 D 6:1 ratio	We have only direct inhibition to accommodation present. ∵ a modified lag must be used ∵ 15Δ ≎ 2.50D most authorities agree that accommoda- tive effect should be decreased by 2/3 ∵ 15Δ ≎ 2/3 (2.50D) 9:1 ratio

Figure 53.

1. hereditary
2. infection history
3. developmental
4. environmental

An example of minus-at-near is when the cross-cylinder test value is in minus (See Figure 54). For example:

#14A	-1.00D.	#14A	-1.00 D.
#15A	6 Exo	#15A	6 Eso
	(LAG 1.00)		(LAG 0.00)
Net #14A	-2.00	Net #14A	-1.00

These examples are not 10 be confused with myopia-at-near. We have the condition of myopia-at-near when the patient has less than standard acuity at near, and with the use of minus spherical lenses the acuity can be improved at near.

The fused cross-cylinder test at near differs from the dissociated test in that convergence is active while we are actively inhibiting accommodation. In the fused cross-cylinder test (#14B) we have:

1. Cross-cylinders, dim illumination, plus spheres inhibit direct accommodation.
2. While the phoria through the lenses of the fused cross-cylinder test (#15B) measures:

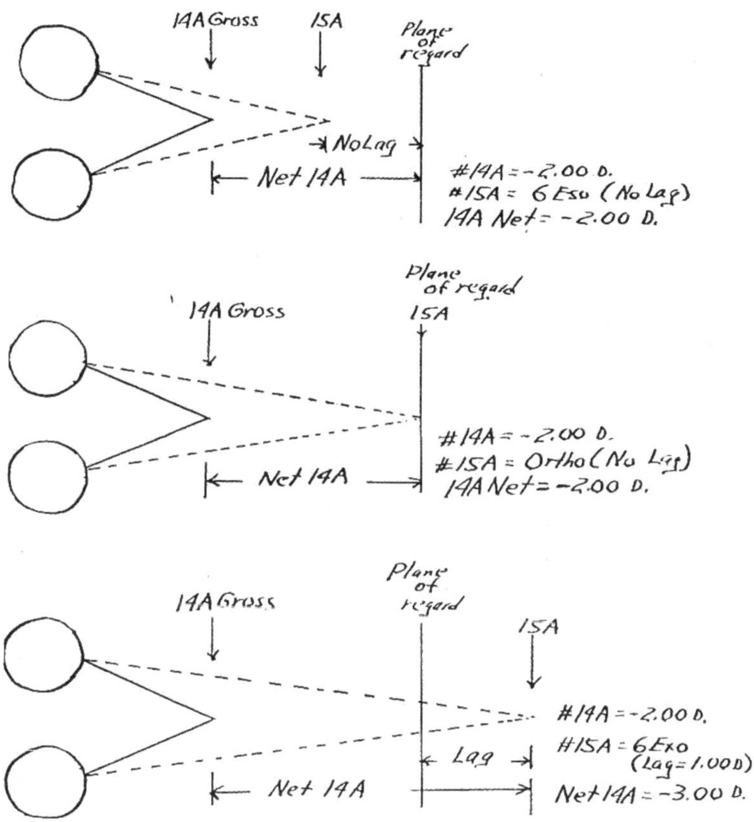

54. The development of myopia at near.

3. Dissociating prisms inhibit direct convergence.
4. Plus spheres inhibit conditioned convergence.

While the fused cross-cylinder test measures the direct inhibition to accommodation the phoria test through these lenses measures the direct and conditioned inhibition to convergence. It is, therefore, obvious that we cannot use a six-to-one relationship in calculating our lag, since under the fused condition the effect of inhibition of conditioned accommodation is not present. Under the fused cross-cylinder conditions that we have, approximately two-thirds of the convergence is stimulated by accommodation, 15 diopters of convergence is thus equivalent to 2/3 x 2.50 D. of accommodation. The maximum lag for the fused cross-cylinder test No.14B) is 1.75 D. (1.67 D rounded off to the nearest 0.25 d. is 1.75 d.). We can state that 9 prism diopters of exophoria is equivalent to one diopter of accommodation.

These two tests, the net dissociated and the net fused cross-cylinder tests (No.14A and No.14B Nets) at near, comprise the *nearpoint subjective*. The nearpoint subjective serves at near in the same manner as the farpoint subjective serves at far. The cross-cylinder nets serve as the basis for the determination of the prescriptable lens at near. The difference between the dissociated and the fused cross-cylinder nets is one of the diagnostic symptoms in determining the degree of embedding. If the No.14B net is lower in plus sphere than No.14A net, we have one of the characteristic symptoms of the disembedded visual pattern. If the No.14B net is greater in plus sphere than the No.14A net, we have one of the characteristic symptoms for the embedded or structured visual pattern.

We obtain the following information from the tests which measure the protection available to the pattern of accommodation.

Test No.	Test Name	What Do The Tests Measure?
#4	Static retinoscopy at far	a. Objective measurement of the amount of accommodation free of convergence at far. b. A measure of the degree of embedding. c. One of the diagnostic symptoms of an A type. d. Objective measurement of anisometropia and astigmia at far.
#5	Dynamic retinoscopy at 20 inches	a. Measurement of negative relative accommodation at 20 inches b. Measure of the intensity and deterioration of the visual problem. c. One of the diagnostic symptoms of a B or a C-type case. d. Objective measurement of anisometropia at near.
#6	Dynamic retinoscopy 40 inches	a. Measures the negative relative accommodation at 40 inches b. Detection of the visual problem at the intermediate test distance.
#14A	Net dissociated cross-cylinder at near	a. The amount of accommodation free of convergence at sixteen inches. b. A measure of the intensity and deterioration of the visual pattern. c. A measure of the degree of embedding of the visual pattern. d. A measure of the recency of the visual problem. e. Measurement of anisometropia at near.
#14B	Net fused cross-cylinder test at near	a. The amount of accommodation free of convergence at near under fused conditions. b. A measure of the degree of embedding of the visual pattern. c. The control lens for nearpoint testing in the presence of low amplitude.

E. Measurement of the potential of inhibition

These tests have been commonly designated as the blur tests. Under the experimental conditions existing while we are performing these tests, we are measuring the ability of the organism to allow inhibition or stimulation of one component of the visual pattern without affecting the other segment of the pattern. These blur tests are:

Test No.	Test Name	Operational Name
#9	True adduction	Base-out to 0.25 D. blur at far
#16A	Positive relative convergence	Base-out to blur out at near.
#17A	Negative relative convergence	Base-in to blur at near
#20	Positive relative accommodation	Minus lenses to blur out at near
#21	Negative relative accommodation	Plus lenses to blur out at near

The true adduction test (No.9) differs from the remaining blur findings in that it is performed at the 20 foot test distance, and the end point of the test is a blur equivalent to that created by a plus 0.25 diopter sphere. The patient must be indoctrinated as to the amount of this blur by demonstration before you start the addition of the base-out prisms. Therefore, before starting the actual performance of the test the following conditions must be present: 1. Subjective to 20/20 V.A. 2. Rotary prisms before each eye and set at the zero point. 3. Fixating the 20/20 Snellen test letters at 20 feet. With these conditions present, the addition of plus 0.25 (diopter spheres before each eye will produce a blur of the 20/20 Snellen test letters. The patient is instructed to inform you as soon as he notices this blur again. The doctor now turns base-out prism slowly until the patient's response of blur is obtained.

Some criticism has been leveled at the true adduction test (No.9) in that the blur noticed in this test is not due to any overt change in the accommodation mechanism, but it is due to the distortion produced by the base out prism. This seemingly has been proven by photographing a ruled line target through a base-out prism. The resulting photograph shows a distortion of the ruled line target. However, if we substitute the human eye for the camera, we obtain a different result. Monocular visual acuity was measured for a number of observers on 20/20 Koenig bars. This monocular acuity was measured through a plano lens and repeated through a six diopter base out prism. The difference between the two measurements was not significant. Thus, the blur experienced by an observer through Increasing application of base out prism is due to an overt change in the accommodative pattern.

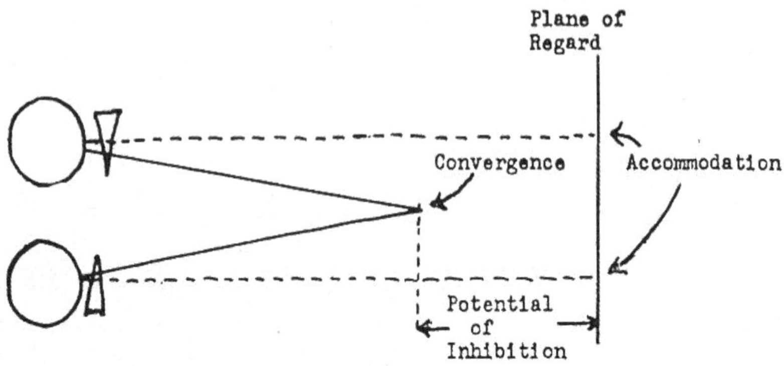

Figure 55. The effect of base out prism on spatial movement.

Figure 55 illustrates graphically the movement in space as we add base out prism before the eyes of a patient fixating a distant test object. Initially, we have both accommodation and convergence at the plane of regard.

As the base out stimulus is applied, accommodation is still at the plane of regard; but now we have convergence moving toward the observer. This stimulation of convergence by the base out prism tends to cause a conditioned stimulus to proceed to the accommodative pattern. The organismic demand is to maintain clear vision, therefore, these conditioned stimuli coming from the resulting stimulus of convergence are inhibited. When the stimulus of convergence (the movement of convergence toward the observer) has reached such a magnitude that the inhibition toward accommodation can no longer be maintained, these impulses will '*spill-over*' and an overt movement of accommodation will occur. The patient will state that the acuity target is now blurred. Therefore, in performing this test, we are measuring a certain range (spatial), latitude or degree of flexibility between the important components of the visual pattern. We are measuring a time-spatial relationship between convergence and accommodation. When this ability is low in magnitude, we have a disembedded or disorganized relationship; when this ability is high, we have an embedded or organized relationship. For a good, efficient functioning of the visual pattern this ability should be at least at its mean or expected value or higher.

The remaining nearpoint blur out tests are designated as the equilibrium tests. These tests measure the potential of inhibition as one component of the visual pattern is stimulated or inhibited to its maximum degree at nearpoint. Positive relative convergence measures the ability of the organism to tolerate the movement of convergence toward him, while accommodation is at the plane of regard. When the range of this movement is of

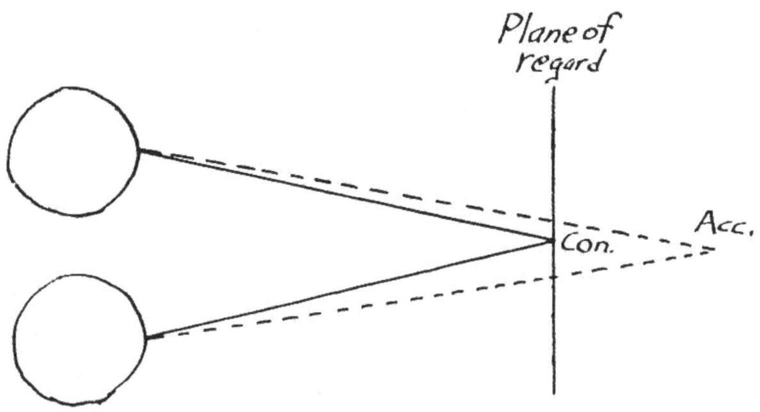

Figure 56. Spatial configuration of a B-type case.

such a degree that the conditioned stimuli arising from convergence can no longer be inhibited, it will 'spill-over'. We then will have the stimulation of accommodation which will result in an overt movement, and the organism will report the letters blurred. Similarly, negative relative convergence measures the ability of the organism to tolerate the movement of convergence away from him, while accommodation is at the plane of regard. When this range of movement is of such a degree that the conditioned stimuli arising from convergence can no longer be inhibited, it will 'spill over' and the resulting inhibition to accommodation will produce a blur. In the same manner, positive relative accommodation and negative relative accommodation represent the range in the accommodative pattern to withstand the stimulation and inhibition of that function without causing an overt movement in convergence. The magnitude of these four ranges are indicative of the presence of an inefficient or disorganized pattern. When the magnitudes of these ranges are low (No.16A 10 d. or less; No.17A 10 d. or less; No.20 -1.50 d. or less; and No21 +1.50 d. or less), the organism does not have sufficient flexibility in the innervational relationships so that it can absorb readily the changes in visual demands because of variations in environmental or physiological factors. These measurements of 'play-between-functions' should be 15 prism diopters for the negative and positive relative convergence; and 2.25 lens diopters for negative and positive relative accommodation. When these ranges are up to these values we have adequate flexibility between accommodation and convergence. Therefore, when we prescribe visual training or lens application, or a combination of both, we must observe carefully not only the relationship between the various measurements of the potential of inhibition, but we must also consider the magnitude of these various measurements. The data that follows illustrates the changes

	Original Values	Four Weeks Later
16A	12	8
17A	18	10
20	-2.50	-1.75
21	+2.00	+1.00

in the equilibrium pattern after a lens application. The rejection of the lens is obvious from the restriction of inhibition ability shown. This rejection is more revealing in the light of the patient's testimony, "I see fine with my new lenses." With this restriction in range, the patient's testimony reveals that he is functioning adequately because of a short period of attention at the task, or he is working on a task which does not require a high demand factor.

The characteristic spatial relationship between accommodation and convergence in a B-type case is for accommodation to be away from the plane of regard and convergence to be closer to the organism. Figure 56 illustrates this spatial relationship between accommodation and convergence in a B-Type case.

You will note that the base-out-to-blur-out (positive relative convergence) and plus-lenses-to-blur-out (negative relative accommodation) allow the same spatial configuration as illustrated in Figure 56 for the B-type case. Thus, in a B-type case, we will characteristically have No.16A and No.21 greater in magnitude than the blur out tests which go in the reverse spatial direction. $\frac{16A - 21}{17A - 20}$ characteristic spatial pattern for B-type.

As the visual problem causes greater changes in the visual pattern we will find that we will get changes in the characteristic spatial pattern. We will have either a reversal in the prism blur out tests, or in the lens blur out tests. After a visual problem has existed for some time we will find: $\frac{16A - 20}{17A - 21}$ or $\frac{17A - 21}{16A - 20}$

If visual care has been neglected and the patient must function in a high demand environment, we then often find a double reversal in the equilibrium tests: $\frac{17A - 20}{16A - 21}$ This double reversal, present in a B-type case, is a sign of rejection of plus lenses and the need for visual training is obvious. The reversal of the arrangement of the configuration of the blur-out tests indicates the fourth stage in the syndrome of deterioration of a B-type case.

Figure 57 illustrates the spatial relationship between accommodation and convergence in a C-type case. You will note that this is the reverse of the spatial configuration of the B-type case.

You will note that in the equilibrium tests base-in-to-blur-out and minus-lens-to-blur-out gives the same type of spatial configuration as shown by

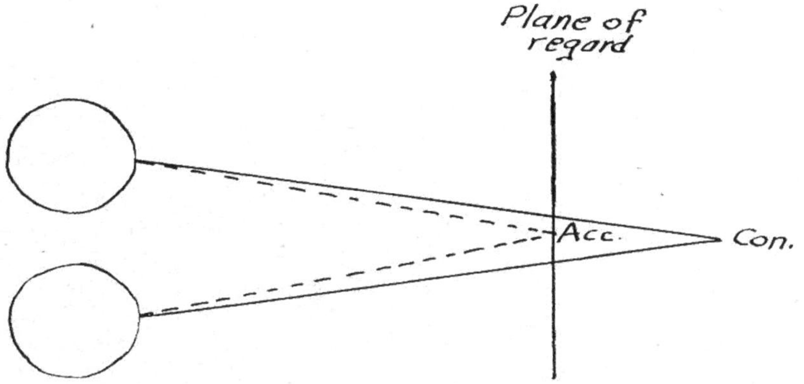

Figure 57. Spatial configuration of a C-type case.

the C-type case. Thus, in a C-type case we would expect to have $\frac{17A - 20}{16A - 21}$ as the pattern of the equilibrium tests. The pattern of the equilibrium tests aid us in arriving at the case typing of the visual pattern

Clinical experience has shown that a patient will not tolerate a lens prescription that reverses the configuration pattern of the habitual relationship of the equilibrium findings. For example, if the habitual equilibrium pattern is $\frac{16A - 21}{17A - 20}$, and the nearpoint cross-cylinder nets give us a pattern of $\frac{17A - 21}{16A - 20}$ or $\frac{16A - 20}{17A - 21}$ then the cross-cylinder nets are rejected, and only that portion of the nearpoint nets can be prescribed which does not reverse the habitual pattern of the patient.

The measurement of the potential of inhibition in the direction of stimulus and inhibition for both convergence and accommodation are significant measures of: 1. the amount of flexibility we have between accommodation and convergence 2. the magnitude of the blur out tests are high enough for the visual activity of the patient; 3. the effect of lens application, visual training progress or combination of these in developing or restricting the visual performance ability of the patient; 4. the deterioration of the B-type case; 5. the acceptance or rejection of the cross cylinder nets.

F. The learned relationship between accommodation and convergence. The tests which explore the extent of the learned relationship between accommodation and convergence are known as the break portion of the duction tests. These tests can be classified in many ways. For example:

I. As to direction
   A. Vertical ductions
      1. Right supra duction
      2. Right infra duction

B. Lateral ductions
    1. Convergences at far
    2. Abduction
    3. Positive fusional reserve
    4. Negative fusional reserve

II. As to type of prism used
  A. Base-in prism
    1. Abduction
    2. Negative fusional reserve
  B. Base-out prism
    1. Convergence at far
    2. Positive fusional reserve
  C. Base-down prism
    1. Right supra duction
  D. Base-up prism
    2. Right infra action

III. As to test distance
  A. Far (twenty-feet)
    1. Convergence at far
    2. Abduction
    3. Right supra duction
    4. Right infra duction
  B. Near (sixteen inches)
    1. Positive fusional reserve
    2. Negative fusional reserve
    3. Right supra duction
    4. Right infra duction

They can also be classified as to the type of stimulus used, either stimulatory to convergence (base-out) or inhibitory to convergence (base in); or as to the type of spatial movement required, base-out tests move convergence toward the observer, base-in tests move convergence away from the observer.

When we break the binocular space lattice by means of a prism we are measuring the magnitude of the learned relationship between the patterns of accommodation and convergence within the central nervous system. It is a spatial exploration of the learned relationship between accommodation under the artificial conditions of the prism probe body. The primary intensity of stimulation or inhibition is placed upon the convergence pattern; but the conditioned or learned relationship between accommodation and convergence creates a stress within the accommodative pattern at the same time. The fact that the accommodative pattern is activated when we stimu-

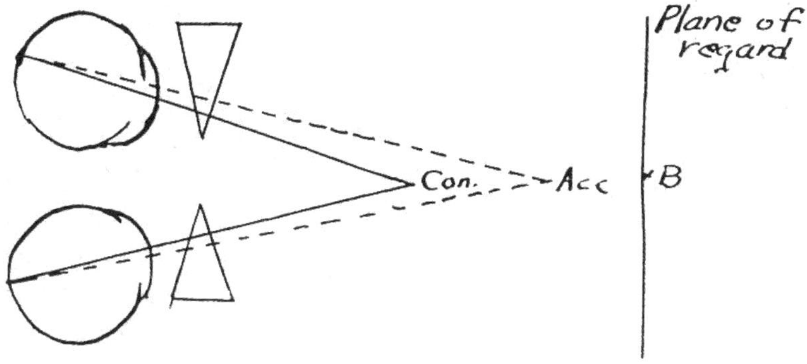

Figure 58. Spatial change induced by means of base out prism.

late or inhibit convergence by the binocular application of prism can be objectively measured by means of retinoscopy.

Figure 58 illustrates the spatial changes in convergence and accommodation when we binocularly apply base-out prism.

When stimulus pattern disparity has reached the functional limit of integration (outer limit of Panum's area) diplopia will ensue. This is recorded as the break point for the particular duction test. This ability to resist diplopia, in spite of the stimulus disparity across retina and the conflict with the contributory kinesthetic pattern, is a learned relationship.

You will note that the movement of accommodation (Figure 58) is from the plane of regard B to position Acc; while the spatial movement of convergence is from the plane of regard B to position Con. It is a matter of conjecture whether the break point or diplopia is reached because of the excessive blurring of the target stimulus pattern due to the conditioned accommodative change and the resultant reduction in fusional desire; or this stage is reached because of the excessive movement of convergence and the stimulus pattern has reached the psycho-physiological limits of Panum's areas. The fusional limits at near are from 21 prism diopters in the base-out direction, 22 prism diopters in the base-in direction, 6 prism diopters in the base-up direction, and 6 prism diopters in the base-down direction. The ability to shift convergence from the plane of regard because of the application of prism is learned. Since it is learned it is highly amenable to training.

Characteristically, we find in the visually unimpaired individual, that these various duction break findings are high; whereas in the visually impaired

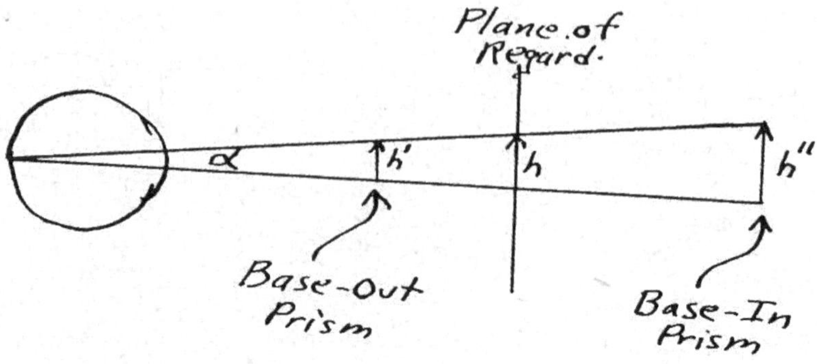

Figure 59. Effect of prism application upon the size of a target.

individual they are usually very low. When the proper visual care has been administered, we should expect these particular tests to increase in magnitude. The degree of the visual problem can be determined by the duction pattern. A simple visual problem, where full plus is accepted at both far and near, will reveal that abduction at far (No.11) and positive fusional reserve (No.16B) are both low. A more intense visual problem will reveal that abduction at far (No.11) and negative fusional reserve (No.17B) are both low. A very intense visual problem, in which we reduce the magnitude of the plus lenses prescribed for both far and near, is revealed when we have convergence at far (No.10) and either of the nearpoint duction tests are low.

For many years it was believed that when we performed a duction test we were measuring the strength of the extrinsic muscle; but a comparison of the statistical average for these tests, with the magnitude of the nearpoint of convergence test, reveals a considerable discrepancy in muscle strength. The usual observer can achieve a nearpoint of convergence of 10 centimeters which for a 60mm p.d., will give us a total convergence of 60 prism diopters. The average of the base-out prism duction test at near (No.16B) will average 21 prism diopters. With our prism probe bodies we are not measuring muscle strength but an artificial measurement of the ability of the organism to move primarily convergence from the plane of regard (since accommodation is also in movement) while interpretation is still on the plane of regard. Since the size of the target (h) at the plane of regard remains constant if the stimulus used is base-out prism, it kinesthetically is informing the subject that the target is moving closer to him, and he must interpret that movement in terms of a decreased target (see Figure 59). If we are using base-in prism in our duction measurement, kinesthetically the patient is informed that the target is moving farther away from him. This movement must be interpreted in terms of the target getting larger (see Figure 59).

It has been expressed as the law of silo or, small in-large out. Therefore, the patient who is not aware of any size change while we are performing the duction tests, has poor kinesthetic awareness. Whenever base-in or base-out ductions are taken, the patient should be informed that we want to know if and when the target moves, doubles, or changes in size. Let us compare the responses of two patients:

	Patient A	**Patient B**
Magnitude of Duction Tests	22 p.d.	22 p.d.
SILO effect	Not detected	Very sensitive to size change

It would be well to prescribe minimum lens values to patient B, particularly if he is older than 20 years of age, because of his silo response; whereas in patient A the full lenses shown prescriptable by the usual means will be accepted. Lenses also change the spatial convergence and will give a silo response.

From the duction tests, we obtain information regarding:

1. The presence or absence of a binocular visual problem.
2. The modification of the prescriptable lens.
3. The intensity of the visual problem.
4. The degree of the kinesthetic-visual integration.
5. The detection and measurement of vertical asymmetry.
6. The embeddedness of the visual pattern.

G. The measurement of the Degree of integration between accommodation and convergence

In performing the duction tests, after we have obtained diplopia and recorded the break point, we begin to reduce the amount of prism, and we record the total prism remaining when the patient has regained single vision. This is the recovery test of the particular duction finding, and it measures the degree of integration between accommodation and convergence. These recovery or reversion to fusion tests are relatively late-comers in the interpretive use of the optometric findings.

They measure the degree of integration (spatially) between accommodation and convergence at both a distant fixation point and a sixteen inch nearpoint fixation distance. The more highly integrated the visual pattern, the sooner the patient will regain single binocular vision, as the amount of prism found at the breakpoint is slowly reduced. The poorly integrated visual-pattern will require a considerable reduction in the amount of prism before single binocular vision is regained. Thus, when the recovery portion of a duction test is high, it surely indicates a performance ability which has existed for a considerable period of time. We say that the performance is "embedded" or "organized." Similarly, if the recovery portion of the duction test is low, it indicates a very inefficient and poorly integrated visual response. For this type of performance, we use the terms "disembedded" or "disorganized." When the recovery finding is low, at any point in space, there is disorganization or disembedding of the visual pattern in that spatial area.

The drive to recapture single vision is a potent one. Survival in a large measure depends upon this ability. Consequently, when conditions were imposed upon the organism that made single vision impossible, the organism moved to recapture single binocular vision as rapidly as possible. When diplopia has been achieved and the amount of prism before the eyeballs is gradually reduced, it would be expected that only a small decrease in the amount of prism would have to be made before the organism would make the necessary integration in order to obtain single vision.

This matter of synthesis of two series of excitations into one perceptual object is a highly complicated, and elaborated organizational activity in the central nervous system. The eyeballs move in the manner observed in the test because of the pull of the synchronous muscles involved.

The recovery of fusion occurs when the undesirable situation of diplopia is within the limits of the organizational ability of the central nervous system to solve the dilemma. On the basis of statistical averages, we expect the recovery values of the farpoint ductions to be at least one-half of the expected break values; while at nearpoint, the recovery for the positive fusional reserve will average two-thirds of the break, and the recovery for the negative fusional reserve test will average three-fourths of the expected break Whenever the break values for the duction tests are higher than their expected values, we expect the recovery values to stay in ratio.

The recovery tests have the following values in visual analysis: 1 Whenever the duction pattern cannot be determined because of the high break values, we can use the recovery values in order to determine the typing. 2 If the recovery values are low, indicating a disembedded situation one can prescribe more plus than when the recovery values are high. 3 One of the important signposts of an efficient visual pattern is a pattern of high recovery values.

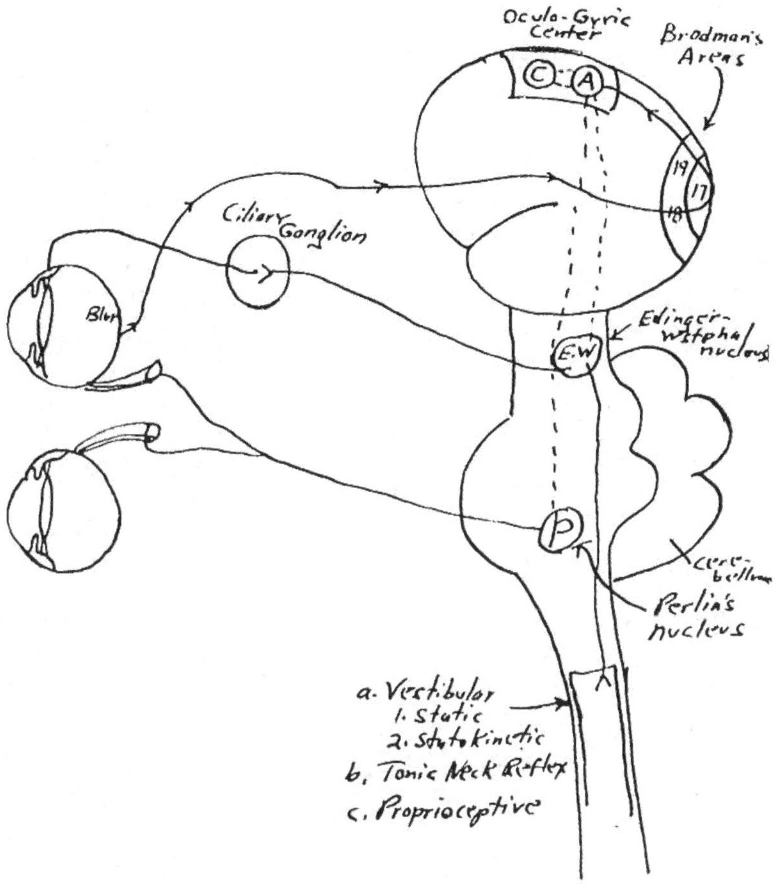

Figure 60.

H. The amplitude of accommodation

The amplitude of accommodation measures the reserve in the accommodative pattern to preserve clear vision in spite of advances in senility. Accommodation amplitude is the range or latitude built into the accommodative pattern to withstand the ravages of advancing age upon clear vision. It is more than just the measure of lenticular accommodation; it is the measure of total accommodation. Total accommodation is the sum total of lenticular accommodation, aberrational accommodation, psychic accommodation and tonic accommodation. Aberrational accommodation provides the same extension (or range) in the focus mechanism that fusional convergence (Panum's areas) provides in the convergence mechanism for single vision.

The total accommodative amplitude of the organism is an important measure of the presence of a visual problem. It has been the clinical experience of the profession that the amplitude must be at least twice the dioptric equivalent of the working distance. If the subject is working at 16 inches a total amplitude of at least 5.00 diopters is necessary. When the measure of amplitude is below five diopters and presbyopia has not intervened, we have the existence of a serious visual problem. The amplitude of accommodation can be increased either by visual training or by increasing the illumination intensity.

The question often arises, in what way is the amplitude of accommodation (No.19) different from positive relative accommodation (No.20)?

	19	20
Target:	0.62 Em type	20/20 Reduced Snellen
Test Distance:	13 inches	16 inches
Lenses in Place:	Subjective	Subjective-hyperope 14B Net-Presbyope Habitual minus-Myope
End Point of Test:	Difficult to read	Complete blur out
Lenses Used:	Minus spheres	Minus spheres

It is obvious that there are considerable points of difference between these two tests. It must also be pointed out that they both measure to some degree the ability to stimulate accommodation with convergence fixed, although at two different test distances. Morgan found that the coefficient of correlation between amplitude of accommodation and positive relative accommodation is +0.8, which is highly significant.

The visual measurements are merely the investigation of the two basic subpatterns of vision-accommodation and convergence. Figure 60 presents our knowledge of the neural-anatomy of accommodation which, because of its slower speed of action, determines the direction of the adaptation.

CHAPTER VIII
The Mechanics of Case Analysis

The following pages contain layers of rules and guidelines for case analysis. They are intended to provide a logical approach to lens prescribing. We suggest that initially you read the chapter through in its entirety. This will allow you to get a sense of the purpose, means and methods of the visual analysis. The following outline can then be used to locate, and study in more detail, the specifics of the subroutines presented here.

The Mechanics of Case Analysis

- Checking the Visual Findings
  - Checking tests 3, 4, 8, 9 & 13
  - Checking tests 5, 6, 14A & 14B
    - Net values for accom. Tests
    - Checking the 14A
- Chaining the Visual finding
  - Informative Sequence
    - Basic finding
    - Case Typing
- Pattern of equilibrium findings
    - Case deteriorations
- C-type case
- 14B Net
- The Equilibrium pattern
- Acceptance of the near nets
    - M.S.D.A.
- The Corrective Framework
  - Fourteen directives for lens application
- Ten Laws of Lens Application
- General considerations
  - Anisometropia
  - Embeddeness

Introduction

This is the portion of visual analysis for which the student has been waiting. Often the introductory chapters have been skipped since the beginning student thinks that they are too theoretical. "Don't tell me what it means, tell me what to do," is the cry of the neophyte as he approaches visual analysis. All methods of visual analysis have developed rules and regulations on how to handle the mass of data we obtain when we perform a visual case study. These rules and regulations are usually relatively simple to learn. This is where the danger arises since the mechanical computations you will be performing will merely give you the framework of the case. The flesh, sinew, and blood of the case must also be applied to this framework in order to arrive at an organismic approach to the solution of the visual problem of the patient.

The Mechanics of Case Analysis will tell us several things about the visual problem of the patient. These are:

1. Is the full plus of the subjective finding at far (#7) acceptable for farpoint activities?
2. Is the full plus of the subjective finding at near (#14A and #14B nets) acceptable for nearpoint activities?
3. Will the lens values tentatively agreed upon create any additional problems for the patient?
4. In order to solve the visual problem will lenses alone be sufficient, or will we have to use a combination of lenses and visual training, or is the problem of such complexity that only visual training can be used.
5. Is the visual problem developed by the patient a recent one, or is it a visual problem of long standing?
6. Is the visual pattern of the patient operating at an efficient level (embedded), or at an inefficient level (unembedded) for that particular adaptation?

When we approach our visual data for the purpose of visual analysis we must be aware that we are measuring a highly dynamic system. The problem of accuracy of data must be considered from a slightly different viewpoint than the viewpoint of a physicist when he is measuring the melting point of some solid. For example, the student will often ask, "Which phoria shall I use? I measured it for the first time (#13A) and it was 6 diopters of exophoria. I repeated the measurement later in the examination (#13B) through the same lens values and now the phoria is 9 diopters of exophoria." The person who approaches the visual system as if it is isolated from the organism would say that one of the measurements is in error and the phoria should be repeated until a constant value is obtained. The practitioner versed in the organismic approach would say that both findings are significant, and the variation in magnitude is highly significant. One interpretation of this variation is that it might tell us how quickly fatigue occurs and the direction in which it shifts. In this case, under fatigue, we have the development of more exophoria. This same problem regarding variation in case data when a different procedure is used will often confuse the student. An example of this occurs in the comparison of the nearpoint induced phoria (#13B) with the phoria computed from the Van Orden Star test (visual skill). The student will ask, "Which phoria is correct?" By comparing these two different methods of measuring the nearpoint phoria, we are determining the effect of body posture and the dynamic use of both hands upon the convergence pattern. Students should recognize that both methods of measurement are accurate for the particular testing conditions of each distinct procedure.

The seasoned practitioner, is concerned not only with the magnitude of the visual measurement, but its variation when conditions are different; when demand is different; and/or when time has elapsed (fatigue factor). We must recognize that the visual system is the most important portion of the total action system of the human organism.

Since this visual system is constantly undergoing dynamic shifts in dominancy because of the various stresses, desires, urgencies and needs of the organism, when we perform our visual test measurements, we are usually attempting to measure one component of this complex system while keeping the remainder relatively constant. In this very act of making the visual measurement we are creating changes in its makeup. If you consider only isolated measurements, they are not nearly as diagnostic as comparisons between measurements made under different conditions or at a later time interval. Knowing that a particular patient has a habitual phoria at near (#13A) of six diopters of exophoria seems to be a normal measurement since it agrees with the statistical average for this measurement. But notice the increased diagnostic significance of the nearpoint phoria test when we consider the effect of the induced fatigue of the visual examination.

(1)		(2)	
#13A	6 exophoria	#13A	6 exophoria
#7	plano	#7	plano
#13B	6 exophoria	#13B	10 exophoria

In case (1) fatigue had little effect upon the convergence pattern. In case (2) fatigue resulted in increased exophoria of a significant amount. When prescribing lenses for these cases, we would tend to prescribe differently for the second case than we would for the first case.

In the visual analysis, from the functional viewpoint, we are interested not only in the actual magnitude of a test measurement but how it compares with a sister measurement as well. We are making these comparisons valid by keeping the procedures as constant as possible, and thus reducing experimental errors.

In approaching the following rules of analysis learn them well. However, in addition, learn to observe the magnitude of the finding, its comparison effect, and the effect of the fatigue of the examination as well.

Checking

Checking is a procedure for designating those analytical findings which vary from a "mean" or "expected" value. The findings that are low are marked with a blue pencil, and those which are high with a red pencil. As an alternative, the high findings can be designated by an "H", and the low findings by an "L." For the purposes of checking the following analytical tests are carefully inspected: 3, 4, 5, 6, 8, 9, 10, 11, 13B, 14A, 15A, 16B, and 17B.

Rules for Checking Tests 3, 4, 8, 9, and 13B

Rule One

Tests 3, 4, 8, 9, and 13B are to be checked high or low by comparison with an expected or mean value for the analytical finding..

a) Test No. 3 (habitual phoria at far) is compared to a mean value of ½ prism diopters of exophoria. If the particular test value for the No. 3 finding is greater than ½ prism diopters of exophoria, it is checked high; if it is equal to ½ prism diopters of exophoria, it is not checked; if it is less than ½ prism diopters of exophoria, it is checked low. The following case data illustrate this procedure for the checking of the No. 3 finding:

#3 ½ exophoria (not checked)
#3 2 exophoria (checked high)
#3 orthophoria (checked low)
#3 1 esophoria (checked low)

b) Test No. 4 (static retinoscopy at far) is compared to the No. 7 or the basic finding. If the No. 4 is in greater plus (or less minus) than the basic finding, the test is checked high; if the No. 4 is equal in lens value to the basic finding, it is not checked; if the No. 4 is in less plus (or more minus) than the basic finding, the test is checked low. The following case data illustrate this procedure for the checking of the No. 4 finding:

Case 1	Case 2	Case 3	
#4 Plano (low)	#4-1.00 D. (low)	#4 +1.00 D.	(not checked)
#7 +0.50 D.	#7-0.50 D.	#7 +1.00 D.	

c) Test No. 8 (induced phoria at far) is compared to a mean value of ½ prism diopter of exophoria. The procedure for checking this finding is the same as for Test No. 3. This is illustrated by the following case data:

#8 ½ exophoria (not checked)
#8 3 exophoria (high)
#8 1½ esophoria (low)

d) Test No. 9 (true adduction at far) is compared to a range in prism magnitude of from seven to nine prism diopters. If the No. 9 test is greater than nine prism diopters, it is checked high; if the No. 9 test is in the range of from seven to nine prism diopters, it is not checked; if the No. 9 test value is less than seven prism diopters, it is checked low. For example:

#9 7 D. (not checked)
#9 5 D. (low)
#9 10 D. (high)

e) Test No. 13B (induced phoria at near) is compared to a mean value of six prism diopters of exophoria. If test No. 13B is more than six prism diopters of exophoria, it is checked high; if the, test magnitude is equal to six prism diopters of exophoria, it is not checked; if the test value is less than six prism diopters of exophoria or is in esophoria, the finding is checked low. For example:

#13B 8 exophoria (high)
#13B 6 exophoria (not checked)
#13B 2 exophoria (low)
#13B 3 exophoria (low)

Whenever one of these tests (No.3, 4, 8, 9, or 13B) is to its expected value we do not check the finding. The test finding checked must be either higher or lower than its expected value. (1)

Check the following case fragments:

Case 1	Case 2	Case 3
#3 1 exophoria (high)	#3 1 esophoria (low)	#3 orthophoria (low)
#4 +0.50 D.	#4 +1.00 D. (high)	#4 +0.25 D. (low)
#7 +0.50 D.	#7 +0.75 D.	#7 +0.50 D.
#8 orthophoria (low)	#8 1 exophoria (high)	#8 2 exophoria (high)
#9 12 (high)	#9 7	#9 4 (low)
#13B 12 exophoria (high)	#13B 6 exophoria	#13 B 4 esophoria (low)

Rule Two

The No. 7 or the basic finding is never checked. The No. 7 test determines the maximum plus that can be prescribed at the farpoint fixation distance. The analysis of the visual data will determine what portion of this finding will be prescribed. (2)

The duction tests are complex test magnitudes since they comprise both a break value and a recovery value. They are, therefore, checked on a double comparison scale. These tests are No. 10 and 11 at farpoint, and 16B, 17B at nearpoint. These tests have the following expected values:

#10 19/10 (recovery must be ½ of the break)
#11 9/5 (recovery must be ½ of the break)
#16B 21/15 (recovery must be 2/3 of the break)
#17B 22/18 (recovery must be ¾ of the break)

Rule Three

A duction test must always be checked either high or low. (3)

Rule Four

If a breakpoint of the duction test is equal to its expected value or higher, and the recovery value of the test is in proper ratio (or higher) with the break, we state that the duction test finding is high.(4)

For example:

#10	20/10 (high)	#10	19/17 (high)	#10	21/19 (high)
#11	9/6 (high)	#11	12/9 (high)	#11	20/10 (high)
#16B	21/15 (high)	#16B	23/16 (high)	#16B	24/16 (high)
#17B	22/18 (high)	#17B	25/20 (high)	#17B	24/18 (high)

Rule Five

If any duction test has a breakpoint below its expected value, or if its recovery point is not in proper ratio with the break magnitude, the test is checked *low*. If the break finding is below its expected value the duction is *low* regardless of the magnitude of the recovery finding. If the break finding is up to its expected value or higher but the recovery finding is not in proper ratio with the break magnitude, the duction is checked low.

For example:

#10	17/15 (low, because of break)	#10	20/5 (low, because of recovery)
#11	9/3 (low, because of recovery)	#11	7 /8 (low, because of break)
#16B	21/10 (low, recovery)	#16B	15/12 (low, break)
#17B	18/17 (low, break)	#17B	30/-2 (low, recovery)

If in any particular case we have both farpoint ductions (#10 and #11) checked low, or both nearpoint ductions (#16B and #17B) checked low, the two tests of the farpoint pair or the nearpoint pair are compared with each other to determine which is the lower of the two, the low-low value.

Rule Six

When both of the far-point breaks, or both of the near-point breaks are low, the designated low finding is the one that gives the lower fraction relative to the expected break for that test. Create a fraction by putting the actual break finding for the test over the expected break finding for that same test. Then compare the resultant fraction computed from the BO values to the fraction computed from the BI values.

For example:
#10 17/11 (break is lower than expected of 19, 17/19)
#11 7/4 (break is lower than expected of 9, 7/9)

We now compare the fraction 17/19 to 7/9. Since 7/9 is the smaller fraction in this example, the No.11 test would be designated as the low-low (LL) finding.

Rule Seven

When both of the farpoint duction tests, or both of the nearpoint duction tests, are low, and one duction test of the pair is low because of a low break value, and the companion finding is low because of a low recovery, then the low-low duction test is the one with the low break value.

For example:
#10 15/10 low (break lower than expected)
#11 10/3 low (recovery lower than expected)

In this example, the #10 becomes the low-low finding.

For example:
#16B 7/6 low (break lower than expected)
#17B 22/14 low (recovery lower than expected)

In this example, the #16B becomes the low-low finding.

The *break finding* portion of the duction test is more diagnostic for the evaluation of the visual status of the case than the recovery portion of the duction test. If however the break finding is higher than the expected value, the recovery portion of the duction test assumes diagnostic importance if it is less than its expected value. Thus, for those cases where the break values of a duction pair at either far or at near are higher in magnitude than their respective expected values, but their recoveries are both low, we utilize the following rule in order to establish the low-low finding.

Rule Eight

If both farpoint duction tests or both nearpoint duction tests are low because of low recovery magnitudes, we compare the ratio of the actual recovery value with the expected recovery value. Remember that the expected recovery values are computed as a percentage of the break value. The fraction computed for each duction is compared, and the duction finding having the smallest fraction is designated as the low-low test.

For example:

#10	20/6 low (recovery less than expected value of 10)
#11	12/4 low (recovery less than expected value of 6)

By rule eight we construct the fraction of measured/expected for each of the duction tests we are comparing.

#10 becomes 6/10,
#11 becomes 4/6

Since 6/10 is a smaller fraction than 4/6, the #10 finding becomes the low-low duction.

For example:

#16B	24/8 low (recovery less than expected value of 16)
#17B	24/10 low (recovery less than expected value of 18)

(The calculated value for the recovery of #16B should be at least 2/3 of break, and the recovery of #17B should be at least ¾ of break.)

The fraction for #16B becomes 8/16,
The fraction for #17B becomes 10/18,

By comparison, 8/16 is a smaller fraction than 10/18, and the #16B becomes the low-low duction.

Utilizing rules three through eight for the ductions, determine the checking for the following case fragments:

	(1)	(2)	(3)	(4)	(5)
#10	12/9	13/8	10/7	12/4	10/6
#11	5/-2	4/1	6/1	8/4	6/2
#16B	10/7	20/14	12/5	30/20	22/12
#17B	12/0	8/6	19/12	11/8	8/2
#10	L	L	LL	LL	LL
#11	LL	LL	L	L	L
#16B	LL	L	LL	H	L
#17B	L	LL	L	L	LL

Rules for Checking Tests 5, 6, 14A and 14B

The checking for tests 3, 4, 8, 9, and 13B were based upon their actual measured magnitude. Checking tests 5, 6, 14A and 14B is done somewhat differently. Before these tests can be checked there must be a conversion from a gross value to a net value. The conversion of a gross value to a net value must be made in order to obtain an accommodative value that we consider relatively free of the effect of convergence.

Definitions:

a) Gross magnitude-- that which is measured.
b) Net magnitude-- that portion of the gross value which is free of the `effect of convergence.
c) Lag -- that which is subtracted from the gross magnitude in order to obtain a net value.
   --the effect of convergence translated into accommodative units.
d) Net Value for the Acc. Test = Gross Acc. Test finding – the Lag

Rule Nine

a) If the No. 15A phoria test is orthophoria or in esophoria, the lag is zero and the gross finding becomes the net value. This is true for tests No.5, 14A and 14B

b) In determining the net magnitude for the dynamic retinoscopy test at 20 inches (#5) we should have a corresponding phoria test taken at this same distance. However, there is a high correlation between the #5 test and the #14A test and for this reason we utilize the #15A phoria test for this purpose. Since the maximum lag we can have for a test performed at 20 inches is two diopters, the 15A phoria test must be modified for this purpose. It is for this reason that we state that the following lag table is loaded or weighted to give us a corresponding magnitude equivalent to a 20 inch test distance.

1 exophoria 0.12 D.	9 exophoria 1.25 D.
2 exophoria 0.25 D.	10 exophoria 1.37 D.
3 exophoria 0.37 D.	11 exophoria 1.50 D.
4 exophoria 0.50 D.	12 exophoria 1.62 D.
5 exophoria 0.62 D.	13 exophoria 1.75 D.
6 exophoria 0.75 D.	14 exophoria 1.87 D.
7 exophoria 0.87 D.	15 exophoria 2.00 D.
8 exophoria 1.00 D.	above 15 exophoria 2.00 D.

c) When the amplitude of accommodation (#19) is less than five diopters the effect of the associated phoria test upon accommodation is lessened, and the lag table must be modified. The product obtained is called a modified lag. We multiply the lag obtained from the lag table by the following decimal fraction in order to obtain the modified lag.

Amplitude	Modification Decimal	Amplitude	Modification Decimal
5.00 D.	1.0	2.50 D.	0.5
4.50 D.	0.9	2.00 D.	0.4
4.00 D.	0.8	1.50 D.	0.3
3.50 D.	0.7	1.00 D.	0.2
3.00 D.	0.6	0.50 D.	0.1

One can also use the fraction of amplitude/5.00 in order to obtain the correction faction whenever the amplitude of the case is below five diopters. These calculations are illustrated by the following examples:

(1)	(2)	(3)
#5 +2.00	#5 -1.00	#5 plano
#15A 6 Exophoria	#15A 18 Exophoria	#15A 9 Exophoria
#19 4.75 D.	#19 3.00 D.	#19 2.50 D.
Lag 4.75/5.00 X 0.75	Lag 3.00/5.00 X 2.00	Lag 2.50/5.00 X 1.25
Lag is equal to 0.75	Lag is equal to 1.25	Lag is equal to 0.62
#5 Net = 2.00 - 0.75	#5 Net = -1.00 – 1.25	#5 Net = plano – 0.62
#5 Net = +1.25 D.	#5 Net = -2.25 D.	#5 Net = -0.62 D.

Note: In computing the lag for the dynamic retinoscopy test at 20 inches (#5), we round off all calculations to the nearest 1/8 of a diopter (0.12 D.).

Rule Ten

The *net value* for the dynamic retinoscopy test at 20 inches (net #5) is now compared directly to the static retinoscopy test at far (#4). If the net No.5 test is higher (more plus) than the No.4 test, we check it in red (high). If the Net No.5 is lower (less plus) than the No.4 test, we check it in blue (low). If the Net No.5 is equal to the No.4 test, it is not checked**.** The following case fragments indicate the checking of the No.5 test:

	(1)		(2)
# 4	+1.00 D.	# 4	+1.00 D.
# 5	+2.00 D. (net +1.25) High	# 5	+2.50 (net +2.00) High
15A	6 Exophoria (lag 0.75)	# 15A	10 Exophoria (lag 1.37 X .35 or 0.50)
#19	6.00 D.	# 19	1.75 D. (mod. dec. 0.35)

The calculation of the net dynamic retinoscopy value:

a) No. 4-Basic objective test value at far.

b) No. 5-An objective nearpoint test to be compared to the basic objective test (No.4); before such comparison can be made it must be modified by a lag based upon a nearpoint phoria.

Gross No. 5 – lag = Net No. 5

c) No. 15A-The phoria used to determine the lag for the No. 5 test. If test is orthophoria or esophoria, the lag is zero. If test is exophoria, determine the lag from loaded lag table. If the amplitude is low (below five diopters), the 1ag must be modified.

Modified lag = lag X modification factor

d) No. 19-If amplitude is five diopters or greater, no modification factor is used. If amplitude is below five diopters, a lag modification factor must be used.

Modification factor = amplitude/5.00

Rule Eleven

The lag for the dynamic retinoscopy test at forty inches (#6) is a constant value of 0.25diopter. The Net No. 6 is checked high if it is greater (more plus) than the No. 4 test; it is not checked if it is equal (same amount of plus) to the No. 4 test; it is checked low if it is less in plus than the No. 4 test. (11)

For example:

#4 +1.00D.	#4 +1.00D.	#4 +1.00 D.
#6 +0.50 (low)	#6 +1.50 (high)	#6 +1.25 (not check)
Net # 6 +0.25	Net # 6 +1.25	Net # 6 +1.00

Rule Twelve

The gross No. 14A must be converted into a net value which is free of the effect of convergence, so that it may be compared to the subjective test (No.7). For this purpose a lag is computed from the magnitude of the No.15A phoria test. If the No.15A test is in exophoria, we determine the lag by dividing the exophoria by six, i.e., 15A = 3 exophoria, lag = 3/6 = 0.50. If the exophoria is excessive (above 15 diopters), any lag above 2.50 diopters is ignored since the maximum accommodative effect you can have at a 16-inch fixation distance is 2.50 diopters. If the No.15A test is orthophoria or in esophoria, the lag becomes zero and the net No.14A is the same as the gross No.14A (12)

For example:

(1)	(2)	(3)
#7 +1.00 D.	#7 +1.00 D.	#7 +1.00 D.
#14A +2.00 D.	#14A +2.00 D.	#14A +2.00 D.
#15A 3 esophoria (lag zero)	#15A 6 exophoria (lag 1.00 D.)	#15A 18 exophoria (lag 2.50
Net #14A +2.00 D.	Net #14A +1.00 D.	Net #14A -0.50 D.

If the amplitude of accommodation (#19) is less than five diopters, the calculated lags must be modified (see modification table under the No.5 finding).

All calculated values of the net No. 14A finding must be carried out to the nearest one-quarter diopter.

The following case fragments indicate the calculation of the No. 14A test:

(1)	(2)
# 14A +2.00 D.	# 14A +2.00 D.
# 15A 6 exophoria	# 15A 15 exophoria
# 19 4.00 D.	# 19 1.00 D.
Lag 6/6 X 4/5 = 0.75	Lag 15/6 X 1/5 = 0.50 D.
#14A Net = 2.00 – 0.75 = 1.25 D.	#14A Net = 2.00 – 0.50 = 1.50 D.

The calculation of the net dissociated cross-cylinder value:

No. 7-Basic subjective test value at far.

No. 14A-A subjective nearpoint test which is to he compared to the basic subjective test (No.7). However, before such comparison can be made it must be converted into a net value which is free of the effect of convergence by the subtraction of a lag which is based upon the associated phoria (No. 15A).

No. 15A-The associated phoria test from which we compute the accommodative lag. If the phoria is in esophoria or orthophoria, the magnitude of the lag is zero. If the phoria is in exophoria, the lag is computed by dividing the exophoria by six. The maximum lag allowable by this computation is 2.50 diopters. However, if the amplitude of accommodation is below five diopters, a lag modification factor is to be computed. Lag modification factor is equal to the amplitude of accommodation divided by five.

No. 19-If the amplitude of accommodation is five diopters or greater, it does not influence the computation of the lag. However, if the amplitude of accommodation is less than five diopters, a lag modification factor must be computed. The lag modification factor is equal to the amplitude divided by five.

The checking of the dissociated cross-cylinder test (No. 14A):

If the net No. 14A is greater (more plus) than the No.7, check No. 14A high and No. 15A low.

If the net No. 14A is less (less plus) than the No.7, check No. 14A low and No. 15A high.

If the net No. 14A is equal to the plus of the No.7, then consider the value of the 15A:

If the 15A is greater than six diopters of exophoria, the 14A and 15A are checked equal and high.

If the 15A is less than six diopters of exophoria, 14A and 15A are checked equal and low.

If the 15A phoria is equal to six diopters of exophoria, the 14A and 15A are equal and not checked.

The checking position of the No. 14A and No. 15A tests when the net No. 14A test is equal in plus to the No. 7 test depends upon the amount of exophoria in the No. 15A test. If it is greater than six diopters of exophoria, they are both checked high; if less than six diopters of exophoria, they are both checked low; if equal to six diopters of exophoria, they are both left unchecked.

A No. 15A test magnitude of six diopters of exophoria becomes our pivot point in checking of the number 14A and 15A tests when the Net No. 14A is equal in plus to the No.7 test.

If the basic finding (No. 7) is in minus (myope), then the No. 14A net is compared with the previously worn minus if the patient has glasses. However, if this previously worn minus exceeds in magnitude the present No.7, than the No. 14A is compared with the present No.7. If the patient has never worn glasses, the Net No. 14A is compared to plano as a control.

If the No. 14A net is in minus and No. 15A is in esophoria, that finding of the two which shows the least stimulation is checked as the higher finding and its mate is thereby checked low. For the purpose of determining the least stimulative test we consider minus one diopter is equivalent to six diopters of esophoria (-1.00 = 6 eso).

For example:

#14A Net -1.50 D. (low)	#14A Net -0.50 D. (high)
# 15A 2 esophoria (high)	# 15A 5 esophoria (low)
(2/6=0.33)	(5/6=0.82)

For the calculations of the accommodative tests that are to be checked, we utilize the sphere associated with the dominant eye. For this purpose, the tests are always written in minus cylinder form and the associated cylinder is ignored.

The following case fragments indicate the checking of the accommodative tests:

Case 1	Case 2 (Patient wears minus glasses)
# 4 +1.00 D. low	# 4 +0.25 D. high
# 5 +2.00 D. (net +1.25) high	# 5 +1.00 D. (net 0.25) not checked
# 6 +1.75 D. (net 1.50) high	# 6 +0.50 D. (net 0.25) not checked
# 7 +1.25 D.	# 7 -0.50 D.
# 14A +2.50 D. (net 1.50) high	# 14A +1.00 D. (net plano) high
# 15A 6 exo (lag 1.00) low	# 15A 9 exo (lag 1.00) low*
# 19 6.00 D.	# 19 3.00 D.

*In this same case if the patient had never worn glasses, it would be checked as follows:

#14A +1.00 D. (net plano) high
15A 9 exo (lag 1.00) high

We have now completed all of the rules for the checking of the various optometric tests. To develop your skill in this ability check the following complete cases:

Case 1		Case 2		Case 3	
#3	1 eso	#3	½ exo	#3	ortho
#13A	2 exo	#13A	15 exo	#13A	5 exo
#4	+1.00	#4	plano	#4	+0.75
#5	+2.00	#5	+0.75	#5	+1.75
#6	+1.75	#6	+0.25	#6	+2.00
#7	+1.00	#7	+0.25	#7	+0.50
#8	ortho	#8	1 exo	#8	½ exo
#9	8	#9	13	#9	4
#10	30/24	#10	20/10	#10	22/15
#11	9/5	#11	7/5	#11	7/2
#13B	4 exo	#13B	14 exo	#13B	5 exo
#14A	+2.00	#14A	plano	#14A	+2.75
#15A	6 exo	#15A	15 exo	#15A	6 exo
#14B	+1.75	#14B	-0.50	#14B	+2.25
#15B	5 exo	#15B	14 exo	#15B	6 exo
#16A	25	#16A	19	#16A	17
#16B	35/25	#16B	23/18	#16B	20/7
#17A	19	#17A	15	#17A	11
#17B	23/4	#17B	25/19	#17B	23/19
#19	8.50	#19	4.00	#19	6.00
#20	-4.50	#20	-3.00	#20	-1.50
#21	+2.25	#21	+2.50	#21	+2.75

Chaining

The previous process of checking has indicated the significance of certain visual tests. However, it is difficult to visualize the relationships between these various tests by merely observing these various high and low designations. Chaining was developed so that relationships between these various high and low designations could more easily be ascertained. Chaining is the process of arranging the significant findings in relationship to a horizontal median line. Those tests which have been checked high are placed above the median line, and those tests which have been checked low are placed below the median line. Those tests which are equal to their respective values, the negative tests, are placed on the median line.

Two different groupings of these significant tests are made: the pathological chain and the psycho-physiological chain. The pathological chain groups those findings which clinical experience indicates the possibility of pathology. All of the tests which have been checked are placed in the psycho-physiological chain.

The following tests are placed in the pathological chain if they are low:

#3 if low
#8 if low
#13B if low
#4 if low
#10 and #11 if both are low
#16B and #17B if both are low

The greater the number of these tests which are present in the pathological chain, the greater the probability of the presence of pathology. If a chain contained:

____
#3 - #8 - #13B - #4 - #10 - #11 - #16B - #17B

we would be more concerned of the possibility of pathology than if the pathology chain contained:

____
#3

In addition to the number of test findings that have been placed in the pathology chain as an indication of the possibility of pathology, one must also consider the significance of the checking, i.e., the lower the magnitude of a particular test finding is in relationship to its expected value, the greater the reliability that the particular test finding is low.

#4 plano (low)	#4 plano (low)
#7 +0.25 D.	#7 +0.75 D.

In these two examples the #4 finding is low in each case and yet, in making our diagnostic decision, we would consider the second case as having greater significance in the pathological chain.

In the physiological chain, we place all of the tests which have been checked. The only exception to this is when we have both ductions at either farpoint, (#10 and #11) or at nearpoint (#16B and #17B) checked low. In these instances we chain the low-low finding only. If at any time we have both ductions at far or at near equally low so that a low- low designation cannot be determined, we place both ductions of the pair in the chain. The greater the number of low test findings in our chain the greater the probability of a serious accommodative-convergence interference. Thus, compare the following two examples of psycho-physiological chains:

(1) 4-5-6-8-9-10-11-13B-14A-16B-17B
———————————————
3- 15A

(2) 15A
———————————————
3-4-5-6-8-9-10-13B-14A-17B

The second example indicates the greater possibility of a serious accommodative-convergence interference than the first example.

From the three complete cases previously given, we would obtain the following chains:

Case 1:

Pathology chain
———————————————
3-8-13B

Physiological chain 5-6-10-11 16B
———————————————14A-15A———————————————
3-8-13B 17B

Case 2:

Pathology chain
———————————————
4-

Physiological chain 8-9-10 13B-15A-16B-17B
——3———————————————6———————————————
4-5-11 14A

Case 3:

Pathology chain
———————————————
3-13B

Physiological chain 4-5-6-10- 14A-17B
——8———————————————
3-9-11-13B-15A-16B

Informative Sequence:

The informative sequence is a shorthand description of the visual problem. The findings which go into the informative sequence are selected from the psycho- physiological chain and from the original case data.

The informative sequence consists of six sections:

(a) the basic finding (#7)
(b) the case typing
(c) the intermediate finding (#6)
(d) the nearpoint finding (#14A and #15A relationship)
(e) the equilibrium pattern (#16A, #17A, #20 and #21)
(f) the amplitude.

These six sections of the informative sequence are arranged on a horizontal line.

(a) The Basic Finding. The position of the No.7 finding on the horizontal control line indicates whether the case is in hyperopia, emmetropia or myopia. If the basic finding is in plus, it is placed above the line, followed by a plus sign; if it is in minus, it is placed below the line, followed by a minus sign; if it is in plano it is placed on the line. Thus, we have:

7+ (above the line)	hyperope
—7— (on the line)	emmetrope
7- (below the line)	myope

(b) The Case Typing. The case typing is a pattern of certain analytical tests. The pattern or case type indicates two things;

(1) the way lenses will be accepted

(2) the direction that the corrective procedures will be given.

The basic case typings are:

A Type $\frac{\quad}{4\text{-}11\text{-}13B\text{-}17B}$

B1 Type $\frac{5}{9\text{-}11\text{-}16B}$

B2 Type $\frac{5}{9\text{-}11\text{-}17B}$

C Type $\frac{15A}{5\text{-}10\text{-}16B}$

The A-type and the C-type have no deviation in the pattern of the findings as given. However, there will often be variations in the pattern of the findings for the B1- and B2-types. In B typings, all variations in the positions of Nos. 5, 9, 10,11, 16B, and 17B must be shown.

In the informative sequence the case typing is always enclosed in parenthesis.

We can never have an A-typing by itself; it will always be in combination with a B2-typing. Whenever the pattern of the case reveals an A-typing, additional information must be obtained in order to ascertain whether it is a true A-typing or whether it is merely an artifact of a B2.

This valuable additional information can be obtained from the case history, ophthalmoscopy, and perimetric field study. In this way a differential diagnosis can be made. If true toxicity is indicated, the patient must be referred for dental and/or medical attention.

(c) The intermediate finding (#6) is placed above, below, or on the line, depending upon its position in the psycho-physiological chain. Thus:

6 (above the line)	More plus at intermediate distance than at far.
6 (on the line)	Same amount of plus at intermediate distance as at far.
6 (below the line)	Less plus at intermediate distance than at far.

(d) The nearpoint finding is the relationship between the dissociated cross cylinder test (#14A) and its associated phoria test (#15A). These two tests are placed in the informative sequence in the same relationship as found in the psycho-physiological chain. We may have:

$\frac{14A}{15A}$ More plus at near than at far.

$\underline{14A\text{-}15A}$

Same amount of plus at near as at far.

$\frac{15A}{14A}$ Less plus at near than at far.

(e) The pattern of the equilibrium findings considers: No. 16A (positive relative convergence), No. 17A (negative relative convergence), No. 20 (positive relative accommodation), and No.21 (negative relative accommodation).

The pattern of these tests is a guide as to whether or not the lens power found in the subjective at far (#7) and the cross-cylinder tests at near (#14A) will create a new problem for the patient.

The equilibrium tests have no expected value for purposes of comparison. Instead we compare Nos. 16A and 17A to each other. The test having the highest numerical value becomes the high value, and its companion is the low finding. In a similar manner we compare No. 20 to 21. The finding with the highest numerical value once more becomes the higher finding, and its mate the low finding.

The relationship of 16A and 17A to each other, and 20 and 21 to each other, are taken directly from the data of the analytical examination. They are recorded above or below the line according to their numerical relationship and separated by hyphens to maintain them as a unit.

If the test for 16A or 17A ended in a "break before the blur" as shown by an "X" in the analytical examination form, the amount of the blur is estimated from the break finding, although it must be realized that this is an approximation.

If 16A and 17A are equal in amounts, they are both placed above the line if they are greater than 15 prism diopters; they are placed on the line if they are equal to 15 prism diopters; and are placed under the line if they are less than 15 prism diopters.

If tests No. 20 and 21 are equal consider their relative values:

- If their values are greater than two diopters, then they are both placed above the line;
- If their values are less than two diopters they are placed below the line;
- If their values are equal to two diopters, they are placed on the line.

The patterning of the equilibrium tests for the informative sequence is illustrated by the following case fragments:

#16A	20	#16A	14	#16A	10	#16A	15
#17A	15	#17A	20	#17A	10	#17A	10
#20	-1.75	#20	-3.00	#20	-2.00	#20	-4.50
#21	+1.75	#21	+2.00	#21	+3.00	#21	+2.50

$$\frac{16A}{17A\text{-}20\text{-}21} \qquad \frac{17A\text{-}20}{16A\text{-}21} \qquad \frac{21}{16A\text{-}17A\text{-}20} \qquad \frac{16A\text{-}20}{7A\text{-}21}$$

If the equilibrium pattern for a B-type is $\frac{16A - 21}{17A - 20}$, it indicates that the control lens has not created any additional problem, and would be in an acceptable range. If however, a reversal in this pattern for a B-type case is found, it is advisable to be more conservative in the plus lenses which are prescribed.

(f) <u>The amplitude of accommodation</u>. If the amplitude of accommodation (#19) is more than five diopters, it is placed above the line; if its value is less than five diopters, it is placed below the line; if the amplitude is equal to five diopters, it is placed on the line. Thus, we may have:

19 (above the line)	Sufficient amplitude present for nearpoint work at sixteen inches.
–19– (on the line)	Minimum amplitude for sixteen inch work.
19 (below the line)	Amplitude insufficient for sustained activity at sixteen inches.

A complete informative sequence might be as follows:

	(a)	(b)	(c)	(d)	(e)	(f)
Above the line	7+	5	6	14A	16A-21	19
Below the line	9-11-16B			15A	17A-20	

In shorthand notation the informative sequence is telling us, "I have a patient who is hyperopic at far; the lens magnitude of this hyperopia is accepted at far and at near; he is a greater hyperope at the intermediate distance than at far; he is a greater hyperope at near than at far; the plus of the subjective does not violate the habitual pattern, and we have sufficient amplitude of accommodation for near-point work."

Typing and Deterioration of the Case

It soon became obvious from the study of case records that very few patients exhibited a typical informative sequence. There seemed to be certain shifts in typical findings with the seriousness (or rigidity) of the case.

- The first change upon the impact of visual stress is the lowering of the net dissociated cross-cylinder test at near (#14A).
- The second type of change noticed is the reversal in the equilibrium findings (#16A, 17A, 20, 21).
- The third type of change is the lowering of the amplitude of accommodation for the non-presbyope.
- The fourth shift is the base-out duction at far becoming low, or the low-low finding.
- The final reaction to visual stress is the lowering of the net dynamic retinoscopy test at 20 inches (#5).

These shifts in findings due to stress occur only for the accommodative type cases and their variations. These shifts in findings, due to stress, have been named *deteriorations*. We recognize seven basic shifts, or deteriorations, in the accommodative type cases.. The sequence in deteriorations in the examples that follow are for B1 hyperopic cases. A similar sequence could be constructed for B2 hyperopic cases by substituting the 17B for the 16B.

Case	Sequence (above line / below line)	
B-1 - 1 (Simple)	7 + (5) 6 14A 16A-21 19 9-11-16B 15A 17A-20	(lens application)
B-1 - 2	7 + (5) 6 14A 16A-21 19 9-11-16B 17A-20	(lens application)
B-1 - 3	7 + (5) 6 15A 16A-21 19 9-11-16B 14A 17A-20	(lens application) (visual training)
B-1 - 4	7 + (5) 6 15A 16A-20 19 9-11-16B 14A 17A-21	(lenses and visual training)
B-1 - 5	7 + (5) 6 15A 16A-20 9-10-16B 14A 17A-21 19	(lenses and visual training)
B-1 - 7	7 + ( ) 6 15A 16A-20 9-5-10-16B 14A 17A-21 19	(visual training)

When we attempt to place all accommodative interference cases (B-types) into one of seven groups, it is obvious that there may be considerable variation in any single group. The higher the deterioration, the greater the variation we may have in any one group. Therefore, in determining the deterioration, it is best to look for the *characteristic* change for each group. The characteristic changes for each group are:

B1 - 7	#5 low
B1 - 6	# 10 low or low-low
B1 - 5	#19 less than 5.00 D.
B1 - 4	Reversal in equilibrium findings $\frac{17A}{16A}$ or $\frac{20}{21}$ or both.
B1 - 3	#15A/#14A
B1 - 2	#14A/#15A (cross cylinder net equal to #7)
B1 - 1	#14A/#15A

As stated, the same sequence can be written for the B2 cases. To illustrate how the informative sequence can look different and yet be of the same deterioration, the following variations in a B2-4 are given:

Sequence (above line / below line)
7 + 5 17A-21 19 9-11-17B 6 14A-15A 16A-20
7 + 5 6 15A 17A-20 19 9-11-17B 14A 16A-21

7+ 5 14A 16A-20 19
9-11-17B 6 15A 17A-21

When you look for the characteristic change for the deterioration, you will note that in each instance we have a reversal in the equilibrium pattern. This places the case in the 4th deterioration. In order to spot the proper deterioration, look for the lowest stage first, and then go down the sequence from seventh stage to first stage.

The A-type and the C-type *do not have any deteriorated changes.* All A-type cases will have a multiple case type such as AB2-deteriorated case.

A characteristic informative sequence for an A-type case might be:

7+ (5) 6 14A 16A-21 19
(4-11-13B-17B) (9-11-17B) 15A 17A-20

This case would be classified as an AB2-1 or an AB2-Simple.

Construct the informative sequence and determine the case typing and deterioration of the case given on the following page.

The Differential Diagnosis of a C-Type case:

Since the B-type case may have certain deteriorations that very closely simulate a C-type case, it becomes important that we can make a differential diagnosis. The informative sequence for a C-Type case is:

7+ 15A 6 15A 17A-20 19
5-10-16B 14A 16A-21

Compare the above with a B1-7 case:

7+ 6 15A 16A-20
5-9-10-16B 14A 17A-21 19

Case 1

4-5	10	13b	14A	17B
3	6-8-9	11	15A	16B

#7	+1.00
#16A	18
#17A	10
#20	-2.00
#21	+2.50
#19	+7.00

Inf. Seq. 7 + (5) 14A 16A-21 19
(9-11-16B) 6 15A 17A-20

- 7: My patient is a hyperope
- (5)/(9-11-16B): of a B1 type full plus acceptted at all points
- 6: Greater hyperope at far than at 40 inches
- 14A/15A: Greater hyperope at far than at 40 inches
- 16A-21/17A-20: Subjective does not violate the habitual pattern
- 19: Type and deter. B1-1
- We have sufficient amplitude for 16-inch work

The differential diagnosis depends upon eight points, which must be carefully considered:

1. In a C-type case the typing must be exactly: 15A/5-10-16B.
2. In a C-type case the equilibrium pattern must not vary from 17A-20/16A-21.
3. In a C-type case the amplitude must be five diopters or higher.
4. In a C-type case the true adduction at far must be equal to its expected value or higher.
5. High exophoria is usually present at both far and near in a C-type case.
6. The binocular amplitude of accommodation is higher than the monocular amplitude for a C-type case. The converse is true for the B-type case.
7. The visual skills show the wide concessions which have been made in the C-type case. We can expect to find extensive suppressions, poor fusion and low stereopsis in these C-type cases.
8. The C-type case will have a case history revealing severe complaints. The patient will usually exhibit several pairs of glasses without obtaining comfort with any of them.

From the following case data determine whether this case is a B- or a C-type:

#3	ortho		
#13A	7 esophoria	#14A	-0.25 D.
#4	plano	#15A	1 esophoria
#5	+1.50 D.	#16A	X
#7	+0.25 D.	#16B	24/16
#8	1 esophoria	#17A	X
#9	15	#17B	28/18
#10	16/2	#19	6.50 (O.D., O.S., O.U.)
#11	8/4	#20	-3.25 D.
#13B	7 esophoria	#21	+2.75

The No. 14B Net:

The fused cross cylinder finding at near (No.14B) must be corrected for the influence of the associated convergence as measured by the No. 15B phoria.

Net 14B = Gross 14B - Lag

The lag is determined by converting the exophoria found in the 15B phoria test into its equivalent lens (accommodative) diopters by dividing by *nine.* That is, nine diopters of exophoria is equivalent to one lens diopter. If the associated exophoria exceeds 15 prism diopters, we use 1.75 diopters as the maximum lag. All calculations for the lag are rounded off to the nearest quarter of diopter.

Whenever the 15B phoria is orthophoria or in esophoria, the 14B gross becomes the net finding: The lag in this case is zero.

If the amplitude of accommodation is less than five diopters, the 15B lag is reduced. There is a proportionately reduced lag since the resultant effect of convergence upon accommodation is lessened (see the modification decimal table for 14A).

The following case fragments indicate the calculation of the No. 14B net:

#14B +1.00D.	#14B +2.00	#14B -1.00
#15B 6Exo	#15B 9 Exo	#15B 2 Exo
#19 5.00 D.	#19 4.00 D.	#19 6.00 D.
Lag: 6/9 = 0.75	Lag: 9/9 X 4/5 = 0.75	Lag: 2/9 = 0.25
14B Net: +0.25	14B Net: +1.25	14B Net: -1.25

The Equilibrium Pattern:

The equilibrium tests are the four blur out tests measured at nearpoint. The equilibrium pattern is determined by comparing the numerical values of

No. 16A directly with that of No. 17A; and comparing No. 20 directly with No. 21 (ignoring signs).

The equilibrium findings are a guide that indicate whether or not the subjective at far, and the net cross-cylinder tests at near, will create a new visual interference.

If the control lens used in taking the equilibrium findings was the No.7, fill in the first column (through #7) with the findings taken from the case examination. If the equilibrium findings were taken through some other control lens, use the proper column on the visual analysis form to record your test amounts.

If a blur finding is recorded as "X" in the case examination, indicating that the patient did not experience a blur, record these findings with the amount of the *break* in parentheses to the right of it. For example:

	#16A X	#16A 21
	#16B 22/18	#16B 22/18
	#17A 23	#17A X
	#17B 26/9	#17B 15/13
	$\frac{17A}{16A}$	$\frac{16A}{17A}$
		#16A 21
recorded as:	#16A X (22)	#17A X (15)
	#17A 23	

To compute the corrected values for the equilibrium tests if taken through other lens powers (other controls), we utilize an ACA ratio of 4:1 for our calculations. That is, four prism diopters of convergence is equivalent to one lens diopter. If the equilibrium tests are taken through one-quarter of a diopter (0.25) diopter more plus, we would expect #16A to decrease 1 prism diopter, #17A to increase 1 prism diopter, #20 to increase one-quarter of a diopter, and #21 to decrease one-quarter of a diopter.

After arriving at the numerical amounts for Nos. 16A, 17A, 20 and 21, the pattern relationship of the findings should be recorded, rather than any numerical amount. This can be done by stating that the test is high, low, or even, whichever fits the existing data. The following data illustrates the determination of the equilibrium:

#7 +2.25
#14A net +2.75
Hab. Rx. +2.00
Control: #7
#16A 26
#17A 14
#20 -1.75
#21 +2.50

	(+2.25) #7	(2.75) #14A	(2.00) hab.
#16A	26	24	27
#17A	14	16	13
#20	-1.75	-2.25	-1.50
#21	+2.50	+2.00	+2.75

Habitual 16A-21
17A-20

14A net 16A-20
17A-21

#7 +1.75
#14A net +3.25
Hab. Rx. +1.00
Control: #14A net
#16A 28
#17A 16
#20 -2.00
#21 +3.00

	(+1.75) #7	(+3.25) #14A	(+1.00) hab.
#16A	...	28	37
#17A	...	16	7
#20	...	-2.00	(+0.25)*
#21	...	+3.00	+5.25

Habitual 16A-21
17A-20

14A net 16A-21
17A-20

The Acceptance or Rejection of the Near Nets (No. 14A and No. 14B):

To determine whether the near nets are acceptable, compare the pattern of the equilibrium tests of each cross-cylinder net with that of the habitual pattern. If they agree, the cross-cylinder nets are marked accepted. If the cross-cylinder net pattern differs from the habitual pattern, mark them rejected. For example:

Habitual Pattern: 16A-21
17A-20

If, 14A net pattern: 16A-21 accepted
17A-20

If, 14B net pattern: 16A-20 rejected
17A-21

If, 14A net pattern: 16A-20-21 accepted
17A

If, 14B net pattern: 17A-21 rejected
16A-20

At times when our control lens is considerably greater than the habitual lens being used, our calculations may give us a value which is impossible. If this occurs, we use parentheses to indicate the unusual magnitude. In this case, the calculations for the No. 20

test give us an impossible plus lens magnitude. This means that the value is so small in the minus direction that it has fallen into the plus range. Therefore, it is considered as very low in magnitude.

If however, at any time, the *habitual pattern* contains elements of the equilibrium pattern that are equal to each other, i.e., if 16A is equal to 17A, or if 20 is equal to 21, and if the near nets give a pattern in the direction of the typing, then it is marked as *accepted.* If under these conditions the near nets give a pattern which is not in the direction of the typing, it is to he marked as *rejected.* The phrase, "in the direction of the typing" refers to an equilibrium pattern of $\frac{16A - 21}{17A - 20}$ for a B-type case, and a pattern of $\frac{17A - 20}{16A - 2}$ for a C-type case.

For example:

Habitual pattern is $\frac{16A-20-21}{17A-20}$, case type is B.

If, 14A net pattern: $\frac{16A-21}{17A-20}$ accepted

If, 14B net pattern $\frac{17A-21}{16A-20}$ rejected

The Maximal Spherical Dioptric Acceptance at Near: (M.S.D.A.)

The "maximal spherical dioptric acceptance" at near, for ease of discussion, is abbreviated as M.S.D.A. The M.S.D.A. at near serves the same function as the basic finding (#7) serves at far. Similar to the basic finding (#7), the M.S.D.A. is the maximum plus that can be prescribed at near-point. Note the use of the word "maximum." Of course, less plus may be prescribed depending upon the associated typing.

1. If both the #14A and #14B nets are *accepted,* the highest value (the greatest plus or least minus) becomes the M.S.D.A.

2. The term "accepted" means that the lens powers do not reverse the arrangement of the blur-out tests (equilibrium findings) as set by the organism (habitual arrangement).

3. If #14A net is rejected and #14B net is accepted (or the converse), the M.S.D.A. becomes the maximum plus which does not reverse the habitual equilibrium pattern. For example:

    #14A net +1.00 D. rejected
    #14B net +0.25 D. accepted

We would normally select as our M.S.D.A. the #14B net; but since we strive for maximum plus acceptance at nearpoint, it is satisfactory to see if +0.75 or +0.50 will give us an equilibrium pattern which is acceptable. For example, if +0.75 is acceptable in the equilibrium pattern, then we would use this value for our M.S.D.A. Since, in the usual case, the #14A net and the #14B net are within 0.25 D. of each other, if one is rejected and the other one is accepted, the accepted cross-cylinder net becomes the M.S.D.A.

4. If neither #14A net nor the #14B net is accepted, that part of the finding which does not reverse the habitual pattern is considered as the M.S.D.A.

5. The M.S.D.A., in the case of a hyperope or an emmetrope, can never be less plus than plano regardless of the magnitude of the near nets. If the near nets are in minus projection, the M.S.D.A. becomes plano. For example:

#7	+1.00
#14A	+0.50 (Net -0.50)
#15A	6 exo (lag 1.00)
#14B	+0.25 (Net -0.50)
#15B	7 exo (lag 0.75)

   The M.S.D.A. is equal to plano

6. For the myope, the M.S.D.A. can never be in more minus than the basic finding (#7), regardless of the amount of minus in the near nets. For example:

#7	-1.00
#14A	-0.75 (Net -1.75)
#15A	6 exo (lag 1.00)
#14B	-1.00 (Net -1.50)
#15B	4.5 exo (lag 0.50)

   The M.S.D.A. is -1.00 D.

The following case fragments indicate the application of these rules:

(1) Case Data

#7 +0.25	Equilibrium	#16A	15
Habitual: Plano	Pattern	#17A	10
14A Net +1.00	Control: #7	#20	-2.50
14B Net +0.75		#21	+1.75

	+0.25	Plano	+1.00	+0.75
	#7	Hab	14A	14B
16A	15	16	12	13
17A	10	9	13	12
20	-2.50	-2.25	-3.25	-3.00
21	+1.75	+2.00	+1.00	+1.25

Habitual Pattern: 16A-20 / 17A-21

14A net pattern: 17A-20 / 16A-21 Rejected (reversal)

14B net pattern: 16A-20 / 17A-21 Accepted

Therefore, M.S.D.A. = 14B Net = +0.75

(2) Case Data

#7 Plano
Habitual: Plano
14A Net +1.00
14B Net +0.75

Equilibrium Pattern #16A 15
#17A 10
#20 -2.50
Control: #7 #21 +1.75

	Plano	Plano	+1.00	+0.75	+0.50
	#7	Hab	14A	14B	
16A	15	15	11	12	13
17A	10	10	14	13	12
20	-2.50	-2.50	-3.50	-3.25	-3.00
21	+1.75	+1.75	+0.75	+1.00	+1.25

Habitual Pattern: 16A-20 / 17A-21

14A Net Pattern: 17A-20 / 16A-21 Rejected (reversal)

14B Net Pattern: 17A-20 / 16A-21 Rejected (reversal)

Therefore, M.S.D.A. = +0.50

The Corrective Framework:

Up to this point we have determined the maximum dioptric acceptance at farpoint (#7) and the M.S.D.A. at near. These maximum plus lens values may or may not be accepted depending upon several factors which we will consider.

1. The corrective framework is the limitation of lens application. This refers to the maximum and minimum lens values that will be acceptable to the patient at far and at near.

2. The controlling factor in the acceptance or success of any lens application is its acceptance at near.

3. When a reduction of plus is demanded by the lens fitting program, the minimum cut is 0.25 D. and the maximum cut is 0.75 D. These magnitudes are based upon clinical observation that the maximum hyperopia that the patient could handle under stress conditions is 0.75 D. The lens value which will be prescribed for any particular case depends upon several additional factors:
   (a) How precise is the maintenance of concentration that is demanded of the patient?
   (b) The multiplicity of working distances demanded of the patient.
   (c) Previous ocular history.
   (d) Chief complaint.
   (e) Organizational status of the case.
   (f) Personality factors--nervous or phlegmatic.
   (g) The social-economic pressures upon the individual.
   (h) Professional judgment: what is your approach to this problem? Prevention, remediation or merely prosthetic.

4. A near net of minus for a patient who is hyperopic at far is called *minus projection.* It is *not* myopia at near. It is an emmetrope at near with minus overtones. It signifies a complete rejection of plus at near. It is an active state of inhibition, and it is highly indicative of an extended visual problem. Minus lenses are contra-indicated, and plus lenses are rejected. Solving the problem with lens application alone cannot be accomplished with any assurance of success.

5. A *myope* is an individual who requires concave lenses (minus) to achieve standard acuity at any point; he is a myope at that point. If a minus lens is necessary to restore standard acuity at far, but the patient has standard acuity at near without any minus lenses, he is a myope at far and not a myope at near. A myopic individual at farpoint, may possess at nearpoint the conditions of hyperopia, emmetropia, minus projection, minus at near, or myopia at near.

6. *Emmetropia* means there is no accommodation free of association with convergence at the point where the measurement is being made. Emmetropia can be found at near, as well as at far. If the net at near is plano or in minus projection, it can be said that the patient is emmetropic at near provided he has standard acuity at near without lenses.

7. Whenever emmetropia is found at far, or near, or both distances, that finding alone is indicative of a visual problem that sooner or later will need plus lenses; and the sooner the better. The presence of emmetropia is not a sign of perfection, but rather an indication that all of the focus range that was free of convergence has been used up under conditions of visual stress. Immediate care is needed to prevent the progression into greater difficulty.

8. Care is required in prescribing plus for "C-type" cases. If occupational demands are for fine concentrated vision, the maximum cut in plus spheres must be made (0.75 D). However, if visual demands are fairly gross, only the minimum cut in plus spheres may be given (0.25 D.).

9. Clinical experience has shown that the student with 20/40 Snellen acuity can meet all of the demands of the classroom for farpoint vision. Therefore, as far as his functional needs are concerned, that amount of minus sphere at far which gives the student 20/40 Snellen acuity is the maximum plus (least minus) that need be prescribed.

10. When *duo focal* lenses are used on a myopic student, they should be set with the top of the segment at about the lower margin of the pupil.

11. Lens limiting factors are the subjective at far and the net cross-cylinder tests at near. They set a maximum limitation on the plus lens power that will be accepted by that individual at these separate distances.

12. Case typings are simply lens fitting procedures based upon the duction pattern.

    (a) $\overline{11 - 16B}$ full plus accepted at far and at near.

    (b) $\overline{11 - 17B}$ full plus accepted at near, cut plus at far.

    (c) $\overline{10 - 16B, 17B}$ cut plus at both far and near.

13. If the prescriptive near net (M.S.D.A.) is less plus than the basic subjective finding (#7), then any single vision lens prescribed for *constant wear* must not exceed the M.S.D.A. This applies no matter what program of lens fitting is indicated by the duction pattern or case type,

14. Establishing the corrective framework for the hyperopic or emmetropic case:

Far:	(1)	$\overline{\text{11-16B}}$	Not Over: #7 Not Under: #7
	(2)	$\overline{\text{10-16B}}$, 17B	Not Over: #7 - 0.25 D.
		$\overline{\text{11-17B}}$	Not Under: #7 - 0.75 D.
Near:	(1)	$\overline{\text{11 - 16B, 17B}}$	Not Over: M.S.D.A. Not Under: M.S.D.A.
	(2)	$\overline{\text{0 - 16B, 17B}}$	Not Over: M.S.D.A. -0.25 D. Not Under: M.S.D.A. -0.75 D.

In the hyperopic or emmetropic case, the duction pattern cannot require that the plus be reduced to the point that the case goes into minus. For example:

	Corrective Framework
#7 +0.50 D. M.S.D.A. Plano	Far: Not Over: +0.25 D. Not Under: plano
Duction pattern: $\overline{\text{11 - 17B}}$	Near: Not Over: plano Not Under: plano

#7 +0.25 D. M.S.D.A. +0.50 D. Far:	*Corrective Framework* Far: Not Over: plano Not Under: plano
Duction pattern: $\overline{\text{10 - 17B}}$	Near: Not Over: +0.25 D. Not Under: plano

15. Establishing the corrective framework for the myopic case:

Far:	(1)	$\overline{\text{11 - 16B}}$	Not Over: #7 (20/40 V.A.) Not Under: #7 (20/20 V.A.)
	(2)	$\overline{\text{10- 16B, 17B}}$	Not Over: #7 (20/20 V.A.)
		$\overline{\text{11 - 17B}}$	Not Under: #7A (Best V.A.)
Near:	(1)	All case typings	Not Over: M.S.D.A. Not Under: M.S.D.A.

Note: In the myopic case, more minus cannot be prescribed at near than at far. If the cross-cylinder nets are in greater minus than the subjective test at far (#7), the M.S.D.A. becomes the same amount of minus as the subjective at far (#7).

For example:

#7 -0.50 D. 20/40 V.A.	*Corrective Framework*
-0.75 D. 20/20 V.A.	Far: Not Over: -0.50 D.
-1.25 D. 20/15 V.A.	Not Under: -0.75 D.
M.S.D.A. plano	Near: Not Over: plano
Duction pattern: 11 - 16B	Not Under: plano

#7 -0.50 D. 20/40 V.A.	*Corrective Framework*
-1.00 D. 20/20 V.A.	Far: Not Over: -1.00 D.
-1.50 D. 20/10 V.A.	Not Under: -1.50 D.
Cross Cylinder Net: -2.00 D.	Near: Not Over: -1.00 D.
Duction pattern: 10 - 17B	Not Under: -1.00 D.
M.S.D.A.: -1.00 D.	

The Ten Laws of Lens Application

1. Never prescribe a lens greater than the amount of accommodation free of association with convergence. This is a basic premise of functional optometry.
   If the lens values we prescribe do not aggravate the existing problem, they will be acceptable. This lens value is the subjective at far. Thus, if the patient is a one-diopter hyperope without a previous correction, when looking at far he must accommodate one diopter without making a change in convergence. He has learned, or perhaps maturationally developed, a certain freedom between the patterns of accommodation and convergence equal to his refractive error. The mechanistically minded will say, "He has created fusional divergence at far equal in amount to the accommodative-convergence stimulated by the accommodative act while looking at far." We are therefore, in agreement, since the fusional convergence (if such an entity exists) is a learned pattern in the central nervous system. If the hyperope has not learned an adequate inhibition pattern between these two systems, he will have diplopia when he looks at far.

2. Never prescribe a single vision lens for constant wear that is greater than the near nets.

Since the great majority of our visual problems arise from near-point stress, the guiding lens value is that which can be worn at near-point. The maximum lens values at near are the cross-cylinder nets. This is the hyperopia at near which is free of association with convergence at near. Therefore, if we have a case in which the subjective at far is +1.00 D. spheres, but the net cross-cylinder is only +0.50 D. sphere, then the lesser plus is the value that can be prescribed for constant wear.

3. When base-out-to-break-and-recovery at far (#10) and base-out-to-break-and-recovery at near (#16) are both low, *cut plus at all points.* This is known as the effect of a "C-typing."

4. When base-in-to-break-and-recovery at far (#11) and base-out-to-break-and-recovery at near (#16B) are both low, *full plus is acceptable at all points.* This is known as the effect of a "B1-typing."

5. When base-in-to-break-and-recovery at far (#11) and base-in-to-break-and-recovery at near (#l7B) are both low, *full plus is acceptable at near; cut plus for far.* This is known as the effect of a "B2-typing."

6. When the base-out break and recovery at far (#10) and base-in to break and recovery at near (#17B) are both low, cut plus at all points. This is a B2-6 typing.

   Whenever we find the duction pattern of both #10 and #17B low, we are dealing with a highly deteriorated B-type pattern, and it is doubtful that full plus will be accepted at farpoint. A spatial inversion has occurred with #10 becoming the low duction at far rather than #11. Such change demands that less plus be used at far.

7. Never prescribe a lens which creates a new interference between the patterns of accommodation and convergence.

   If the tentative prescription creates a change in the phoria values of more than two diopters, the amount of plus should be reduced by 0.25 diopter. For example, the habitual phoria at near (#13A) is 4 exophoria, tentative near Rx is +1.00, and the resultant induced nearpoint phoria (#13B) is 8 exophoria. It is better not to prescribe more than +0.75 diopters for nearpoint wear. From a lens fitting standpoint, it is best not to make changes in gross amounts when the visual pattern of the patient is too responsive to test lenses.

8. Never prescribe a lens that reverses the equilibrium pattern findings (blur-out tests at near).

   The blur findings measure the ability of the organism to inhibit one component of the visual system while we probe the other component. Therefore, the relative relationship between these blur findings indicates the direction in which the greatest degree of flexibility exists. If the lenses should change this relationship, visual difficulty would ensue.

9. Only that part of the near nets that is considered "acceptable" according to the balance in the equilibrium findings can be prescribed at near. It becomes the maximal acceptance.

   If the net values for the dissociated cross-cylinder test (14A) and the fused cross-cylinder test (14B) create a reversal in the habitual pattern of the equilibrium findings, then that portion of the nets which does not give this reversal becomes "acceptable" at near.

10. All of these laws are based on a change in posture of the focusing mechanism by a lens.

The Problem of Anisometropia

In determining the corrective framework for the case, if we have no anisometropia or if the anisometropia is the same at far and at near, we have no problem in arriving at the lens value for the non-dominant eye.

For example:	#4	+0.25	
		+0.50	
	#7	+0.25	We have 0.25 diopter of anisometropia
		+0.50	with the maximum plus before
	M.S.D.A.	+1.00	the left eye.
		+1.25	

But what if the amount of anisometropia is highly variable, what values would we use in our corrective framework?

For example:	#4	+0.25
		+0.50
	#7	+0.50
		+0.50
	M.S.D.A.	+0.75
		+0.50

For this type of case some professional judgment must be exercised. When the indicated anisometropia is highly variable, consider these general rules:

1. If the patient has never worn a previous correction and is of school age, the minimum amount of anisometropia should be prescribed.

2. If the nearpoint anisometropia disagrees with the farpoint anisometropia, maximum attention should be paid to the nearpoint data since visual problems stem from this activity. To verify nearpoint anisometropia (besides using #5 and #14A), repeat the negative relative accommodation test at near (#21) under monocular conditions.

3. If the patient is wearing an anisometropic correction, and some of the values I have determined agree with the habitual correction, this would aid in prescribing the amount of anisometropia.

4. The amount of anisometropic correction to be prescribed is also a function of the amount of associated sphere. For example:

(1)	(2)
#7 plano	#7 +1.50
+0.25	+1.75

Case (1) The anisometropia may be a factor in the analysis.

Case (2) It is doubtful that the 0.25 diopter difference has any optical meaning.

5. The older the patient, the less change should be made in the habitual anisometropic correction. This can be violated if the patient is to have visual training.

Old Rx:	-1.00
	+1.75
Corrective Framework	+1.00
	+3.00

It would be well to hedge on the initial Rx and prescribe only one-half of the change and the remaining portion in six months.

The Consideration of The Embeddeness of The Case.

Just as any behavior pattern can be organized or integrated at a higher level of performance, the visual pattern of a particular patient may be at a poorly organized or "non-embedded" stage. Also, in some cases the visual pattern may be at an organized, or "embedded" stage. A normal two-legged individual may have a poor ability for balance on a narrow board while another person may have excellent balance ability. In a certain manner we may say that the first individual, in spite of the presence of a good total behavior pattern, has a poor ability for balance, i.e. it is poorly organized, or "non-embedded". In the case of the second individual, who also has a good total behavior pattern, we have an individual with excellent balance, i.e. this skill is well organized, or "embedded". In the same way we may have a one-legged individual who has no balancing ability, but another handicapped individual may have considerable balancing ability. Again, in spite of the constriction in total behavior due to the loss of a limb, one individual has no ability to balance (non-embedded), while the second individual has developed considerable ability for balance (embedded). At any level of total behavior we may have an individual with an embedded pattern, or a non-embedded, pattern of behavior.

Similarly, at any level of the visual pattern we may have a well organized pattern (embedded) or a poorly organized pattern (non-embedded). Perhaps we can think of the stages of deterioration (B-type case) as the type of visual space volume available to the individual. We are not considering distance (or visual acuity) but operational volume. In this context, the B1-1 deterioration patient has a greater operational space volume than a B1-7 deterioration. Yet within these restrictions in visual pattern, one person can embed his performance and thereby gain efficiency in spite of the visual deterioration.

Typically the embedded pattern resists change, and therefore, we must prescribe the minimum plus possible. However, if the case has a non-embedded pattern, it is constantly in a state of change, and maximum plus may be used. The embedded case will usually have few symptoms of discomfort, while the non-embedded case will usually have many subjective symptoms for inventory. Clinical research has revealed that the following visual findings shift when a binocular pattern that is well integrated is subjected to a stress environment or is given prolonged monocular visual training, i.e., #4, #7, #9, #10, #11, #14A, #14B, #16B (#17B for the B2-case), #19 and #20.

The Syndrome of the embedded Case	**The Syndrome of the non-embedded Case**
1. #4 equal to or greater than #7 in plus.	1. #4 lower than #7 in plus.
2. #9 up to its mean value or higher.	2. #9 excessively low; except in myopia when #9 will be high.
3. #10 break low, but recovery above or equal to its mean.	3. #10 recovery excessively low.
4. #11 break and recovery up; recovery to mean or higher	4. #11 break and recovery excessively low.
5. #14B net equal to or in excess of. #14A net	5. #14B net lower than the #14A net.
6. #16B break lower; the recovery at mean or higher.	6. #16B recovery excessively low (B2-case; #17B recovery low).
7. #19 and #20 are not both low; one high and the other low.	7. #19 and #20 both excessively low.

A symptom is classified as non-embedded when its numerical value is at least three prism diopters or more from its expected value, or when the accommodative value differs from the expected by 0.50 D. or more.

Case examples:

1.	#4 +1.00 D. #7 +1.00 D. *embedded*	#4 +0.75 D. #7 +1.00 D. *embedded*	#4 +0.50 D. #7 +1.00 D. *non-embedded*
2.	#9 10 *embedded*	#9 8 *embedded*	#9 4 *non-embedded*

3. The recovery magnitude is the key symptom for classification. The break magnitude is the secondary factor. If the #10 break is at the mean level or lower, but the recovery is three diopters less than its expected value, then the finding is designated as *non-embedded.*

#10 18/9 *embedded*	#10 19/8 *embedded*	#10 17/5 *non-embedded*

4. If the break is excessively low (three diopters low), and the recovery is less than normal, we consider the #11 finding as being non-embedded.

#11 9/5 *embedded*	#11 9/3 *embedded*	#11 6/3 *non-embedded*	#11 6/5 *embedded*

5.

#14A+1.00 D. #14B+1.00 D. *embedded*	#14A +1.00 D. #14B +0.75 D. *embedded*	#14A +1.00 D. #14B +0.50 D. *non-embedded*

6. For non-embeddedness, the #16B break is not excessively low, but the recovery is excessively low. Whereas for the embedded condition, the

#16B break is excessively low with the recovery at about its mean value or better.

	#16B 21/11	#16B 15/5	#16B 18/12
	non-embedded	*non-embedded**	*embedded*
7.	#19 5.00 D.	#19 3.00 D.	#19 6.00 D.
	#20 -5.00	#20 -1.00	#19 -1.50
	embedded	*non-embedded*	*embedded*

It is rare to find a case in which all of the symptoms that indicate either an embedded (structured) or a non-embedded (disorganized) pattern are present. As a rule, whenever five or more of the symptoms indicate that a particular syndrome is present, we diagnose the case as having that particular syndrome. For example:

(1)

5 symptoms indicate non-embeddedness
2 symptoms indicate embeddedness
Visual pattern is judged as being non-embedded

(2)

4 symptoms indicate non-embeddedness
3 symptoms indicate embeddedness
Visual pattern status is indefinite

(3)

3 symptoms indicate non-embeddness
4 symptoms indicate embeddedness
Visual pattern status is indefinite

(4)

2 symptoms indicate non-embeddness
5 symptoms indicate embeddedness
Visual pattern is judged as being embedded

* Where both the break and recovery are excessively low we consider the finding as being non-embedded.

The following case fragments indicate the method of determining the embeddedness of the visual pattern:

Visual pattern exhibiting complete non-embeddedness		Visual pattern exhibiting complete embeddedness	
#4	-0.50 D.	#4	plano
#5	+1.25 D.	#5	+2.00 D.
#7	plano	#7	plano
#9	4	#9	7
#10	19/15	#10	19/10
#11	5/1	#11	9/4
#14A	Net +1.00	#14A	Net +1.00
#14B	Net +0.50	#14B	Net +1.00
#16B	20/10	#16B	20/17
#17B	22/10	#17B	24/20
#19	5.00 D.	#19	8.00 D.
#20	-1.50 D.	#20	-2.00 D.
#21	+2.25	#21	+1.75 D.

Whenever the visual tests indicate a non-embedded pattern, then the maximum plus as indicated in the M.S.D.A. may be used.

For example:

	Corrective Framework		
#7 +1.00 D.	Far:	Not over.	+0.75
10 - 16B		Not under	+0.25
M.S.D.A. +1.00	Near:	Not over.	+0.75
		Not under	+0.25

If the case is considered a non-embedded pattern, we would prescribe the maximum plus indicated in the M.S.D.A. of +0.75 D. O.U.

Whenever the visual tests reveal an embedded pattern, then the minimum plus as indicated in the M.S.D.A. should be used.

In the previous case fragment, if the syndrome indicated a well embedded visual pattern, minimum plus would be prescribed. In this case, an Rx of +0.25 D. O.U. might be suitable. The more embedded the visual pattern, the less amenable it is to attack by lenses alone. Visual training either at the office or at home must be utilized.

In addition to the other guidelines presented in this chapter, the organizational status of the case gives us another tool in evaluating the type of visual program to be utilized.

CHAPTER IX
Case Examples

Introduction

The more statistically significant your data is, the greater the certainty as to your diagnosis. Thus, we may have:

Case a	Case b
#10 19/18 (Low)	#10 16/5 (Low)
#16B 20/18 (Low)	#16B 17/8 (Low)
10 - 16B	10 - 16B

In both of these cases, we have the mandate of cut plus at both far and near since we have the duction pattern of #10 and #16B both lower than the expected value. It is obvious that the mandate is much more significant in Case b than in Case a. Therefore, do not lose sight of the actual magnitudes of your test values when you perform the checking and chaining operations. A test may be checked *low,* but is it significantly low, or is it within the experimental error margin? Some practitioners are using an arrow to indicate if a certain value that has been checked differs significantly from the expected values. For example:

Case a	Case b
#3 1 Exo	#3 3 Exo
#4 +0.50	#4 plano
#7 +0.75	#7 +0.75
3	3↑
4	4↓

One can become so mathematically minded that he forgets the purpose of the checking and chaining, which is to determine a significant syndrome pattern for diagnostic purposes.

The following case examples illustrate this technique of visual analysis.

Case One:

Name: F. A. Age 49. Occupation: plasterer. Physical and dental condition excellent.

Complaint: “Things aren’t bright when reading; I can tell that my glasses need changing.” No headaches or ocular pain.

Handedness: Right. Dominant eye: Right.

Old Rx: 1 ½ years ago (for reading, but lately wearing continuously)

O.D.	+0.50	20/20	unaided VA	20/20
O.S.	+0.50	20/20	unaided V.A.	20/20
O.U.		20/20	unaided VA	20/20

#1 negative — 5 14A ___ ___
#2 no astigmia — 3 8-9-11 -15A 13B 16B
#3 1 eso #13A 1 eso — 7 5 14A 16A-21
#4 +0.75 -.25 X 90° — 9-11-16D 15A 17A-20 19
+0.75
#5 +2.50 -.25 X 90° — type and deterioration: B1-1 (simple) presbyope
+2.50
#6 not taken
#7 +0.75 20/20
+0.75 20/20 — +0.50 +2.00 +2.00
#8 ortho — Hab. 14A 14B
#9 5
#10 19/10 — #16A H 12 12 Habit. 16A-21
#11 7/1 — #17A L 11 11 Pat. 17A-20
#12 neg. — #20 (+0.50) -1.00 -1.00
#13B 2 exo — #21 +3.00 +1.50 +1.50 14A and 16A-21
#14A +2.75 — 14B 17A-20
+2.75 — net #14A accepted
#15A 10 exo — net #14B accepted
#14B +2.50 — M.S.D.A. +2.00
+2.50 — +2.00
#15B 9 exo — corrective framework
Control: 14B net — far: not over: +0.75
#16A X — +0.75
#16B 12/4 — not under: +0.75
#17A 11 — +0.75
#17B 22/5 — near: not over: +2.00
#18 neg. — +2.00
#19 2.00 — not under: +2.00
+2.00
#20 -1.00 — organizational status of the case: organized
#21 +1.50
Net #5 +2.00 -.25 X 90° — prescription: +0.75 add + 1.25
+2.00 — +0.75
Net #14A +2.00 — diagnosis: organized B case who needs increased
+2.00 — plus at near because of presbyopia.
Net #14B +2.00
+2.00

Case One: Questions and Answers

1. Why did you type the case as a B1-1 presbyope, instead of a B1-5? *As soon as the patient enters the age range of from 36 to 40 years, we expect to find lowered amplitude of accommodation. We, therefore, classify these individuals as presbyopes. The case is, therefore, typed as a B1-1, since all other relationships within the informative sequence show this simple relationship.*

2. If the age of the patient in this case had been 25, how would you have typed this case? *Since the lowered amplitude does not correspond with his age, the drop in amplitude must be due to an adaptation caused by impact with his environment. In this case, we would type him as a B1-5.*

3. What would have been the difference in the corrective framework if 17B had been the low-low duction at near?

corrective framework:

far:	not over:	+0.50
		+0.50
	not under	plano
		plano
near:	not over	+2.00
		+2.00
	not under	+2.00
		+2.00

4. What would have been your prescription if 17B had been the low-low duction in this case? The prescription under these conditions would be:

   O.D. +0.50
   O.S. +0.50 Add: +1.50

5. How did you determine which duction was the low-low at near?

   #16B 12/4 low (low because of a low break)
   #17B 22/5 low (low because of a low recovery)

Rule: If one duction of a pair is low because of a break finding and one is low because of a recovery finding, the low-low finding is the test with the low break.

Therefore, in this particular case: 16B low-low.

Case Two:

Name: E.C. Age: 22. Male. Occupation: student. O.S. dominant.
Health: Present health is excellent; polio at seven, right side musculature is affected.
Complaint: Patient fails to see as well with his right eye as he does with his left eye. After reading for one hour, print tends to double.
Ocular history: Has worn glasses for 10 years; five lens changes, each change to stronger lenses. Present Rx is one year old.

Uncorrected V.A.	Old Rx	Corrected V.A.
11/200	-3.75 -.25 x 90°	20/30
12/200	-4.00 -.25 X 90°	20/15 +2
11/200	-4.00 -.25 X 90°	20/15

#3 1 eso; 13A 10 eso
#4 -4.75 -.75 X 105°
-4.25 -.50 X 90°
#5 -3.50 -.75 X 105°
-3.25 -.50 X 90°
#6 not taken
#7 -4.00-.50 X 90° 20/20
-3.75-.50 X 80° 20/20
#8 1½ exo
#9 8
#10 30/20
#11 10/3
#12 ortho
#13B 7 eso
#14A -2.75 -.50 X 90°
-2.50 -.50 X 80°
#15A 2 exo
#14B -2.75 -.50 X 90°
-2.50 -.50 X 80°
#15B 2 exo
Control: #7
#16A X
#16B 36/28
#17A X
#17B 24/6
#19 13.25
#20 -4.50
#21 +2.25

Net #5 -3.75 -.75 X 105°
Net -3.50 -.50 X 90°
Net #14A -3.00 -.50 X 90
Net -2.75 -.50 X 80
Net #14B same as 14A

5-8 10 / 3-4 — 14A 16B / 11-13B 15A-17B

5 / 7-4-11-13-17B — 14A / 15A — 16A-20 19 / 17A-21

case type AB2-4

-3.75	-4.00	-2.75	-2.75
#7	hab.	14A	14B

#16A	36	37	32	32
#17A	24	23	28	28
#20	-4.50	-4.25	-5.50	-5.50
#21	+2.25	+2.50	+1.25	+1.25

habitual pattern 16A-20 / 17A-21 — net #14A and 14B pat. 16A-20 / 17A-21

net #14A: accepted. net 14B: accepted
M.S.D.A. –3.00 .50 X 90
-2.75 -.50 X 80
Corrective framework
far: not over: -4.00 -.50 X 90
-3.75 -.50 X 80
not under: #7 to best V.A.
near: not over: -3.00 -.50 X 90
-2.75 -.50 X 80
not under: -3.00 -.50 X 90
-2.75 -.50 X 80
Organizational status of case: disorganized
Prescription: -4.00 -.50 X 90
-3.75 -.50 X 80
add: 1.00 D

Diagnosis: Disorganized myope who needs less minus for near so that he can become an organized B case.

Case Two: Questions and Answers

1. Why was his case classified as a disorganized case, when it seems to be organized?
   I am primarily calling this case disorganized because of the subjective complaint of the patient that he tends to have diplopia after he studies for awhile, No. 4 definitely less plus than No. 7, and the very low recovery on No. 17B.

2. What will the less minus at near tend to do for this student? *As indicated by the static retinoscopy test, this case will continue into more minus unless it can be stabilized. The plus add at near will tend to aid this stabilization.*

3. Would any other treatment be advisable for this case? *This case could use plus binocular training at near to speed up this stabilization process.*

4. Why would a patient who has such a high amplitude need a bifocal? *The purpose of the bifocal is not to make print at near any clearer nor to aid his accommodation so that he will have sufficient amplitude for near work. Rather, the less minus at near will change spatial projection so that now accommodation will project away from the plane of regard with convergence at the plane of regard. This is the pattern sought by the B case.*

5. What is the meaning of the A typing found in this case? *Case history is negative, so fields were taken. They were also negative. Therefore, the A typing is an artifact of the B2 typing. This was borne out by the progress report made in four weeks, which gave a B2 typing only.*

Case Three

Name: F.P.D. Age: 6. Occupation: 2nd grade of school.

Complaint: None, mother thought it would be a good idea to have a checkup.

#3	1 eso	5-6 14A					
		3 4 8-9-11-13B-15A-16B					
#13A	2 eso	7+ 5 6 14A 17A-20					
#4	-0.50	9-11-16B 15A 16A-21 19					
#5	+2.25	Type & deterioration: B1-4					
#6	+2.00	+0.75	plano	+1.25	+0.75	+0.25	
#7	+0.75	#7	hab.	#14A	#14B		
#8	5 eso	#16A	18	21	16	18	20
#9	3	#17A	19	16	21	19	17
#10	19/3	#20	-4.50	-3.50	-5.00	-4.50	-3.75

#11	4/-2	#21	+3.25 +4.00	+2.75 +3.25 +3.75	
#13B	2 exo	habitual pattern:		16A-21	
				17A-20	
#14A	+2.50	14A net pattern:		17A-20	rejected
#15A	8 exo			16A-21	
		14B net pattern:		17A-20	rejected
#14B	+1.50			16A-21	
#15B	6 exo	M.S.D.A. +0.25			
#16A	X	Corrective framework			
#16B	18/3	far:	not over:	+0.75	
#17A	19		not under:	+0.75	
#17B	24/18	near	not over:	+0.25	
			not under:	+0.25	
#19	4.75	Organizational status: disorganized			
#20	-4.50	Prescription:	+0.75		
#21	+3.25		+0.75		

Diagnosis: Disorganized B-type case, needs plus acceptance training. (In order to accept +0.75 at near)

NETS: #5 +1.25
#14A +1.50
#14B +1.00

Case Three: Questions and Answers

1. Does this case have minus projection?
   Yes, we have minus projection at far and hyperopia at near, since #4 is in minus and #7 is in plus.

2. What are the symptoms of visual disorganization present in this case?
   This case presents the perfect pattern of a disorganized visual pattern. We have #4 less than #7; #9 is low; #10 recovery low; #14B net less plus than #14A net; #16B recovery is low and the presence of low esophoria.

3. How can you prescribe +0.75 spheres when the case shows an acceptance of only +0.25 for near?
   We can prescribe plus outside of the acceptance pattern if the case shows definite signs of disorganization. Usually disorganization must be done by means of visual training, since the case is already disorganized the prescription of plus will aid stabilization.

4. What made you decide on +0.75 spheres for this case, why not +0.50 spheres?
   The amount of plus you can prescribe in a particular case showing symptoms of disorganization depends upon the following factors: (a) the maximum plus acceptable at far; (b) age of patient; (c) degree of disorganization; (c) type of additional care being

prescribed. Since this patient will receive visual training and all other factors indicate ready acceptance of the extra plus, it was prescribed for this case.

Case Four:

Name: E.C. Age: 9. Occupation: 3rd grade of school.
Complaint: Can't see at far. V.A. @ far 20/30.

#3	2 exo
#13A	7 exo
#4	+0.50 -0.50 X 90°
#5	+1.25 -0.50 X 90°
#6	+1.00 -0.50 X 90°
#7	+0.50 -0.50 X 90°
#8	2 exo
#9	8
#10	12/10
#11	8/4
#13B	8 exo
#14A	+2.25-0.50 X 90
#15A	15 exo
#14B	+1.75 -0.50 X 90°
#15B	16 exo
#16A	14
#16B	17/12
#17A	12
#17B	19/17
#19	6.00
#20	-3.25
#21	+2.25

3 6 8 13B 15A
4-5 9-10 14A-16B

7+ 6 15A 16A-20 19
5-9-10-16B 14A 17A-21

Type & deterioration: B1-7
M.S.D.A. plano -0.50 X 90°
20/20

Corrective framework

far:	not over:	+0.25 -0.50 X 90°
	not under:	plano -0.50 X 90°
near:	not over:	plano -0.50 X 90°
	not under:	plano -0.50 X 90°

Organizational status: organized
Prescription: +0.75
+0.75

Diagnosis: Highly organized pattern especially when we consider the age of the patient. B1-6, Complete rejection of plus at all points. Above Rx can only be prescribed if patient has visual training.

NETS: #5 -0.75-0.50 X 90
#14A -0.25-0.50 X 90
#14B plano-0.50 X 90

Case Four: Questions and Answers

1. Does this case have minus projection?
We have signs of minus projection at near. The net cross cylinder tests are -0.25 for 14A, and plano for 14B.

2. How do you get a net of plano for the 14B?
The lag for 14B is computed by using 15B/9. This formula holds because we never use more than 15 diopters for the phoria value. Therefore, in spite of having an exophoria of 16 diopters, the lag is 15/9 or if we

round off to the nearest 0.25 dioptor, we have a lag of 1.75. The gross #14B minus the lag is equal to the net #14B. Therefore, +1.75 - 1.75 = plano.

3. What are the symptoms of organization present in this case?
   The data indicating an organized pattern are: #4 equal to #7, #9 up to expected value; recovery on #10 high; #11 break and recovery almost up to expected value; #16B recovery is in ratio with the amount of break; #19 and #20 high, and the presence of high exophoria at near.
4. How can you justify the application of plus 0.75 spheres in this case?
   The application of plus spheres is a must for this case. The only question is the amount of plus sphere. If we consider the age and the completely distorted visual pattern, we must use sufficient plus to aid in the training room. It is, therefore, possible to use +0.75 spheres for this case even though it violates the lens application mandate, but only if visual training is given.
5. How would you have modified your prescription if the patient did not take visual training?
   I would prescribe +0.50 spheres with instructions to the patient that they are to be worn intermittently at all near work. I would also prescribe monocular home training.

Case Five:

Name: Miss S.F. Age: 15 yrs. Occupation: Sophomore in high school, has fair grades. Complaint: "Her eyes have been bothering her for several years, especially when reading." She further complains of burning, itching and watering of the eyes when reading. She has frequent frontal and a supra-orbital headache particularly after some sustained reading, and is right eyed and right handed . Visual skills are good. She failed nearpoint of convergence and second degree fusion at near.

#3	1 exo; #13A 8 exo
#4	+1.00
	+1.00 - .37 X 180°
#5	+2.25
	+2.00 -.37 X 180°
#7	+0.75
	+0.75 -.50 X 5°
#8	2 exo
#9	9
#10	22/8
#11	4/1
#13B	9 exo
#14A	+1.25
	+1.25 w.c.
#15A	10 exo
#14B	+1.25
	+1.25 w.c.
#15B	10 exo
#16A	X
#16B	6/5
#17A	20
#17B	24/19
#19	5.00
#20	-5.00
#21	+3.25

3 4 8 13B 15A
5 11 14A 16B
7+ 15A 17A-20
5-11-16B 14A 16A-21 19

Case type & deterioration: B1-7

14A net: -0.50

14B net: +0.25

	+0.75	+0.25	Plano
	#7	14B	Habitual
16A	6	8	9
17A	20	18	17
20	-5.00	-4.50	-4.25
21	+3.25	+3.75	+4.00

Habitual pattern: 17A-20 / 16A-21

14B net pattern: 17A-20 / 16A-21

Therefore: M.S.D.A. +0.25

Corrective Framework

far:	not over:	+0.75
	not under:	+0.75
near:	not over:	+0.25
	not under:	+0.25

Organizational status:

3 symptoms disorganized

4 symptoms organized

Diagnosis: We have a normal farpoint hyperope with very little plus acceptance at nearpoint. The visual pattern is highly deteriorated. The organizational status of the case will not allow prescribing plus outside of the pattern, and still this patient is in need of plus for her nearpoint activities. The prescription to be used in this case depends upon the objective of the practitioner. If glasses alone are to be prescribed, then the Rx would be +0.25 spheres O.U. If visual training is to be prescribed, we can anticipate the changes which will occur and prescribe +0.75 O.U. Unfortunately the practitioner reasoned that since we have 11-16B low, the mandate is full plus to be prescribed. He, therefore, prescribed +0.75 for constant wear. This particular practitioner has no facilities for visual training. Case 6 is the visual examination of this same patient three months after receiving her glasses.

Case Five: Questions and Answers

1. Would you say that this case is organized or disorganized?

   Although three symptoms indicate disorganization while only four symptoms indicate organization, the status of the case is indefinite.

2. What is the significance of the low amplitude of accommodation found for this 15-year old youngster?

   At age 15 we would expect to find 12 diopters of accommodative amplitude ; this drop to five diopters indicates a reaction of the accommodative pattern to the stress situation. The highly significant decrease in ability to change focus forces the youngster to work at the very limit of her range. Is it any wonder that she has such drastic symptoms of complaint?

3. Is the number five finding significantly low?

   We have #5 + 2.00

   #15A 10 exo (Lag is equal to 1.37)

   Therefore, net #5 = +0.62 (+2.00-1.37)

   This value is compared in magnitude with the #4 test value; which in this case is +1.00. The difference is greater than 0.25 diopter, and we would consider that the dynamic retinoscopy test value is significantly low.

4. Why didn't you use the net 14A in determining the M.S.D.A.?

   The net #14A was a minus. Whenever the cross cylinder nets are in minus and the subjective is plano or in plus. We cannot go below plano for the M.S.D.A. This is based on rule 5 under the maximal spherical dioptric acceptance at near.

5. Do we have minus projection in this case?

   We do not have minus projection at far. At near, we do have the dissociated cross-cylinder test in minus projection.

6. Upon what diagnostic clues did you determine that this case is of the seventh deterioration?

   The key symptom for a seventh deterioration is a low dynamic retinoscopy at 20 inches. In this particular case we do have a low #5.

Case Six

Name: Miss S.F. Age: 15 years. Three months after prescribing +0.75 O.U. the practitioner attempted to have patient return for a progress study. Patient was very reluctant to return since she was completely satisfied. Her headaches were gone, and she could read with comfort. Visual skills were not as good as previously, patient failing second degree fusion at both far and near, and failing lateral phoria at near with a high exophoric response.

#3	2 exo; #13A 7 exo
#4	+0.75
	+0.75 - .25 X 180°
#5	+2.25
	+2.25 w.c.
#7	+0.50
	+0.75 -.25 X 180°
#8	1 exo
#9	11
#10	16/8
#11	6/2
#12	2 right hyper (4/2; 2/1)
#13B	7 exo
#14A	+1.25
	+1.00 w.c.
#15A	14 exo
#14B	+0.50
	+0.25 w.c.
#15B	6 exo
#16A	& #16B suppresses O.S.
#17A	X
#17B	4/-12
#19	9.25
#20	-2.75
#21	+4.00

3 4 8 9 13B 15A

5 11 14A 16B?

7+ 9 15A 17A - 21

5-11-16B? 14A 16A? -20 19

Case type & deterioration: B1-7

14A net: -1.00

14B net: -0.25

Therefore, M.S.D.A.: plano

Corrective framework

far:	not over:	+0.50
	not under:	+0.50
near:	not over:	plano
	not under:	plano

Organizational status:

2 symptoms disorganized

5 symptoms disorganized

Diagnosis: Patient has achieved visual comfort by visual simplification of pattern. Patient is now suppressing her left eye for nearpoint activities. The plus originally supplied merely forced her to find another solution to her dilemma. The minus projection at near has increased in spite of the use of plus sphere for her nearpoint work. Patient needs visual training.

Case Six: Questions and Answers

1. What function did the previously prescribed plus serve?

   It started a desired pattern of having accommodation project away from the plane of regard while convergence is at the plane of regard. Unfortunately, this case did not have the acceptance of this situation, and therefore it simplified this pattern to the ultimate use of one eye only. If visual training had been incorporated in the visual care program the desired aims would have been achieved.

2. How do you account for the decrease in the astigmatism found in the left eye after wearing plus spheres for three months?
   It is often found that prescribing spheres will result in a decrease in the amount of the astigmatism. It is for this reason that the rule has emerged that a cylinder should not be prescribed unless it creates a desirable situation.

3. What is the organizational status of the case?
   The patient is now exhibiting a majority of the symptoms indicating organization. This would indicate that the suppression of the O.S. will progress and spread to farpoint performance.

4. How do you determine the characteristic duction pattern for this case?
   Since the patient exhibits suppression at near in the base-out direction, we would conclude that this finding is at zero level. Therefore, we would consider 16B as the low duction test value at near and #11 the low value at far.

5. What is the significance of the appearance at 2 right hyper at far in this case?
   This is just another indication of the stress under which the patient is functioning. It merely improves the possibility for the patient to develop a deeper suppression pattern.

CHAPTER X
Myopia

Historical

The term "myopia" is derived from the two Greek words "myo", to shut or half-close, and "ops", the eye. The term thus describes a reaction of many myopes who half-close their eyes in order to improve their distant visual acuity. This condition was well known in the 1600's but Donder's (1866) was the first to establish myopia as a clinical entity and prescribed minus lenses for the improvement of distant visual acuity. Since that time, the most frequent solution to the myopic problem has been to supply the amount of minus spheres that will restore distant acuity.

It was the optometrists who noted that although they seemingly had corrected the myopia by means of minus spheres, it was only a very short period of time before the patient would return with the complaint that distant vision was once again blurred. In fact, many optometrists reported that the prescription of the minus spheres for the restoration of distant vision seemed to increase the rate of myopic progression. The attempt to find a better approach to the solution of the myopic problem was initiated by Skeffington and his associates in the 1930's. They began to realize that myopia, the *symptom,* was the loss of distant visual acuity, and myopia, the *cause,* was a nearpoint adaptation to visual stress.

Introduction

Myopia began to be defined as that condition in which minus spheres were necessary to restore distant visual acuity. One of the first questions to arise was, "How much minus spheres?" The fact that this is not an easy determination is illustrated by an experience reported by Rasmussen in the preface to his book *Myopia Control.*

> *A father consulted us about his nine-year-old daughter who possessed several pairs of glasses that had been prescribed over the past few years. The parent was worried by the girl's constant asthenopia and fatigue. My colleague and I agreed to examine independently and not reveal the findings for the time being. In addition we sent the girl, at our expense, to eleven different ophthalmologists-German, British, French, American, Russian, Japanese, and an Armenian of European schools. Each gave a prescription separately and unknown to one another. The result was eleven different prescriptions ranging from -2.50 D. to -14.00 D. sphere, and cylinders ranging from -0.00 D. to -1.75 D. About six had been obtained*

> *under full cycloplegia, and three apparently under partial cycloplegia. Both eyes were given identical spheres in a minority, but wide differences in others. Our own findings averaged under -5.00 D. with fractional cylinders, the total differing by- 0.50 D."*

Our position is that when performing the subjective finding at far (#7), it is essential to make the patient try to identify the 20/20 Snellen letters through the minimum minus. Since the myopic patient has given up trying to identify detail at farpoint, it is necessary for the refractionist to encourage the patient to try to see the letters and not to add any additional minus sphere until such effort has been made.

Also, it is wise not to assume that another practitioner was in error in the Rx prescribed since the conditions of visual stress prior to the other examination may have been different than for the present examination. For example, the original examination may have been made immediately after a week of scholastic examinations, and the present examination may be at a time just prior to the student returning to school after a summer vacation. These situations would likely present with different findings.

A careful case history is an essential tool in the analysis of the myopic visual problem. We will often have educators refer school children for visual examinations because of low visual acuity, and yet at the time of the exam, we may find that standard visual acuity is present. Rather than inform the parents that the school was in error in their visual acuity measurement, it is advisable to consider this a warning symptom of the first stage of beginning myopia. At this point we want to initiate remedial measures immediately.

Etiology

Numerous theories have been advanced as to the cause of myopia. Some of the more prominent ones are: congenital; hereditary; pathological; developmental; and acquired or functional theory.

1) *The Congenital Theory*: Every day there is evidence that deviations in growth are present in small numbers for almost every portion of the human body. The eye is no exception, and we will at times find a young child of three or four that will reveal a high myopia. This type of myopia is undoubtedly present at birth. Fortunately, this type of high myopia is rare. One authority reported one case out of 3,200 babies possessed myopia.

2) *The Hereditary Theory*: The study of statistic relations between parents and their offspring indicates that a significant relationship is present. When both parents are highly nearsighted, there is some likelihood that

more of their children will be myopic than if both parents are hyperopic. Although this relationship is significant, the magnitude of the relationship is still low, and does not account for the high percentage of myopia found clinically. It seems that we inherit a tendency for the condition rather than the myopia itself. Therefore, any given child may or may not develop myopia depending upon the intensity of the nearpoint environment.

3) *The Developmental Theory*: The normal development of the child is not a simple linear process. There are periods when the child is outgoing, and exploring space actively. There are other times when the child is ingoing, and is seemingly assimilating previous experiences. Vision develops in a similar manner. There are times when book retinoscopy reveals that the child is projecting away into space, and there are times that a myopic reaction is present. It would, therefore, seem possible, that if cultural restraints are present at the developmental time when the child is moving inward (against motion present while doing book retinoscopy), that the visual development may stay at this level and the child would remain myopic. We would expect this type of myopia to be present at an early age, and to be associated with other immature or absent motor skills. We sometime see this type of myopia at the four to five year age level. Again, this does not account for the great number of myopes which appear later.

4) *The Acquired or Functional Theory*: It was Skeffington, in the late thirties, who pointed out that most myopia starts at about the third grade and increases each year thereafter. He called this “acquired myopia” since these children had entered school with normal visual acuity. Betts coined the name “adventitious myopia” to describe this occurance.

In the Journal of the AOA, March 1950, Hendrickson published a statistical study of the retinoscopic findings for 1,000 school children in the Pasadena area. The following is a summary of this data:

Grade	No. of Children	Percent Myopic	Average Refractive Condition
1	150	1.6%	+0.75
2	169	7.2%	+0.53
3	145	9.6%	+0.48
4	172	5.8%	+0.44
5	128	8.5%	+0.44
6	100	18.5%	+0.52
7	95	16.8%	+0.29
8	45	25.9%	+0.06

The results clearly show an increasing incidence of myopia as children progress through elementary school. The same pattern of an increasing number of myopes is also found at the college level when we compare freshmen vs. seniors, and also for industrial workers when we compare the new employee with the worker of several years of experience at tasks requiring nearpoint concentration within a limited area.

How do we know that these youngsters of school age are "developing" or "acquiring" myopia? Perhaps the appearance of myopia at this scholastic level may be due to other causes. Insights into this issue were made possible by the development of the technique of "Book Retinoscopy" by Getman.

Getman performed nearpoint retinoscopy on school children while they were reading material of increasing difficulty. He noticed a very interesting phenomena. As the child read easy material, Getman found a "with" motion. As the reading material was increased in difficulty, the retinoscopy motion changed to "neutral". With very difficult material the retinoscopy motion became an "against" motion. This objective appearance of the "against" motion tells us that under stress (difficult reading material) the child is using more accommodation than the fixation distance requires, and thus we have the appearance of a myopic retinoscopic reflex. It seems that under visual stress the organism is moving accommodation toward himself, thereby, increasing the magnitude of the accommodative effort in relationship to the amount of convergence. Since the child is holding the reading material from eight to ten inches when we obtain a definite "against" motion, the child is exhibiting a considerable degree of myopia. Typically, the child does not report that the print is blurred.

The magnitude of the shift into "myopia" under visual stress varies with the age of the subject, initial refractive condition, heredity, growth, environmental experiences, etc. Murroughs (private communication) reported his observations of a young infant. Murroughs observed that when the child was nursing, the reflex was approximately two diopters of hyperopia, but when the child was wet and crying, the reflex indicated 10 diopters of myopia.

Kephart reports his observations of grade school children from the Lafayette area. Kephart noted that as he presented reading material of increasing difficulty, the child would make one of the following responses: (1) the child quits; (2) the child increases his nervous activities such as wiggling in the chair, swinging arms or legs, rubbing nose, eyes or ears, scratching the head; or (3) the child continues to move in closer to the reading material as its difficulty increased. Furthermore, when they used the technique of "Book Retinoscopy" with this third group of children, they found that the reflex had a magnitude of about three diopters of "against" motion as the reading material reached the difficult level.

We have clinically observed that as the child approaches the task of silent reading, which occurs between the second and third grade of school, we have our first significant increase in the percent of myopia. As the intensity of the educational, industrial and socio-economic demands increase, we find that the percentage of myopes in the group will also increase.

By similar reasoning, we would expect that if the environmental stress is reduced, we will have a decrease in the percentage or magnitude of the myopia present. Such a decrease in myopia was found by Luckiesh and Moss in their study of the ocular changes in school children during the fifth and sixth grades (American Journal of Optometry *16*, 443 [1939]), Kephart and Unger also made significant observations when they studied the changes in static retinoscopy for a group of school children from the fourth through the eighth grade for both a rural and an urban school (American Journal of Optometry *30,* 635 [1953]). Kephart and Unger not only found a decrease in myopia over the summer vacation, but also less of a decrease in myopia from the rural school (children lived on farms). They reported *(Note: negative numbers here represent less myopia and are a decrease in the amount of myopia measured.):*

Rural school	-0.008 diopters of myopia
Urban school	-0.607 diopters of myopia
Spring (end of school year)	-0.385 diopters
Fall (after summer vacation)	-0.231 diopters

They stated that the difference between the rural and urban schools is significant at the one percent level. The decrease in myopia found after the summer vacation is also significant at the one percent level.

The functional theory assumes that myopia develops under the stimulus of environmental stress, and that to some extent it is reversible. Also, since it develops under the stimulus of visual stress, a lens application designed to minimize this stress should result in some: (1) reduction of the magnitude of the myopia; (2) stabilization of the myopia; (3) slowing of the progression of the myopia. The application of the functional philosophy to the visual analysis of the myopic case has been most fruitful in determining this.

Where Is The Myopia?

The clinician who has been saturated with his study of physical and geometrical optics is often puzzled by the functional viewpoint. For some reason this type of clinician will readily admit that through physical exercise various organs of the body may be modified. However, when we consider the eye, it becomes a different category and inviolate to change. To this type of clinician the myopic eye is the mathematical reduced eye of more than 60 diopters. To this clinician, parallel rays of light striking such an eye would come to a focus before they strike the retinal plane.

The first thing that one must keep firmly in mind is that the mathematical reduced eye is a theoretical construct that does not exist in reality. For example, if we construct the mathematical reduced eye for a one-diopter myope, we can show (mathematically) that a minus one-diopter sphere placed before such a diagram would result in the reduction of the total plus power of the system so that light rays from infinity striking such a surface would come to a focus at the retinal plane. But let us instead consider an actual one-diopter myopic eye and how it differs from the mathematical construct described.

Some of the points of difference are:

(1) The actual eye has chromatic aberration.

(2) The center of curvature of the physical structures is at an angle to the point of fixation.

(3) The actual refracting surfaces are not on a common optical axis.

(4) The curvature of the surfaces is not perfect.

(5) The various refractive surfaces are not homogeneous.

I am certain there are several other differences. The point is, however, that the effect of these aberrations, present in the living physiological eye, creates a conoid of light rays rather than a point focus. When I place a minus one-diopter lens before the mathematically myopic eye it is easy to show that light rays meet at a point focus at the retinal plane. However, when I consider the actual living eye, and attempt to determine the change in conoidal optics due to the placement of the one diopter minus lens, it becomes very difficult to account for the improvement in visual acuity due solely to refinement in focus position.

We must also consider that there are the psychological changes induced by the placement of the minus one diopter lens. These psychological effects are undoubtedly as important as the changes in physical optics of the eye.

These include the change in image size change due to the minus sphere lens, the shift in the accommodative convergence relationship, and the spatial distance shift. Additionally, because of the psychological shifts created by the minus lens, we have certain shifts in the dual innervation going to the ciliary muscle. These produce changes in its poise, and result in a change in the curvature of the lens itself. We should realize that the mere interposition of a minus lens before the myopic eyeball is a very complex action. It involves not only activities in the eyeball, but also certain central neurological shifts as well.

The ten-diopter myopic eyeball is undoubtedly larger in size than the ten-diopter hyperopic eyeball. Size however, is not the total change involved. Before final structural alteration in the eyeball occurs, we have certain functional changes which occur, and these *simulate* actual structural modification. Every organ in the body is modified by functional activity and it seems that the eyeball is no exception. In the initial stages, the adaptation process can be reversed by merely changing the functional activity. However, if the stress is very rigorous or is prolonged, we begin to have structural modifications which are not easily reversed.

There are seemingly three stages in this adaptation process to visual stress:

1) *Functional stage*: The subject acts and behaves as *if* he were myopic, but may refract emmetropic, or even low hyperopic.

2). *Functional-structural stage*: Certain irreversible changes have occurred which result in structural changes whose magnitude varies considerably from day-to-day.

3) *Structural stage*: We have a stabilized myopic condition.

Functional Stage: The following example demonstrates the functional stage of myopia change. Consider the following case fragment and how it reacted to a prescription of a plus one-diopter sphere (+1.00) for all near work.

Original Examination	Eight Months Later	Two Years Later
#3 1 Eso	#3 4 Eso	#3 1 Eso
#4 -1.25	#4 +0.50 –0.50 X 180	#4 +0.25 -0.25 X 180
#5 +0.75	#5 +2.00	#5 not taken
#7 -0.75 20/20	#7 +0.50 –0.50 X 180	#7 plano 20/20

Functional-structural Stage: The following example demonstrates the functional-structural stage of myopic development.

Original Examination	One Year Later	Two Years Later
Male, 17yrs., "Can't see too well in the distance. Headaches in the afternoon	"I've been having headaches lately."	"I thought I would come in for a checkup."
V.A. 20/40 O.D., O.S., O.U.	V.A. 20/70 O.D., 20/60 O.S.	V.A. 20/30 O.D., O.S., O.U.
#4 -1.50	#4 -1.75	#4 -1.25
#5 +0.25	#5 plano	#5 plano
#7 -0.75 20/20	#7 -1.25 20/20	#7 -0.50 20/20
#8 ortho	#8 1 Eso	#8 1 Eso
#13B 8 Eso	#13B 12 Eso	#13B 4 Eso
#14A +0.75	#14A +1.00	#14A +0.25
#15A 1 Eso	#15A 7 Eso	#15A 0 Eso
#19 4.75 O.U.	#19 4.25 O.U.	#19 4.50 O.U.
Rx prescribed: -0.75 O.U.	Rx prescribed: +1.50 clipovers to fit over old Rx.	Rx prescribed: -0.75 with 1.50 add.

Some reversal in the magnitude of the myopia was achieved by means of the plus lenses prescribed, but the embedded structural modifications present could not be reversed by the lenses used. When one considers that only lenses were used, it is remarkable that even this magnitude of change was obtained.

Structural Stage: As an example of the complete structural stage of myopic development consider the following case fragment:

Male, age 16, has been wearing his present Rx for two years. No visual complaint of any type. Broke his frame, wants a checkup.

N.V.A. 20/200
Old Rx: -3.25 O.U. 20/20
#4 -3.50
-3.25
#5 -2.50
-2.25
#7 -3.50 20/20
-3.25 20/20
#8 2 Exo
#13B 6 Exo
#14A -2.50
-2.25
#15A 6 Exo
#19 8.00 D. O.U.
No change in Rx, replace old frame.

It is obvious that often we cannot be certain as to the precise etiology of a particular myopia. However, the functional approach has been most fruitful in the prevention, alleviation and stabilization of myopia. It is for this reason that this approach is emphasized.

The Stages in The Development of Myopia

The development of myopia starts with hyperopia and its continuous erosion under the impact of environmental stress. Eventually, all the hyperopia is lost, and the appearance of myopia is evident. Clinically we find that any child with less than one diopter of hyperopia at age five is destined to become a myope before graduating from the school system unless a preventive program has been initiated.

The stages in the development of myopia are:

1. The low hyperope who has less hyperopia in the evening than in the morning.
2. The emmetrope who will show some low hyperopia in the morning.
3. The daily recurrent myope whose myopia appears during the day, but has normal acuity (emmetropia) return by morning.
4. The "transitional" myope whose blur at far is maintained daily although the magnitude of the myopia will fluctuate considerably.
5. The fixed myope who exhibits all of the visual symptoms of more myopic progression to follow.
6. The final stabilized myope where the progression has finally reached a level of equilibrium with the demands of the environment, and we have an equal magnitude of myopia at far and at near.

It should be apparent by reviewing this sequence that *the greatest amenability to prevention is to attack the visual adaptation in its beginning stages.*

Myopia Prevention

The only way that myopia can be completely prevented is to block the myopic adaptation while the patient is still hyperopic, or at least is emmetropic at far. The sooner the proper lens application is utilized the better the chances for the prevention of the development into myopia.

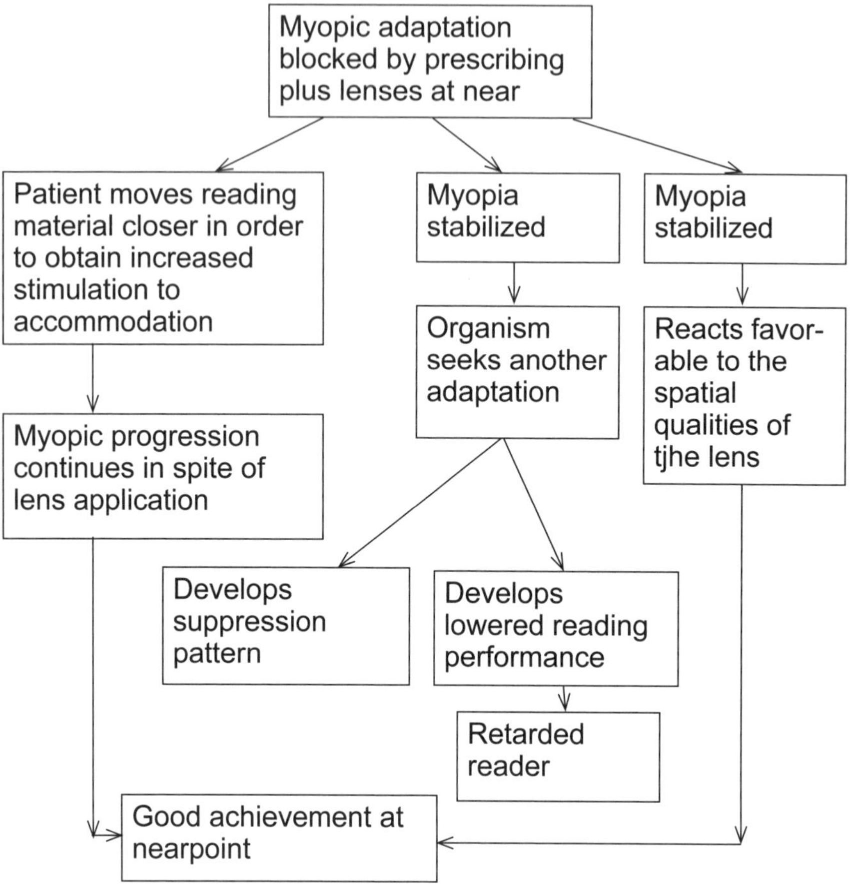

Figure 62.

The lens application for this purpose must be within the acceptance pattern of the patient. If not, then visual training must be utilized in addition to the plus lens application. Visual training will allow the patient to obtain the necessary plus acceptance for the prevention of myopia.

Since patients often do not experience any acuity improvement with the plus lenses, they may not be aware of the purpose of such lenses. It is important to carefully indoctrinate patients and their parents as to the purpose of the lens application. When the parents and patient are unaware of the importance of the preventive program and fail to wear the lenses, the result will be the development of myopia. Case 7 will illustrate this.

CASE 7

Age 11, Female, "Eyes hurt"	Age 17, "Can't see too well in the distance." Headaches in the afternoon. **Never wore her glasses.**
N.V.A. 20/25, 20/20, O.U. 20/20	
#3 1 Exo	#3 ortho
#13A 4 Exo	#13A ortho
#4 +0.25	#4 -1.50
#5 +1.25	#5 +0.25
#7 +0.75	#7 - 0.75 - 0.25 x 60°
#8 1 Exo	#8 ortho
#9 6	#9 18
#10 16/7	#10 26/14
#11 10/4	#11 16/0
#12 1 R.H.	#12 ortho
#13B 5 Exo	#13B 8 Eso
#14A +1.75 Net 14A +0.75	#14A +0.75 Net 14A +0.75
#15A 5.5 Exo	#15A 1 Eso
#14B +1.50 Net 14B +0.75	#14B +0.50 Net #14B +0.50
#15B 6 Exo	#15B ortho
Control Lens: #7	Control Lens: #7 (wrong control lens used, should be plano)
#16A 32	#16A 34
#16B 36/16	#16B 38/14
#17A 28	#17A X
#17B 34/9	#17B 19/-4
#18 1 R.H.	#18 ortho
#19 6.50 O.U.	#19 4.75
#20 -2.50	#20 -2.25
#21 +2.75	#21 ~~+2.50~~
Informative Sequence	Informative Sequence
7+ 16A-21 19 5-9-1017B 14A-15A 17A-20	5 - 9 14A 16A - 21 7- 11 - 17B 15A 17A - 20 19
Case Type: B2 - 7	Case Type: B2 - 5
M.S.D.A. +0.75	M.S.D.A. +0.75
Max plus at far +0.50	Max plus at far ~~plano~~
Min. plus at far plano	Min. plus at far -0.50
Max. plus at near +0.50	Max. plus at near +0.75
Min. plus at near plano	Min. plus at near -0.75
Rx. prescribed +0.75	The doctor decided that the patient could not be indoctrinated into the preventive or stabilization program of myopia

In this case, the practitioner examined an 11-year-old girl who had complained of some visual discomfort. Plus spheres O.U. were prescribed for her nearpoint problem with the instructions that they were to be worn in school. The child conveniently lost her glasses since, as she stated it, “I could see as well without them.” The result, as you can see from the comparative examination taken six years later, is the development of myopia. In addition, the practitioner now decided that this person could not be indoctrinated into a proper program of visual care, and he merely prescribed the distant subjective finding (#7) of -0.75 D. This gave the patient the distant acuity that she desired.

The preventive program for this patient failed because the patient and the parents were not properly indoctrinated into the purpose and function of the prescribed lenses. Other segments of the healthcare field have this same difficulty making patients take advantage of preventive measures. As you can see from the second Rx prescribed, the doctor was discouraged as to the possibilities of using a preventive approach with this patient.

Sometimes the patient comes to the practitioner at the proper time for a preventive myopic program, but the practitioner does not recognize the symptoms. Case 8 illustrates such a case where the youngster was aware of a loss of distant visual acuity in the afternoon.

Case 8

Age 11, Female “I can’t see too well faraway. I see good up close.” No previous Rx. or examination. Right handed.

In this case, the youngster was in the daily recurrent myopic stage. A plus lens application for all near work would have, in all probability, blocked the subsequent movement into myopia. When this particular youngster was once again seen by the practitioner, it was because the school insisted that the child could not see the chalkboard. Nine months later, the practitioner found that the child had shifted from 0.75 diopters of hyperopia into 0.75 diopters of myopia.

Case 8

Age 11, Female. “I can’t see too well far away. I see good up close.”
No previous Rx or examination. Right handed.

#3	3 Exo		
#13A	6 Exo		
#4	+0.50 - 0.50 x 180		
	+0.75 - 0.75 x 15		
#5	+2.00 - 0.50 x 180	Net #5	+0.75 - 0.50 x 180
	+2.25 - 0.75 x 15		+1.00 - 0.75 x 15
#7	+0.75 20/20		
	+0.75 20/20		

$$\frac{7+ \quad 5 \qquad\qquad 15A \;\; 16A \; - \; 20 \;\; 19}{9\text{-}11\text{-}17B \qquad 14A \;\; 17A \; - \; 21}$$

#8	ortho	
#9	4	
#10	18/12	
#11	8/4	
#12	ortho	
#13B	3 Exo	
#14A	+2.00	Net +0.50
#15A	9 Exo	
#14B	+1.25	Net +0.75
#15B	4 Exo	
#16A	X	
#16B	26/16	
#17A	X	
#17B	20/12	
#18	ortho	
#19	5.50 O.U.	
#20	-4.00	
#21	+1.25	

Case Type: B2 - 4

	+0.75 #7	plan hab	+0.75 14B	+0.50 14A
#16A	(26)	(29)	(26)	(27)
#17A	(20)	(17)	(20)	(19)
#20	-4.00	-3.25	-4.00	-3.25
#21	+1.25	+2.00	+1.25	+1.50

M.S.D.A. :+0.75 O.U.

FAR	NOT OVER	O.D. +0.50 O.S. +0.50
	NOT UNDER	O.D. Plano O.S. Plano
NEAR	NOT OVER	O.D. +0.75 O.S. +0.75
	NOT UNDER	O.D. +0.75 O.S. +0.75

Initiating Myopia Prevention

Whenever we are fortunate enough to have the opportunity to examine a youngster prior to myopic development, it is essential that we test carefully in order to determine the best course of action for the patient.

Those cases showing low amounts of hyperopia should have preventive lenses to prevent the transition into myopia *when:*

1. *Case History reveals some of the following:*
   - A. The patient complains of blur at far although visual acuity is standard.
   - B. The parent reports that the child has been doing better at school the past few weeks.
   - C. The child is going to be exposed to increasing environmental demands.
   - D. The child insists on watching television at a close distance although he does not resist when the parent moves him further back.
   - E. The child who is bookish, ignores all other activities, and becomes sedentary.
   - F. The parent or teacher reports that the child has a very close reading distance.
   - G. The school screening program reports that he failed the visual acuity test.

2. *Preliminary Observations and Tests reveal:*
   A. The child becomes immersed in reading as soon as he enters the reception room.
   B. The child's reading distance is more than two inches inside the Harmon norm (distance from the tip of elbow to knuckle)
   C. The child acts shy in shaking hands, or in meeting the doctor.
   D. The child has a downward head posture (looking toward the ground), as he walks toward the doctor.
   E. The child is hesitant about answering questions and expresses no interest in the testing situation.
   F. Spontaneous Drawing (make a house)
      1) Drawing is relatively small in comparison to the size of the paper.
      2) Excessive detail in the drawing for his age level.
      3) Adds numerous extraneous objects of small size to the drawing.
      4) When he signs his drawing the letters are small for his age level.
      5) His working distance while doing his drawing is less than the expected Harmon norm.
   G. Van Orden Star performance indicates an esophoric projection (The pattern is separated less than 65 mm.)
   H. Cheiroscopic drawing indicates high esophoric projection (less than 70 mm.)
   I. Visual Skills Tests
      (1) Lateral phoria test indicates esophoria.
      (2) The right and left eye visual acuity tests indicate less than 100% at farpoint

3) *Analytical Examination reveals:*
   A. #4 is less plus than #7.
   B. #7 is low in hyperopia (+0.75).
   C. Esophoria is found at near.
   D. The net #5 is less than +1.50 D.
   E. The net #10 is the low duction at far.
   F. Phoria at near is ortho or in esophoria.
   G. The cross-cylinder nets are in low plus or even minus projection.
   H. The #19 O.U. is less than 6.00 D.
   I. The #19 O.U. is definitely lower than either O.D. or O.S. #19.
   J. #17B is the low duction at near.
   K. The #20 finding is higher in magnitude than the #21 test finding.
   L. The #21 test finding is less than 2.00 D.

Do not expect to find all of these symptoms and observations in a single case. The mere presence of several of these responses in a low hyperope of a B2 type at a young age is sufficient reason to start a preventive program. If the low plus magnitudes are acceptable at far and at nearpoint, the prescription may be in a single vision form. Since most of these cases are of a B2 type, a bifocal form may be required for the prescription. When the bifocal form of the Rx is resisted by the patient, parent or the mores of the community, you may prescribe a distant Rx, and combine it with plus sphere fitovers that the patient can use for study time.

In addition to the lens application, it is essential that home visual training be utilized in order to assure that the new visual demands of the lens application are being integrated into the visual pattern.

The home training must build the visual skills of:

1. Peripheral awareness - the patient practices seeing all of the objects in the field of view while fixating on a single object;
2. Accommodative rock - to establish flexibility in the accommodative pattern for quickly inhibiting or stimulating the focusing operation.
3. Whenever the preventive program has *not* been found effective in preventing the transition into myopia, we have found one or more of the following causes:
4. The patient had neglected to wear his glasses for all nearpoint activities.
5. The patient had not increased his reading distance to the Harmon norm distance but rather had *decreased* his distance.
6. The home visual training program was not done, or was not parent supervised.

Since the patient can often see as well, or better, at far without his plus lenses, it is essential that the parents and the child be thoroughly indoctrinated into the concept of the purpose of these lenses.

Consider that from the child's previous experience, when the target size increases it means that the target is moving closer. If the child has not been properly indoctrinated regarding the proper reading distance, he may mechanically respond to the size increase created by the plus lens by bringing the book closer to his eyes. It is therefore imperative that you demonstrate the proper reading distance to the patient and parent, and emphasize the importance of maintaining this distance.

We can eliminate most adventitious myopia if we start a preventive program while the patient is still hyperopic or at least emmetropic. I am certain that some practitioners will be aware that we may be placing reading glasses on some hyperopes who would not have become myopic. Consider however, that these particular cases will be better off with their low hyperopic corrections because they will have an improvement in visual efficiency. In addition, these lenses will prevent this type of hyperopic case from taking the retarded reader route. *Protective lenses serve all children to meet the demands of our modern educational environment.*

Myopia Stabilization

In the normal course of events, with our present levels of environmental stress, we can expect that approximately 30 to 40 percent of all children will be myopic by the time they graduate from high school. The ultimate fate of this myopic development for one-fourth of these individuals will be progression to a level of five diopters or more. In addition, we will find an increasingly greater loss of visual acuity with the degree of progression. This, in turn, will preclude certain occupations and job opportunities for these people. We should also consider that some doctors propose that myopia is associated with introversion. If this is true the greater the amount of the myopia, the higher the degree of personality changes present.

Unfortunately, most of the children we see in our offices have already started the actual development of myopia. Therefore, it is highly desirable to initiate a program to stabilize the myopia when the analysis of the case data indicates the probability of further progression.

The uncorrected one-diopter myope that has a 16-inch reading distance, utilizes 15 prism diopters of convergence associated with one and one-half diopters of accommodation. When corrected with a minus one-diopter lens, he now utilizes 15 diopters of convergence associated with two and one-half diopters of accommodation. Also, the minus lenses make the print seem smaller. To compensate for this minification, the patient may bring the print closer, with the net result of increased demands upon both convergence and accommodation. Since certain elements of his old pattern are still present, he may start to reduce the accommodative demands by building more myopia.

The first step in the solution of the myopic problem is the recognition that the corrective demands for farpoint are usually different than the corrective demands at nearpoint.

Case 9 illustrates the late starting myope who is having his first complaint.

Case 9

Age 14, Male. "I am having trouble with my eyes for the first time. I have some blur at far in the afternoon. Fatigue after reading for awhile."
N.V.A. O.D. 20/40; O.S. 20/40; O.U. 20/33

#3	2 Eso	
#13A	2 Exo	
#4	-1.00	
#5	+0.50	Net +0.50
#7	+0.75 20/20	
#8	3 Eso	
#9	15	
#10	20/15	
#11	3/1	
#12	Negative	
#13B	ortho	
#14A	+0.75	Net +0.75
#15A	ortho	
#14B	+0.75	Net +0.50
#15B	2 Exo	
Control lens: Plano		
#16A	X	
#16B	23/8	
#17A	10	
#17B	13/3	
#18	Negative	
#19	6.00 O.U.	
#20	-2.50	
#21	+1.75	

	5	-	9	14A	16A	-	20	19
7-	11	-	17B	15A	17A	-	21	

Case Type: B2 - 4

	#7	plano hab	+0.75 14A	+0.50 14B
#16A		23	20	21
#17A		10	13	12
#20		-2.50	-3.25	-3.00
#21		+1.75	+1.00	+1.25

M.S.D.A. :+0.75 O.U.

FAR	NOT OVER NOT UNDER	-0.25 O.U. -0.50 O.U
NEAR	NOT OVER NOT UNDER	+0.75 O.U +0.75 O.U

Embeddedness

#4 less #7	Disemb.	
#9 high	Disemb.	
#10 rec. high		Emb.
#11 Br. & rec.	Disemb.	
#14B & #14A	Disemb.	
#16B rec. low	Disemb.	
#17B rec. low	Disemb.	
#19 & #20		Emb.

In this case, the myopia found at far is not reflected in the nearpoint findings. In fact, this patient presents as a three-quarter diopter hyperope at near. Enough minus sphere was prescribed at far to restore his distant visual acuity to a poor 20/20, and sufficient plus sphere was given to match the plus three-quarters of a diopter of nearpoint hyperopia. A progress report in six weeks, and a re-examination one year later, showed no further increase in myopia. The boy had discontinued the wearing of his glasses outdoors, and was wearing them only in the classroom and when he drove his car at night.

We have found that good results are obtained if the patient exhibits less minus acceptable at near than at far (cross-cylinder nets in less minus sphere than the subjective at far). Case 10 illustrates this situation.

Case 10

Age 13, Male. “I see things blurred at far in the afternoon.”
Parents - “Can’t something be done to prevent these constant changes in glasses?”
N.V.A. O.D. 20/200 O.D., O.S., O.U.
Old Rx O.D. -2.75 20/20
O.S. -2.25 20/20’

#3 2 Eso
#13A 7 Eso
#4 -3.25 O.U.
#5 -1.00 Net -1.00
#7 -2.75 20/20
-2.50 20/20
#8 2 Eso
#9 15
#10 30/10
#11 8/2
#12 Ortho
#13B 7 Eso
#14A -1.75
#15A 9 Eso
#14B -2.00
#15B 7 to 10 Eso
Control lens: #7
#16A 22
#16B 35/10
#17A 12
#17B 24/8
#18 Ortho
#19 7.50 O.U.
#20 -1.75 (diplopia)
#21 +2.75

5 - 9 14A 16A - 21 19
7- 11 - 17B 15A 17A - 20

B2 - 1 (Simple)

	-2.75 #7	-2.75 hab	-1.75 14A	-2.00 14B
#16A	22	22	18	19
#17A	12	12	16	15
#20	-1.75	-1.75	-2.75	-2.50
#21	+2.75	+2.75	+1.75	+2.00

M.S.D.A. -2.25 O.U.

FAR	NOT OVER -2.75 O.U. NOT UNDER -2.50 O.U
NEAR	NOT OVER -2.25 O.U NOT UNDER -2.25O.U

Embeddedness

#4 IOW #7	Disemb.	
#9 high	Disemb.	
#10 rec. low	Disemb.	
#11 Br. & rec.		
#14B & #14A	Disemb.	
#16B rec.	Disemb.	
#17B rec.	Disemb.	
#19 & #20	.	Emb.
Variable PhoriA	Disemb.	

In this case, the parents brought in their young son for an examination with the presenting complaint that even though his eyes had been examined every year since he was in first grade, he was given a stronger pair of glasses each year. He was told to wear his glasses all of the time because it would help to strengthen his eyes. His present pair of glasses were only six months old and already he has begun to note a little blur at far. The parents contend that instead of helping to strengthen his eyes, the glasses have actually made them worse.

The present examination indicates that there is a possibility of further progression since the static retinoscopy (#4) is -3.25 D. with the subjective at far (#7) having less myopia. The presence of esophoria is another clue to the possibility of a further increase of myopia. The presence of a simple B2 typing is also helpful. In addition, the decreased minus found in the cross cylinder tests (#14A & #14B), and in the dynamic retinoscopy, indicate that an add will be required.

Favorable indications for going beyond the framework of the case in prescribing decreased minus at near is the disembedded visual pattern, and the high value (+2.75) found for the negative relative accommodation at near (#21). The presence of esophoria deemed it advisable to incorporate some base-in prism into the Rx. The patient was instructed to maintain a normal reading distance at all times. Peripheral awareness was to be used at all times. He was to eat all of his meals without glasses. Visual re-examinations over a four-year period have shown no further increase in myopia.

The indications of further myopic progression as gathered from the case study are as follows:

1. *Case History*
   - A. Patient reports that he has had frequent visual examinations with stronger glasses prescribed each time.
   - B. When all of the patient's activities (educational, social and occupational) emphasize nearpoint requirements.
   - C. Patient is a good student but has trouble seeing what has been placed upon the chalkboard.
   - D. Age is below 20.

2. *Preliminary Observations and Tests*
   - A. Downward head posture as he walks toward you.
   - B. Handwriting is small.
   - C. Introverted characteristics.

3. *Analytical Examination*
   - A. #4 test is in higher minus than the #7.
   - B. #7 is in more minus than his old Rx.
   - C. Patient requires more minus for obtaining standard farpoint acuity than his loss of visual acuity would normally require, i.e. Old Rx -1.00, V.A. 20/40; takes -2.00 to obtain 20/20.

D. Phorias are in esophoria.

E. Gross #5, #14A, or #14B are equal to or exceed the minus found in the #7.

F. #19 is low for his age.

C. Equilibrium pattern is #20/#21.

When the case findings indicate that the patient is a progressive myope, the application of bifocal lenses is essential for the stabilization of the myopia. When possible, the magnitude of the plus add should exceed the magnitude of the myopia present in order to have some plus remaining for the nearpoint activities. The smallest add that may be prescribed is +0.75, and the maximum add is +3.50. The following data may be used as an approximate guide as to the magnitude of the add with regard for the minus Rxed at distance:

Distance Rx	Add
-1.00	1.00 to 1.50
-2.00	1.50 to 2.50
-3.00	2.50 to 3.00
-4.00	3.00 to 3.50

If the patient has worn a previous minus prescription, the nearpoint lens mandate may be violated if the patient will take visual training to build plus acceptance at nearpoint. If the case is disembedded, we may consider prescribing additional plus for nearpoint. In any case, the bifocal application for the myope will be of little use unless the patient is properly indoctrinated in using the bifocal. In many instances the bifocal may actually speed up the progression of myopia unless the patient makes an effort to maintain: (a) peripheral awareness; (b) maximum possible nearpoint working distance.

If the case is in esophoria, the distance Rx should be decentered out in order to introduce some base-in prism. In some cases where the minus power is low, decentering the lenses will not introduce sufficient base-in prism. In these cases incorporate at least one-half diopter base-in with your Rx.

Miles (Missouri Medicine, p. 1152, Dec. [1957]) has reported on the effectiveness of the bifocal lens application for stabilization of myopia. He states, "Of 10 cases of increasing myopia treated with bifocals before the age of 13, six showed an immediate and sustained decrease in myopization rate." In addition, Miles reports that one case had the bifocals removed for a four month period and the myopia increased 1.25 diopters. Introducing the bifocals once again, the youngster has shown no further increase in myopia over a four month period. In a later article on progressive myopia (American Journal of Ophthalmology, 1962;54:111) Miles reports, "...on the average, before bifocals, the myopia was increasing about 0.75 diopters per year from the age of six to 14 years. After bifocals, in the same group of children, on the average, the myopia was increasing about 0.40 diopters per year from the age of eight to 16 years..."

When we rechecked 50 of our myopic cases that had not stabilized, we found that the patients were doing one or more of the following:

1. Reading at excessive close distances (in one case at six inches).

2. Were not practicing peripheral awareness.

3. Were looking over the top of the bifocal when reading (avoid this possibility by placing segs about two millimeters higher than normal).

4. Reading in dim illumination.

5. Lying on the floor while looking at television.

In our experience, when the practitioner has supplied a bifocal application for the progressive myope, and has indoctrinated him thoroughly into the development of proper visual habits, we find that there is no further progression in 70 percent of the cases. In 20 percent of these cases there is a slowing down of the rate of myopic progression, and in 10 percent of these cases the lens application has little or no effect on the rate of progression.

For proper visual care, the myopic patient must be seen at regular intervals in order to evaluate not only visual changes, but also any changes in environmental demands. Young children must be checked at six month intervals, and high school and college students should be scheduled for yearly case studies. If the visual changes remain constant, but the environmental demands increase, the patient may need a greater plus add in the bifocal to maintain a stabilized condition.

The Stabilized Myope

The stabilized myope is handled clinically in the same manner as any other refractive problem. The M.S.D.A. and the corrective framework will reveal that a single vision lens will meet the visual mandates of the case. However, if the patient will be exposed to increased environmental demands, it is well to consider the application of a low bifocal add for visual protection against progression.

The stabilized myope can be recognized from the following criteria:

1. The present subjective refraction is in close agreement with the previous refraction.
2. The #4 and the #7 have almost equal amounts of myopia.
3. The net #5, net #14A and the net #14B are in close agreement with the #7.
4. The phorias are in exophoria and are of normal magnitudes.
5. The duction breaks are usually high and a simple B2 typing is present.
6. #19 and #20 are usually high.

Case 11 illustrates such a stabilized myopic case.

In this case, there is no need to make any changes in the prescription. The stabilized myope is the easiest type of refractive problem to handle, and at the same time this very simplicity can make us careless in our case study. As an example, consider the following incident. A young college instructor had been a stabilized myope for over five years. He decided that he wanted to return to college and obtain a law degree. Since he had a number of children he decided to build a study nook in his basement where he could pursue his legal study with a minimum of family interference. In constructing his desk he made it two inches higher than his regular desk. After spending 18 weeks studying at this new and closer working distance he began to notice an afternoon and evening blur at far fixation distances. A visual examination at this point revealed that he had resumed his former progressive visual pattern and his subjective had increased another -0.75 diopters. This increase in myopia may have been avoided if the patient had been thoroughly indoctrinated into the importance of proper nearpoint working distance. If a myope changes his job, and his nearpoint working distances, and/or the visual stress demands are different, he should be advised to have frequent visual checkups to prevent any recurrence of the progressive state.

Case 11

Age 16, Female. Five previous visual examinations since third grade. Last visual examination two years ago, at which time the doctor told her that only a slight change was needed.

N.V.A. O.D. 20/20, 20/20, 20/20 Right handed, right eyed.

Old Rx O.D. -3.25 20/20
O.S. -3.25 20/20'

5 9 14A 16A - 20 19
7- 11 - 17B 15A 17A - 21
B2 - 4

#3 2 Exo
#13A 4 Exo
#4 -3.50
-3.00
#5 -2.50 Net -3.25
-2.00 -2.75
#7 -3.50 20/20
-3.25 20/20
#8 2 Exo
#9 8
#10 25/18
#11 7/4
#12 Neg.
#13B 4 Exo
#14A -2.50 Net -3.50
-2.25 -3.25
#15A 6 Exo Net -3.50
#14B -2.50 Net -3.50
-2.25 -3.25
#15B 9 Exo
Control: -3.25
#16A X
#16B 24/18
#17A 14
#17B 26/14
#18 Neg.
#19 9.00 D.
#20 -4.50
#21 ≠2.25

	-3.25 Hab.	-3.50 #14A	-3.50 #14A
#16A	24	25	25
#17A	14	13	13
#20	-4.50	-4.25	-4.25
#21	≠2.25	≠2.00	≠2.00

M.S.D.A. -3.50
-3.25

FAR	NOT OVER	-3.50 -3.25
	NOT UNDER	-3.50 -3.25
NEAR	NOT OVER	-3.50 -3.25
	NOT UNDER	-3.50 -3.25

Embeddedness

#4 = #7		Emb.
#9 (expect)		Emb.
#10 rec. high		Emb.
#11 Br. & rec.		Emb.
#14B & #14A		Emb.
#16B rec.	Disemb.	
#17B rec.		Emb.
#19 & #20		Emb.

Summary

Most myopia can be avoided if we prescribe acceptable protective lenses while the patient is still hyperopic or emmetropic. In addition, most progressive myopia can be avoided and the condition stabilized by the prescription of proper bifocal lenses. The progressive myope must be indoctrinated to the proper visual habits of peripheral awareness and maintaining proper nearpoint working distances. The stabilized myope can maintain his uniform farpoint refractive condition if he realizes the importance of the environmental factors of good illumination, proper working distance, and peripheral awareness. We can ensure the effectiveness of our lens application in preventing and stabilizing myopia by utilizing elementary visual training procedures.

CHAPTER XI
Esophoria

Introduction

The mere presence of esophoria is an immediate signal to the optometrist that the patient is operating under tension. The typical visual complaints of these patients are:

1. "My glasses make me nervous." (He often reports that he sometimes wears his glasses but that he has to take them off after a short period of time.)
2. Holds books close when he reads. When he does desk work his dominant eye may be only four inches from the work-surface.)
3. Sits unusually close to the television set.
4. Blurred vision at far. (Although he may exhibit 20/20 Snellen acuity at far.)
5. Eyes hurt and/or tire when I read.
6. Severe headaches. (At times he has had headaches for so long that he no longer describes them as headaches, but rather as a dull ache.)
7. Grades slipping. (This type of youngster frustrates the instructor. His initial performance tests indicate good potential. His initial examinations may fulfill this potential, but then he begins to fade scholastically. He is often accused of not studying, and he may drop from the course.
8. Cannot concentrate on any particular task for an appreciable time.
9. Nervous (this observation particularly prevalent with the thin body type.)
10. Diplopia at times. (Present while riding a bicycle, hanging laundry outside) driving a car at night, and whenever the visual field contains the minimum of peripheral cues.)
11. Facial tic.
12. Excessive blinking.
13. Distance judgment is poor. (He tends to underestimate size and distance.)
14. Carsickness.

Esophoria is both an elementary and an intricate visual problem. This plurality of aspects stems from the ease with which we can measure the lateral posture of the eyes while under dissociation, and the complexity of considering what causes the eyes to assume this inward deviation under dissociated conditions. The measurement of esophoria is performed peripherally (outside of the skull) while the cause of this movement is central or cortically located. No muscle moves unless a neurological command has been issued from the central nervous system. Thus the measurement of esophoria may be similar for two different cases, i.e., they may both have one diopter of esophoria, and yet the cause (why the central nervous system is issuing this type of command) may be different for the two cases. To illustrate, in one case we may have one diopter of esophoria present because the patient is an uncorrected hyperope; whereas, in the second case the patient has the one diopter of esophoria because of the presence of a toxemia. To complicate the situation even more, we may have the same magnitude of esophoria present in a single case over an extended period of time and yet the cause of the esophoria may be different or at least seem different from time-to-time. For example:

(1)		(2)	
No previous Rx		Has worn +1.00 for one year	
#3	1 Eso	#3	1 Eso
#13A	3 Exo	#13A	Ortho
#7	+1.00 D.	#7	+1.00 D.
#8 1	Exo	#8	1 Eso
#13B	4 Exo	#13B	Ortho
Rx prescribed: +1.00			

In the original examination *it would seem* that the cause of the esophoria is due to the one diopter of uncorrected hyperopia. The proof of the correctness of the diagnoses would seem to be proven when we applied the one diopter of accommodative inhibition by means of plus lenses and the resultant phoria shifted to one diopter of exophoria. Yet either this explanation is too simple, or there is a different process in action because when the patient returned for his re-examination in one year we found that the esophoria had returned. If the esophoria was due to a simple accommodative cause, the inhibition to accommodation applied by means of the plus lenses should have maintained the exophoric posture originally obtained.

There have been many theories advanced to account for the presence of esophoria. Two of these have been prominent, namely: (1) accommodative, and (2) toxic.

The accommodative theory as to the cause of esophoria has been applied to two types of cases: (a) the uncorrected hyperope who is in esophoria and when corrected by the farpoint subjective moves the phoria into exophoria; (b) the uncorrected exophoric myope who when corrected by the farpoint subjective shifts the phoria tests into esophoria. It is obvious, in these two types of cases, that the higher the ACA ratio the greater the immediate phoric shift. The accommodative cause as to the shift in the habitual phorias is mechanically logical since we can observe these immediate changes. Yet, when we recheck these patients after a few months of wearing these Rx's, what do we find? The hyperopic case that was shifted into exophoria by means of the plus lenses will begin to show the return of the original esophoria through the prescribed plus spheres; the myopic case that was shifted from exophoria because of the prescribed minus sphere lenses will upon re-examination several months later show a return toward the original exophoric condition. Thus the mechanical accommodative explanation is perhaps of some value in understanding the immediate shift in the type and magnitude of the phorias found. However, it has not been fruitful in the understanding of the what and why of esophoria.

The toxic esophore can be recognized from information obtained during the case history, particularly the health history portion of the interrogation. The presence of a positive ophthalmoscopy or perimetric findings indicates that the esophoria found is of the toxic type. The presence of a significant A-case-typing is a signal for a more complete health history investigation. Furthermore if all of the duction findings are low and the patient has not received a complete dental or medical checkup in the previous year, a recommendation should be made to the patient to have this done.

The most fruitful approach to the understanding of esophoria has been the functional concept. The functional viewpoint regards esophoria as an emergency situation for the protection of the convergence pattern against prolonged stress. Therefore, it is advisable that you reread and study Section 3, Chapter VII, *The Measurement of The Protection Available to The Pattern of Convergence.* Upon the impact of prolonged and continuous visual stress it is found, clinically, that the exophoria will decrease and finally shift into esophoria. When this shift from exophoria to esophoria occurs, the patient, from a spatial standpoint, is shifting from a projection beyond the lane of regard to a projection toward himself. When this shift into esophoria occurs, the patient has increased incidence of visual complaints and/or intensity of these complaints. Since we have increased incidence of suppression with the appearance of esophoria, some of these cases may escape symptoms of discomfort. There is a definite shift in the type of visual performance of the patient when the esophoric organismic spatial shift occurs. This seems a curious phenomena at first, since we ask ourselves what can possibly be the difference between a patient having one diopter of exophoria or one diopter of esophoria; there is merely a change of one prism diopter from orthophoria. The difficulty in understanding the significance of this spatial shift lies in thinking in terms of equal physical units (one prism diopter) and not in the psycho-physiological changes induced by this spatial movement. The exophoria-orthophoria-esophoria scale is a simple linear scale and units at any position of the scale are equal to units at some other position. For comparison, let us consider another simple physical linear measuring device such as the Centigrade thermometer. On this Centigrade scale, what is the difference between plus one degree and minus one degree on this scale? They are both equal distance from the zero point, so what is the big difference? The error in our thinking is that we are considering the measuring device in isolation from the system which it is going to measure. For example, if we consider the thermometer immersed in water at plus one degree and reduce the temperature of the system to minus one degree, the physical state of the system has changed and we now have a solid (ice) present. Just this small change through the zero point of the measuring device has produced a radical change in the property of a system. It has changed from liquid to solid. In a similar way, when a phoria shifts from one diopter of exophoria to one diopter of esophoria we have a complete shift in the level of protection received by the convergence pattern to a higher cortical level, and therefore it is inefficient. Exophoria and esophoria both operate as a protective device to enable the convergence pattern to maintain single vision under prolonged stress, but the manner in which they operate is completely different. Exophoria, as a protective device, operates at a relatively low cortical level, whereas, esophoria operates at a much higher cortical level. The very presence of any magnitude of esophoria is always indicative of the presence of impaired visual performance and suitable remedial measures must be instituted. In addition the normal considerations of functional analysis as outlined in Chapter VIII we must consider the following factors for the successful solution of the esophoric problem

1. The difference between the habitual and the induced phorias.
2. The cross-cylinder tests.
3. The embeddedness of the case.
4. The case typing and deterioration.
5. The age of the patient.

Let us now consider the effect of each of these factors in detail.

The Difference Between The Habitual and The Induced Phorias

Rule 7 of the Ten Laws of Lens Application states: "Never prescribe a lens which creates a new interference between the patterns of accommodation and convergence." Thus, if the lenses which are going to be prescribed create abnormal or greater magnitudes of phoria measurements, it is usually best to reduce the magnitude of the prescribed lenses. Therefore, in considering the prescribed lenses, it is important that we also compare the habitual and induced phorias at both farpoint and nearpoint fixation distances in order to determine if this change in accommodation induced by the lenses is undesirable. Whenever the subjective at far (#7) or the subjective at near (#14A or #14B net) increase the drive toward esophoria or increase an already existing esophoria, a more modest Rx should be utilized. For each three-diopter increase in the phoria, the prescribed lenses should be reduced by one quarter of a diopter. Let us consider some examples:

Case 12

Original examination. No previous Rx, failed school screening test. No visual complaint.

#3	Ortho
#13A	6 Exo
#7	-1.50 O.U. 20/20
#8	5 Eso
#13B	4 Eso

Based on this case fragment, it would be advisable to reduce the farpoint minus to the minimum farpoint demand of a poor 20/30 and consider additional application of plus at near as indicated by the cross- cylinder tests.

Case 13

Original examination. No previous Rx, failing in school, not aware of farpoint blur. However, does experience some doubling at near while reading.

#35	Exo
#13A	12 Exo
#7	-1.00 O.U. 20/20
#8	1 Exo
#13B	6 Exo

Since the subjective test at far (#7) provides us with normal magnitudes for both the farpoint and nearpoint phoria tests, we would tend to use this as our basic lens for application. This must also be considered in relationship to the remaining test data.

Case 14

Original examination. No previous Rx. Holds reading material close, aware of doubling at times.

#3	2 Eso
#13A	6 Eso
#7	+2.00 D.
#8	3 Exo
#13B	1 Exo

This is surely a very desirable phoric shift in the desired direction. However, one would hesitate to prescribe this full amount unless the patient is willing to do at least home visual training and to return for visual retests at frequent intervals. The esophoric traces (memory traces in the central nervous system) do not erase this easily, and we may find if careful visual supervision is not followed that we will have a gradual return to the esophoric condition through the prescribed plus spheres. If the patient is not willing to perform the home visual training chores, it is advisable to include in your prescription at least one diopter of base-in prism.

The Cross Cylinder Tests

The gross cross cylinder tests are measures of the maximum inhibition to accommodation that the patient is willing to initiate under minimal target demand conditions at nearpoint. The phorias taken through these lens magnitudes tells us what has happened to the convergence pattern because of this accommodative inhibition. The cross cylinder net values are that amount of accommodation available at near that will not cause any additional interference in the convergence pattern. Thus the cross cylinder net values are the nearpoint subjective values and have the same status at near as the farpoint subjective has at far. In the normal hyperopic exophoric case we have no problem with the cross cylinder findings. However, with the appearance of esophoria we have two types of visual analysis difficulties; namely, the hyperopic case with esophoria at near, and when the cross cylinder values are in minus and associated with esophoria. In considering these cases we must remember that we have no lag value when the associated phoria is ortho or eso. To illustrate the problem with the first type of case (hyperopic-esophore), consider the following case fragments:

(1)	(2)
#14A +1.00	#14A +1.00
#15A 1 Eso (lag 0.00)	#15A 10 Eso (lag 0.00)
Net #14A +1.00	Net #14A +1.00

The magnitude of the net cross cylinder tests for both examples are the same (See Case 12). However, I am sure it is obvious that while the inhibition to accommodation in both instances is the same, the effect on the convergence pattern is radically different. Since there is a reciprocal flow between accommodation and convergence, the greater extent of the esophoria in the second case will make it less amenable to lens therapy. Therefore, in prescribing for esophoric cases of this type, the following rule should be kept in mind:

The greater the magnitude of the esophoria associated with the cross-cylinder test, the more drastic the reduction in plus is required.

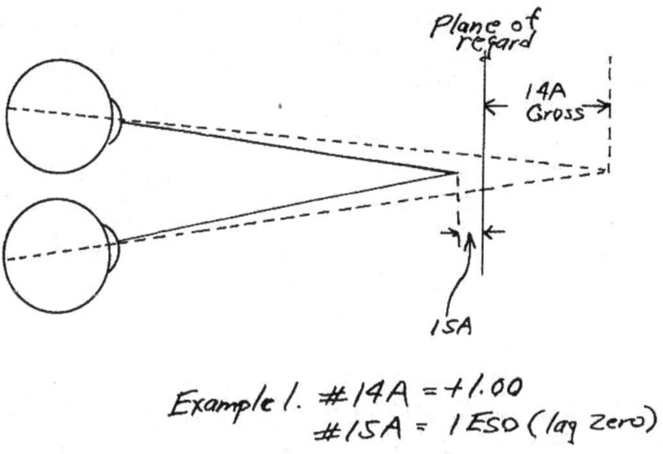

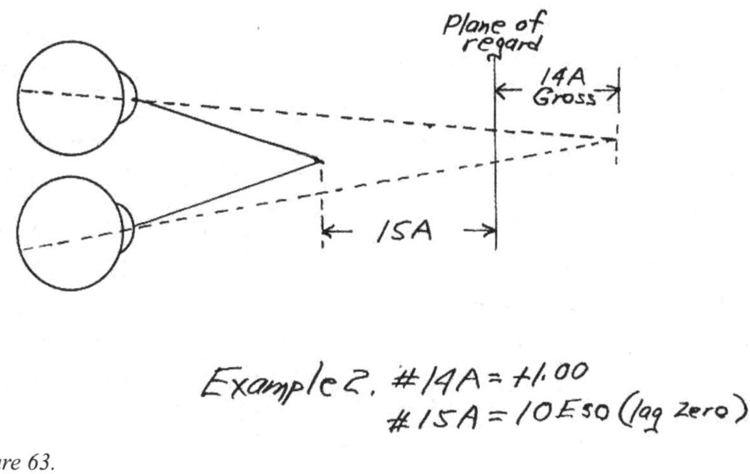

Figure 63.

In Figure 63, example 1, the maximum plus found in the corrective framework at near could be prescribed, whereas, in example 2, the minimum plus in the corrective framework at near can be prescribed (and in many instances it should be reduced arbitrarily below this amount).

There is a normal tendency to prescribe excessive plus (above the magnitude of the cross-cylinder test values) because of the immediate decrease in the esophoria that is measurable. Unfortunately, there is a rebound from this situation, and within a short period of time the patient will show this same original magnitude of esophoria through this increased plus. From a subjective viewpoint, in many instances this increased plus at near may result in an immediate decrease in subjective symptoms, but only to have these same symptoms return after six to nine months. In some instances the elimination of the subjective complaints are found because the increased plus has allowed the patient to learn how to suppress.

The application of plus spheres tends to embed the esophoric pattern and therefore, it should be judiciously applied.

The Embeddedness of the Case

The embeddedness of the case is determined from those characteristics of the visual pattern which indicate how deeply the distorted visual pattern is ingrained into the central nervous system. The measures of the degree of embeddedness depends upon the following factors:

1. The relationship of the magnitude of the #4 test to the #7 test.
2. The magnitude of the #9 test.
3. The recovery magnitude of the #10 test.
4. The break and recovery values of the #11 test.
5. The relationship between the #14B net and the #14A net.
6. The magnitude of the recovery of #16B (#17B for B2 case type).
7. The comparison relationships of #19 and #20 tests.
8. The magnitude of the ACA ratio.

In the case of the esophores, we have two additional clues as to the embeddedness of the visual pattern, namely:

9. The phorias are consistent as to magnitude and pattern for the embedded case; usually variable for the disembedded case. To illustrate the variable condition:

(a)	(b)	(c)
#3 1 Exo	#13A 2 Eso	#3 ortho
#7 +0.50	#14A +1.00	#7 -1.00
#8 1 Eso	#15A 3 Eso	#8 1 Exo

10. The greater the number or intensity of subjective complaints, the greater the certainty that the visual pattern is disembedded; when the patient expresses no subjective complaints in spite of the presence of a visual problem, the more certain we can be that the visual pattern is embedded.

As with all visual problems, the more embedded the visual problem, the less amenable it is to attack by only lenses. The less embedded the visual problem the greater the likelihood that it will respond in a desirable manner to lenses. In addition, the greater the dis-embeddedness of the visual pattern the more we can violate the lens mandate of the case and prescribe additional plus lenses. To illustrate this approach with the esophoric case, let us consider cases 15 and 16.

Case 15 is a disembedded B2 type case which is approaching myopia (low #7, #4, in minus, eso at near, low #19). The plus lenses of the cross-cylinder nets at near reverse the habitual equilibrium pattern. However, because of the disembedded pattern present in this, case, we can, with a greater degree of certainty as to its effect, prescribe the plus which is necessary to block the transition into myopia, and in addition, carry the pattern back into exophoria with its more efficient functioning. The magnitude of the plus and the associated program of visual care depends upon the desires of the patient, after a careful explanation has been made regarding the visual problem. This may take the course of (a) +0.50 D. O.U. for all nearpoint use and progress examination in six weeks in order to determine if this minimum care is giving the desired visual changes; (b) +0.75 D. O.U. for all nearpoint use and a home program of visual training; (c) +1.00 D. O.U. with lenses decentered for nearpoint use with a program of home and office training.

Case 16 is an embedded hyperopic esophore that is in the beginning stages of presbyopia. The patient obviously needs additional plus lenses for her nearpoint work. However, if this additional plus is prescribed for this case it will only tend to more deeply embed the existing esophoric pattern and make it more difficult to provide adequate visual care. The practitioner has three choices: (1) Make no changes in the present Rx but prescribe some fitovers containing 4 D. B.I. for each eye (total 8 diopters). These are to be worn over her glasses while doing nearpoint task for at least two hours daily. When the esophoria has disappeared, a normal presbyopic Rx may be prescribed. (2) Prescribe an Rx of + 2.00-0.50 x 180 with a 1.00 add to include a program of home and office training. The use of the bifocal will act as a disembedding technique and with the base-in emphasis of the home and office training, will transfer the pattern into exophoria. (3) Make

Case 15 Female, 19 years old, no previous Rx. Discomfort in the afternoon at work. It has been getting worse lately. Secretary and some bookkeeping.	**Case 16** Female, 40 years old, received her present glasses three years ago for reading. Lately has been wearing them continuously. She has been feeling nauseated when she reads. Distant vision worse. Old Rx. +2.00 O.U., 20/20, 20/20
#3 ortho	#3 3 Eso
#13A 1 Exo	#13A 5 Eso
#4 -0.25	#4 +2.50
#5 +1.00	#5 +4.00
#7 plano 20/20, 20/20	#7 +2.50 - 0.75 x 180°
#8 ortho	#8 3 Eso
#9 23	#9 9
#10 35/9	#10 24/12
#11 5/0	#11 8/3
#12 negative	#12 negative
#13B 3 Eso	#13B 4 Eso
#14A +0.50 Net +0.50	#14A +3.25 - 0.75 x 180°
#15A 3 Eso	#15A 3 Eso
#14B +0.25 Net plano	#14B +3.75 - 0.75 x 180°
#15B 3 Exo	#15B 3 Eso
#16A X	#16A 20
#16B 21/14	#16B 21/15
#17A 17	#17A 23
#17B 21/18	#17B 28/13
#18 negative	#18 negative
#19 7.50, 7.50, O.U. 5.50	#19 3.00, 3.00, O.U. 3.00
#20 -0.75	#20 -0.50
#21 +2.25	#21 +2.75
B2 - 1 Esophoric indications at near	B2 - 4 Presbyopic esophore
Embeddedness	Embeddedness
#4 lower #7 Dis.	#4 lower #7 emb.
#9 high emb.	#9 high emb.
#10 rec. low Dis.	#10 rec. high emb.
#11 Br. & rec. Dis.	#11 Br. & rec. emb.
#14 Bnet & #14A Dis.	#14 Bnet & #14A emb.
#17B rec. Dis.	#17B rec. Dis.
#19 & #20 Dis.	#19 & #20 Dis.
Phorias Dis.	Phorias emb.
Complaints Dis.	Complaints Dis.
We would consider that this patient has a disembedded pattern and should react well to plus lens therapy.	This case is more embedded that disembedded. Therefore, it would be wise to utilize the minimum of magnituude of plus lenses combined with visual training.

no change in Rx at present, start immediate program of home and office base-in visual training. When esophoria has been eliminated proceed to normal bifocal application as indicated by the case data.

The more embedded the visual pattern of the case, the less amenable it is to attack by the mere application of plus lenses. The greater the embeddedness of the visual pattern, the more conservative you should be in prescribing plus lenses. The more embedded the visual pattern, the greater the certainty that some form of visual training will be essential. In the embedded case, when the patient will not do either home or office training, it is advisable to include a small amount of base-in prism (for large lens values this may be obtained by decentration, for small lens values incorporate one-half to one diopter of base-in prism in your prescription).

The more disembedded the visual pattern of the case, the greater the latitude you have in prescribing the necessary plus lenses. The more disembedded the visual pattern of the case, the greater the likelihood that no visual training will be necessary. In the disembedded case, it is usually not necessary to prescribe base-in prism, but in writing your prescription, be certain to use the actual nearpoint inter pupillary distance of the patient.

The Case Typing and Deterioration

As esophoria first develops we will normally find that the base-in ductions at far and at near are low. However, if the stress situation persists for some time there will be a disintegration of all ductions at both far and at near and the determination of the low-low duction of a pair may be just a mathematical computation with little reality to the total situation. The greater the collapse in the magnitudes of the positive and negative fusional reserves at both far and at near, the greater the acceptance of plus lenses beyond the corrective framework of the case. A B1-typing will respond more readily to plus lens therapy than a B2-type. In addition, the higher the deterioration of the case, the less amenable the case is to plus lens attack. The lower the deterioration, the newer the visual problem; the higher the deterioration, the older the visual problem.

If the deterioration is: -1 through -3 plus lens application.
-4 through -5 plus lens application with base-in prism, home visual training.
-6 through -7 minimum plus lenses (maximum minus if possible) and vigorous home and office visual training.

The Age of The Patient

For the same magnitude of esophoria present, the younger the patient, the more radical we may be in prescribing plus lenses outside the corrective framework of the case. The older the patient, the more conservative we must be in the plus lens prescription and the greater reliance placed upon the incorporation of base-in prism into the Rx. To illustrate this situation let us consider the following case examples:

Case 17: The patient is a 14-year-old female who reports squinting when she tries to see at far. She also complains of blurred vision at far and at near. She has had no previous visual examination or Rx. The presence of a B2 typing indicates that plus is essential for nearpoint use. In addition, the presence of against-the-rule astigmia which improves the distant visual acuity indicates the necessity for some lens aid for farpoint vision. However, the presence of a high deterioration with esophoria at both far and at nearpoint indicates that if a lens prescription is used, it should be in conjunction with visual training. The patient stated that since she is already scheduled for dancing lessons and piano that it is impossible for her to come in for visual training. It was therefore decided to use the weakest plus lens prescription and in addition, incorporate some base-in prism for all her close or nearpoint activities at school and at home. The lens application was to act as a disembedding device to disrupt the esophoria. The prescribed Rx was:

O.D. +0.50 -0.50 X 90°, with 1 diopter base in prism
O.S. +0.25 -0.75 X 75°, with 1 diopter base in prism

In addition, a home visual training procedure for accommodative rock was prescribed. The patient was to return in two months for a progress checkup. However, the patient did not return until she received her recall appointment one year later. She stated that she had never done her home training because she was so comfortable in her glasses. The case data for this examination is prescribed as Case 18.

Case 17

Age 14, Female. Squints a lot. She complains of blur at far and at near. No previous Rx.

#3	2 Eso	
#13A	4 Eso	
#4	-0.25	-0.50 x 80
	plano	-0.75 x 75
#5	+1.50	-0.50 x 80
	+1.75	-0.75 x 75
#7	+0.75	-0.50 x 90
	+0.75	-0.75 x 75
#8	1 Eso	
#9	12	
#10	16/14	
#11	8/2	
#12	ortho	
#13B	2 Eso	
#14A	+1.50	-0.50 x 90
	+1.25	-0.75 x75
#15A	2 Eso	
#14B	+0.75	-0.50 x 90
	+0.50	-0.75 x 75
#15B	2 Eso	
#16A	X	
#16B	36/18	
#17A	14	
#17B	22/6	
#18	Neg.	
#19	6.50 O.U..	
#20	-1.75	
#21	+2.75	

+7	5 9	14A	16A - 20 19
	10 - 17B	15A	17A - 21

B2 - 6

	+.75 #7.	(plano) Habit.	+1.50 #14A	+0.75 #14B	+1.25
#16A	36	39	33	36	34
#17A	22	19	25	22	24
#20	-1.75	-1.00	-2.50	-1.75	-2.25
#21	+2.75	+3.50	+2.00	+2.75	+2.25

:. #14A rejected
:. #14B accepted

M.S.D.A. O.D. +1.25 - 0.50 x 90
O.S. +1.00 - 0.75 x 75

Corrective Framework

FAR	NOT OVER	+0.50 -0.50 x 90 +0.50 -0.75 x 75
	NOT UNDER	plano -0.50 x 90 plano -0.75 x 75
NEAR	NOT OVER	+1.00 -0.50 x 90 +0.75 -0.75 x 75
	NOT UNDER	+0.50 -0.50 x 90 +0.25 -0.75 x 75

Embeddedness

#4 lower #7	Dis.	
#9 high		Emb.
#10 rec. high		Emb.
#11 Br. & rec.		Emb.
#14B net & #14A	Dis.	
#17B rec. low	Dis.	
#19 & #20		Emb.
Phorias		Emb.
Complaints		Emb.

Case 18

One year later, 15 yrs. of age, "Eyes seem to hurt when reading. My eyes tire rapidly. My eyes sometimes pain. Headaches after reading for thirty minutes."

#3 4 Eso
#13A 2 Eso
#4 +0.50-0.75 x 90
+0.50-0.75 x 80
#5 +1.50-0.75 x 90
+1.50-0.75 x 80
#7 +1.00-0.75 x 90
+1.00-0.75 x 75
#8 4 Eso
#9 12
#10 19/8
#11 14/0 5
#12 ortho
#13B 1 Exo
#14A +2.00-0.75 x 90 (Net + 1.00)
+2.00-0.75 x75
#15A 6 Exo
#14B +1.50-0.75 x 90 (Net + 1.25)
+1.50-0.75 x 75
#15B 2 Exo
#16A X
#16B 16/4
#17A X
#17B 8/4
#18 ortho
#19 7.50 O.D. & O.S., 5.75 O.U.
#20 -4.00
#21 +2.50

7+ 5 - 9 / 11 - 17B   14A - 15A   16A - 20 19 / 17A - 21
B2 - 4

	+1.00 #7.	+50 Habit.	+1.00 #14ANet	+1.25 #14BNet
#16A	(16)	(18)	(16)	(15)
#17A	(8)	(6)	(8)	(9)
#20	-4.00	-3.50	-4.00	-4.25
#21	+2.50	+3.00	+2.50	+2.25

M.S.D.A. O.D. +1.25 - 0.50 x 90
O.D. +1.25 - 0.50 x 75

Corrective Framework

FAR	NOT OVER	+75 - 75 x 90 +75 - 75 x 75
	NOT UNDER	+25 - 75 x 90 +25 - 75 x 75
NEAR	NOT OVER	+1.25 - 0.75 x 90 +1.25 - 0.75 x 75
	NOT UNDER	+1.25 - 0.75 x 90 +1.25 - 0.75 x 75

Embeddedness

#4 lower #7	Dis.	
#9 high		Emb.
#10 rec. high		Emb.
#11 Br. & rec.	Dis.	
#14B net & #14A		Emb.
#16B rec. low	Dis.	
#17B rec. low	Dis.	
Phorias	Dis.	
Complaints	Dis.	Emb.
#19 & #20		

Case 18: The lens prescription has served its purpose well. The case is still of a B2 type but the deterioration is less than in the original examination. The esophoria is gone from nearpoint and more plus acceptance is present. The case is well disembedded at near and will therefore accept additional plus for nearpoint use. The prescription at this point was modified into dual achievement lenses (bifocals) and once again the home training procedure for accommodative rock training was explained. This time the patient promised to follow instructions. The Rx prescribed was:

O.D. +0.50 -0.75 X 90°
O.S. +0.50 -0.75 X 75°
Add: 0.75

The next progress checkup in six weeks revealed that all traces of esophoria were gone and the binocular accommodative amplitude was now eight diopters.

Case 19: In this instance we have a male child of eight years of age who has never experienced any visual difficulty. The patient was brought in for a case study at this time on the suggestion of his third grade teacher because he was barely passing and she had noted that he tended to hold his book very close when he was reading As you can observe from the case data, he has a very inefficient visual pattern. The case reveals a fifth deterioration with less plus available at nearpoint than at farpoint. In addition, we have esophoria present at the end of the examination which undoubtedly indicates that as the school day progresses he has greater difficulty. This was demonstrated to the parents by means of the Van Orden Star and the Brock String tests, which revealed very high esophoria. Since the visual pattern was well disembedded and a home visual training device was to be used, the Rx prescribed was outside the framework of the case.

O.D. +0.50
O.S. +0.50

In addition, the minus cylinder with-the-rule was not incorporated since in this type of case it indicated the presence of considerable nearpoint effort. The progress case study revealed the presence of simple hyperopia with the complete elimination of the esophoric pattern. His school teacher reported that he was making excellent school progress.

Case 20: In this instance we have a male college student of 21 years of age. His college grades have been decreasing each semester and, at present, he is in danger of failing. He has severe asthenopia when he tries to study for longer than 15 minutes. His visual efficiency score is 52 (based on 20 visual skills tests) and a score of 85 is needed for college work. His

Case 19

Age 8, Male. No previous eye examination. No visual complaints. Mother thought he should have a checkup. Just barely passing in his school work.

O.D. 20/20-; O.S. 20/25; O.U.20/20-

#3	1 Eso
#13A	2 Exo
#4	+0.25-0.50 x 180 +0.50-0.50 x 180
#5	+2.25-0.50 x 180 +2.50-0.50 x 180
#7	+0.75 sphere +1.00-0.25 x 180
#8	2 Exo
#9	4
#10	14/3
#11	6/0
#12	negative
#13B	5 Eso
#14A	+0.25 +0.25 - 0.25 X 180
#15A	5 Eso (lag 0.00)
#14B	+0.50 +0.50 - 0.25 X 180
#15B	4 Eso (lag 0.00)
#16A	20
#16B	24/11
#17A	8
#17B	14/0
#18	negative
#19	4.00 O.U.
#20	-2.25
#21	+1.25

7+ 5 15A 16A - 20 19
9 - 11 - 17B 14A 17A - 21
B2 - 5

	+.75 #7.	(plano) Habit.	+.25 #14A	+.50 #14B
#16A	20	23	22	21
#17A	8	5	6	7
#20	-2.25	-1.50	-1.75	-2.00
#21	+1.25	+2.00	+1.75	+1.50

14B net is rejected
14A net is rejected

∴ M.S.D.A. +0.25
+0.25 - 0.25 X 180

Corrective Framework

FAR	NOT OVER NOT UNDER	+0.50 +0.75 - 0.25 x 180 Plano +0.25 - 0.25 x 180
NEAR	NOT OVER NOT UNDER	+0.25 +0.25 - 0.25 x 180 +0.25 +0.25 - 0.25 x 180

Embeddedness

#4 lower #7	Dis.	
#9 low	Dis.	
#10 rec. low	Dis.	
#11 Br. & rec.	Dis.	
#14B & #14A		Emb.
#17B rec. low	Dis.	
#16B rec. low	Dis.	
#19 & #20	Dis.	
Phorias	Dis.	
Complaints		Emb.
ACA ratio (high)		Emb.

The pattern is considered as disembedded.

visual acuity was 20/25, which was improved slightly with minus sphere (20/20-). Drastic action was needed and the patient was highly motivated for the program of training lenses and visual training. A training Rx of -0.50 O.U. was supplied and he was to use them at all times.

The home and office training emphasized base-in training through the minus Rx Accommodative rock training was also included. The second examination was taken six weeks later. A significant visual change had occurred. His visual efficiency score had advanced to 91. He reports that he is able to study for two hours at a time without visual discomfort, and that his grades are better. His Rx was changed at this point to +0.75 O.U. for all nearpoint study and his visual training was continued. The base-in training was continued through plus which tends to embed the pattern. Increased emphasis was placed upon perceptual training. This boy finished his college studies as a B student.

Drastic measures were used in this case because of the age of the patient, and the necessity to improve visual performance quickly. There was some danger of producing myopia because of the lenses utilized and the base-in training emphasized. However, the subject was carefully tested each training period to avoid this possibility.

Type of Refractive Error

For the uncorrected myope with habitual phorias in exophoria and with the induced phorias in esophoria, it is advisable to prescribe the minimum minus at farpoint with an add of sufficient plus to restore the original exophoric condition. However, if the patient is already wearing a minus correction and both the habitual and induced phorias are in esophoria, minimum minus sphere changes should be made and at least one diopter of base-in prism prescribed. For extremely embedded cases one may utilize slipovers with the back surface of the slip-over ground to correspond to the front surface of the wearing Rx and incorporating from 4 to 6 diopters of base-in prism before each eye. These should be worn for all nearpoint work with a change each hour as follows: O.D. only, binocular, O.S. only. This cycle should be repeated at least three times daily for maximum effectiveness.

For the uncorrected hyperope whose habitual phorias are in esophoria and induced phorias are exophoria the maximum plus in the corrective framework and home training of a base-in nature should be prescribed. However, if the induced phorias are still in esophoria care must be taken not to over prescribe in plus spheres since this will tend to embed the existing esophoria. It is wise in a case of this type to prescribe the minimum plus

Case 20

Original Examination	Progress Examination
#3 6 Eso	#3 ortho
#13A 2 Eso	#13A 4 Exo
#4 +0.25 +1.25	#4 +0.25 +0.50 - 0.50 x 135
#5 +1.75 +2.25	#5 +2.25 +2.50 - 0.50 x 135
#7 -0.75 -0.50 x 90 20/20 -0.75	#7 plano 20/20 + plano 20/20 +
#8 4 Eso	#8 ortho
#9 X	#9 10
#10 24/16	#10 26/12
#11 14/1	#11 9/3
#12 ortho	#12 ortho
#13B 3 Eso control:Plano	#13B 2 Exo control:Plano
#14A +0.25 +0.50	#14A +0.75 +1.00
#15A 4 Exo	#15A 5 Exo
#14B -0.25 plano	#14B +0.75 +1.00
#15B 6 Exo	#15B 5 Exo
#16A 14	#16A 24
#16B 16/12	#16B 33/12
#17A 16	#17A 19
#17B 28/4	#17B 26/10
#18 ortho	#18 ortho
#19 5.00 O.U.	#19 10.00, O.U.
#20 -0.50	#20 -6.00
#21 +1.50	#21 +2.75
Visual efficiency score 52%	Visual efficiency score 91%
#14A Net -0.50 -0.25	#14A Net plano +0.25
#14B Net -1.00 -0.75	#14B Net +0.25 +0.50
B1 4 Type and Deterioration	B1 4 Type and Deterioration
Training Rx: -0.50 O.U.	Training Rx: -+0.75 O.U.

found in the corrective framework and, in addition, vigorous home and office base-in type training.

Summary

In determining the immediate prescription for the esophoric patient the normal rules regarding visual analysis must be followed. However, the very presence of esophoria is a danger signal to the doctor that this patient is operating in his visual space world at a high cortical level. Therefore, this individual cannot maintain or reach his true potential unless adequate visual care is received. It has been the clinical experience of the profession that to attempt to erase this esophoric posture by merely "crowding" plus lens application results in the return of the patient with the same symptoms and the esophoria. No esophoric problem is ever solved unless we completely erase the esophoric posture. To merely be satisfied that by means of a traditional lens application we have reduced the esophoria from an original magnitude of eight diopters to the present value of four diopters, is to do a disservice to the patient. We should continue our visual care program with vigor until all traces of the esophoria are gone and the patient has regained the normal exophoric posture.

By judicious use of base-in prism and reduction in the magnitude of prescriptable plus, many of the esophoria type cases can be solved. However, in the older patient, the patient that is already wearing a maximum plus correction, and/or the embedded visual pattern you will find that a more vigorous approach must be followed if the esophoria is to be eliminated. In these cases, slip-overs, containing base-in prism will have to be prescribed while doing home chores, office work, etc. for several hours daily. In addition, home and office training devices may have to be utilized. In every instance however, the patient must be informed as to the importance of, and the necessity for, eliminating the esophoria. The patient should have the opportunity to decide on the depth of the visual program he will undertake. It is, therefore, imperative that the esophoric posture be demonstrated. The best means of doing this is by the Brock string test. The esophore will give the "X" response instead of the normal "V" response, which means that as he is observing his thumb with one eye, the other eye is looking at some closer position. The esophore will readily understand that if this type of positioning is going on while reading, for example, it must be slowing down his work. In addition, the patient should be aware of the necessity for periodic visual examinations (in one to two months) in order to make certain that his visual gains have been maintained and to inaugurate remedial measures if the patient has lost any of his visual performance.

CHAPTER XII
Glossary and Questions and Answers

Ability-Developed capacity.

Acceptable-The net spherical lens value as determined from the dissociated and fused cross-cylinder tests must not reverse the order of the blur (equilibrium) findings as they have been arranged by the organism.

Accommodation-The mechanism of focusing, designated in its postural set-up by the measurable light value brought to a focus congenial to interpretation.

Accommodative amplitude-The patient's response to minus lens stimulus upon 0.62 em size target located at 13 inches. It measures the change taking place in the relationship between accommodation and convergence, due either to advancing years or any other cause. It is one of the latitudes of performance within the visual pattern which the organism can absorb in the task of maintaining single and clear vision as long as possible, despite changes in total behavior brought about by sensibility.

Accommodative "rock"-A visual performance test designed not to study the amount of accommodation, but rather for study of the flexibility of the accommodative response. A study of the ability of the patient to change the posture of accommodation quickly within a standard range of ability (about two diopters). Significant information is yielded when this ability is hampered, slowed or cancelled in a degree. It ascertains if there is any interference in integration slowing the radiation of the impulses that should excite the motor centers and, thus, bring about a change in the accommodative mechanism.

Acuity-The ability to respond to faint sense-impressions or to distinguish slight differences between stimuli.

Adaptation-The point where a mediator establishes a level between stimulus and response. The three major pathways of adaptation the organism may explore are: adventitious myopia, adventitious squint and lowered achievement. It is the distortion of abilities, without the elimination of meaning.

Adaptive process-The maneuvers (conscious or unconscious, automatic or voluntary) by which the individual attempts to make his fit as comfortable and as gratifying as possible within the demands of his environment.

Adjustor-Another name for a nerve center. It consists of a collection of neurons in synaptic relation with each other. It is a terminal for incoming and outgoing fibers. Impulses from receptors are received and transmitted to effectors or other centers.

Adventitious-Acquired. A refractive error or tropia that is not congenital, or due to trauma or infection but occurs because of environmental impact.

Afferent-efferent arc-It is one of the circuits conveying inward a sensory stimulus to the central nervous system, its radiation across the same and the resulting discharge outward of a motor impulse to the control mechanism of an end organ and the confirmatory feedback arc to the central nervous system.

Afferent fibers-Nerve fibers which carry impulses from the sense organs to the nerve centers.

Aggregate-Total.

Alignment-It is the placing of the retinal quadrants of the eye so that the light stimulus is equally distributed on all four quadrants. This is the "pointing" or "bomb sighting" of the ocular mechanism.

Analysis-A scientific procedure for dividing a complex experience into simpler constituents.

Analytical examination-The 21-point optometric examination. Each point is a measurement of performance of a visual behavior pattern. These measurements, made through the application of prism and sphere, show the absorption of the potential of inhibition, measure the existing learned associations between patterns and probe for the degree of organization existing in the visual pattern.

Anomaly-Any striking deviation from typical or normal.

Area-A region set off from its surrounds by contour; a portion of the total performance of the organism.

Area of compensation-The "delay in time" between the accommodation and convergence "areas" of the visual behavior patterns to absorb the changes wrought by altered distance, measured as exophoria and hyperopia.

Atomism-The assumption that any whole is a derivative of pre-existing parts.

Attention-The total adjustment of the organism that facilitates the reception of stimuli and the appropriate response.

Autonomic nervous system-That section of the nervous system that regulates the internal organs; consists primarily of ganglia connected with the brain stem and spinal cord, and it may be subdivided into the sympathetic and parasympathetic systems. It is primarily concerned with controlling the internal environment of the organism.

"B" case-The individual who makes the characteristic response to the near-centered task of a drive to center nearer in space than the localization of identification. The direction of interference is from the pattern of accommodation towards that of convergence.

B1-typing-A characteristic organism response to a restricted near-point environment which requires full lens power for both far and near.

B2-typing-Essentiallv a distortion of a B1-case. It is an intensification of the near-point problem, resulting in a "reversal phenomenon," when transferred to the other areas of the visual performance, far-point for instance. It demands a reduction in the applicable lens power at far, with full plus accepted as near.

Background-An unpatterned surface lying beyond and not perceived as belonging to the figure or object; ground.

Backstroke-The sum total of all the afferent impulses which arise in the proprioceptors located in or about the muscles and glands, which are activated in the consummation of any movement.

Ballistiform movements-Movements performed on a low cortical or reflex level. They are movements so completely removed from the executant levels that the organism is unaware of the process.

Basic finding-The subjective; it is the lens power that alters light rays entering an eye and causes a change in the focusing mechanism in the greatest degree without causing a subjective detected alteration in the convergence mechanism.

Behavior-The reaction of the individual to his environment. All types of muscular and glandular response of the organism to stimulation.

Behavior pattern-The combination of behavior elements into a more stable combination or complex act; the evolution of the visual pattern. A functional integration of discriminable parts, which operates or responds as an unitary whole; an enormous complex action in the central nervous system to bring about some certain activity desirable to the organism.

Binocular Vision-The resultant cortical integration of innervational patterns received from the photoreceptors when they are both aligned on the target.

Blocking-Inhibition.

Blur-It is significant of the "potential of inhibition" between the patterns of accommodation and convergence. When the full potential of inhibition has been reached (because of the probe bodies-lenses or prisms), when all of the inhibition of associative impulses that the organism can muster has been used (lens), the pattern of accommodation will change, the mechanism of accommodation will change and a blur will result; (prism) the pattern of convergence will change, the mechanism of convergence will change and a blur will result.

Blur points-Equilibrium tests; limitations on the amount of lens power which the optometrist may prescribe for his patient.

Book retinoscopy-The application of the retinoscope to the study of perception. The ability to determine the intellectual grasp of the observer to the stimulus situation by objective retinoscopy.

Break point tests-Amounts of prism base-in or base-out which will disrupt the fusional pattern of the individual. They are directions for the quantity of lens fitting. They are significant of the extent of the "learned association" between the patterns of accommodation and convergence.

C-type-The change in the pattern of convergence is of a degree that the associative change in the pattern of accommodation would cause blurring; the direction of the interference is from the pattern of convergence towards the pattern of accommodation.

Cancellation-Suppression; the cancellation of a visual skill signifies that the organism has ceased to use that skill. The failure on the part of the organism to perform some phase of the seeing act.

Capacity-Potential or latent ability.

Case analysis-A study of visual performance.

Case record-Profile of a visual performance.

Case typing-A study of relations between the adjustor patterns of accommodation and convergence.

Caustic (light)-Gullstrand's term for the total area of excitation on the retina produced by a single beam of light passing through the optical mechanism of the eye.

Centering-It is the selection of some area of space for attention and meaning. A covert process of knowing where an object is in relationship to other objects. The computing process of "where is it?"

Chaining-The process of arranging the significant findings in relationship to a horizontal median line, placing findings which are relatively "high" above the line and those which rate as being relatively "low" below the median line. It is the compilation of symptoms into a syndrome.

Checking-The process of designating analytical findings which vary from the "mean" or "expected" value by marking those which are low with a blue pencil and those which are high with a red pencil; a method of determining symptoms.

Concession-Ignoring any of the energy transmission that has been instituted in the interest of maintaining an effective association in the central nervous system between the patterns of accommodation and convergence. It is the elimination of manifest perceptual meaning.

Converge-Direct toward the same point in space.

Convergence-Bilateral alignment. It is the overt positioning of the visual axes so that the alignments touch one another at the point of interest. Any change or maintenance of the posture of eyes in orbit.

Corrective framework-The listing of the range of acceptable lens findings- the "not over" and "not under" at far, intermediate and near.

Corrective syndrome-Same as informative sequence.

Correlation-The tendency for certain paired measures to vary concomitantly. Two variables are said to be positively correlated when an increase in one is likely to be accompanied by an increase in the other. Things are negatively correlated when an increase in one variable is likely to be accompanied by a decrease in the other variable. The maximum or perfect relationship is 1.0; whereas, no relationship between variables is expressed as 0.0.

Cortical-Within the central nervous system.

Cortical level-Conscious level.

Defect-Any impairment of performance forced on the organism from whatever cause.

Degeneration-Same as deterioration.

Deterioration-The stages of erroneous behavior constitute what is known as the deterioration or degeneration of a B-type case. Certain definite changes occur in the visual pattern with time. These are: (1) the dissociated cross-cylinder net has more plus than the basic finding; (2) the dissociated cross-cylinder net is now equal to the basic finding; (3) the dissociated cross-cylinder net is now in less plus than the basic findings; (4) a reversal in the equilibrium findings; (5) the amplitude of accommodation is below five diopters; (6) convergence at far becomes the low distant duction test; (7) the dynamic retinoscopy net is in less plus (low) than the static retinoscopy test.

Development-The modification of growth by the activities and experiences through which the organism goes at various times.

Diagnosis-The procedure by which the nature of disease or disorder is determined by study of its origin, its evolution and the signs and symptoms manifested by it.

Discomfort-The subjective complaint of the patient that is due to dissatisfaction with his level of visual achievement.

Disorganize-To destroy the regularity or systematic structure of a process. The organism is performing at cortical levels.

Disorganize-It produces the greatest decrement in achievement, but the pattern has the greatest amenability to lens application, even when the lens power is not acceptable in the cross-cylinder nets or violates the equilibrium pattern. The "recovery" tests are the yardsticks of the degree of disorganization, in the area of visual behavior where taken. In the first impact of the impairing task "recoverics" drop significantly, the "break" tests drop below the statistical expected values, but only in the direction of the interference. The pattern of disorganization is indicated when: (1) static retinoscopy test is in less plus than the subjective; (2) true adduction at distance is below its statistical expected value; (3) the recovery portion of the convergence at far test is below its expected ratio with the break portion of the test; (4) the break and recovery of the abduction at far test is below its statistical expected value; (5) the fused cross-cylinder net is lower than the dissociated cross-cylinder net; (6) the recovery of the positive ratio with the break value of the test; (7) the amplitude of accommodation and positive relative accommodation tests are excessively low. If in a particular case all seven factors indicate disorganization, the patient would be completely disorganized visually; if only four of the factors reflect signs of disorganization, the patient would be considered as indicating disorganization.

Disorganized-The organism is performing at cortical levels.

Dissociation-Destroying the binocular space lattice. Devices which create this condition are: prisms, Maddox rod, double prism, anaglyph glasses, polaroid glasses or a septum device (stereoscope).

Duction-It is a signal of the degree of interference between the patterns of the mechanisms of accommodation and convergence in the central nervous system. The higher the test value, the less the existing interference.

Dynamic-Active; tests performed at close working distances.

Effector-It is an organ which receives excitations from the nervous system and as a result of such excitations performs activity of some sort, i.e., any organ which yields a response to a stimulus.

Effector patterns-Those behavior patterns in the central nervous system which control a particular mechanism in relationship to the environment.

Efferent fibers-Nerve fibers which carry nerve impulses from the nerve centers to the muscles or glands. Motor fibers.

Egocentric locus-The individual. The center from which all activity goes out. The body as a reference point.

Embedded case- (see "structured" or "organized") A visual problem in which structure (visual mechanism or its attachments or cortical mechanism) has been changed to conform to the adverse type of activity being demanded, so that the organism need not expend energy to overcome the stress.

Emmert's law-The size of an object changes as the second power of the distance. That is, an object moved twice as far away will have one-fourth the size (optically).

Emmetrope-An individual who has standard acuity (20/20) without concave lenses and who refuses plus lenses.

Emmetropia-It is significant of a stress between the behavior patterns. The area of compensation (exophoria) for the protection of the interpretive pattern and posture of accommodation has been absorbed.

Environment-It is the aggregate of all external conditions and influences affecting the life and development of an organism. That which surrounds the individual; the sum total of the physical-chemical, biological and social phenomena, which surrounds man.

Equilibrium findings-These are the near-point analytical blur tests of positive relative convergence, negative relative convergence, positive relative accommodation and negative relative accommodation. They are a guide as to whether the spherical lens power found in the subjective at far and the net subjective at near will or will not create a new visual problem if prescribed.

Erroneous behavior-Any behavior that is non-characteristic of the response of the organism to energy.

Esophoria-It is significant of "an active state of inhibition" between patterns of accommodation and convergence to prevent blurring or doubling.

Etiology-The study of casual relations.

Examination, analytical-A term applied to the visual examination known as the "Twenty-One Point" technique.

Excursions-Indications of complete integrity of response to a stimulus moved in the cardinal directions without interference.

Executant-Cortical.

Exophoria-A relationship between the patterns of accommodation and convergence to protect the integrity of the convergence performance; it is measured by the amount of prism base-in required to align two dissociated images. A developmental or maturational relationship within the visual behavior pattern between areas of that pattern, operationally active to preserve the integrity of performance of the convergence mechanism.

Exophoria, maturational-That amount of exophoria which is normal (statistically) for the race.

Exophoria, structural-The exophoria (high amounts usually) resulting from the effects of a visually unacceptable task.

Expecteds-The statistical average of the optometric tests for the general population.

Experimental world-The organism's awareness of himself and of objects in the surrounds and of certain relationships between them. This is the "real" world to most human beings.

Exteroceptors-They are the sense organs of touch, smell, hearing, taste and sight. They inform us of changes in our external environment.

Fatigue-A decreased ability of performance on the part of an organism, or some member or muscle, resulting from prolonged activity, boredom or other causes.

Feedback-When a portion of the effector impulse pattern re-enters the input system in order to maintain control. It is the confirmatory and modifying input that is the resultant of the final common motor pattern output, altering, modifying, elaborating or inhibiting original input.

Field-Dispersions or distributions of energy in space forming a pattern or structure. A contour arrangement of energy in space.

Figure-A group of impressions derived from a single sense, which is perceived as an object; object of regard; that which has meaning for the observer. It is discrete-opposite of ground. An aggregation of objects or processes segregated from their surrounds.

Figure-ground-A general dual characteristic of perception first emphasized by Rubin. When a total field is so structured that different parts exhibit varying degrees of integration, the most highly articulated ones are called "figures" while the simpler and more homogeneous areas are called "grounds."

Fixation-A manipulatory investigation of the behavior of the convergence mechanism in making quick and accurate response to fixation from far-to-near and from side-to-side (cardinal directions). The inability to make quick change from far-to-near fixation smoothly and promptly shows a high correlation with lowered visual achievement.

Focus-The pattern of light energy distribution on the retina.

Frustration-A behavioral reaction precipitated by the inability to accomplish some task deemed important by the organism.

Functional analysis-A method of influencing the conditions under which an event occurs for the sake of determining the factors essential to the event.

Functional approach-A hypothesis which asserts that the neuropsychological processes constitute the dynamic and determining factors in the functioning of the organism.

Fusion-The synthesis of excitation from the two sense receptors into a single percept.

Gestalt-Form, shape or configuration. All those organized units of experience and behavior which have definite properties not traceable to parts and their relations.

Gradient-A rate of change; any magnitude which slopes from a high to low value by steps or degrees instead of maintaining a uniform value of varying inequality.

Gross-Refers to near-point accommodative tests which have not been corrected for the influence of convergence. The gross test amount minus the lag is equal to the net test value.

Groundal-Supporting.

Growth-The process of completion of a certain portion of the size and structure of the bodily systems through biochemical activity that has been biochemically initiated by virtue of the incompleteness of those structures.

Holistic-A systematic approach to science involving the study of the whole or total configuration; the view of the organism as a unified psycho-physiological being inextricably immersed in a socio-cultural-economic environment.

Homeostasis-Organisms by their own activity tend to restore physiological balances. The organism tends to maintain a constant state.

Horoptor-The sum total of points in space which can be seen singly by the two eyes.

Hyperopia-A relationship between the patterns of accommodation and convergence to protect the integrity of the accommodative performance. It is measured by the change in accommodation induced by means of a plus lens without producing an undesirable change in the pattern of convergence. It exists in the central nervous system. It is an ability of the organism to manipulate space away from the plane of regard.

Identification-It is the totality of the process that uses the light distribution on the retina, the integrative process with other modality information and past experience with the resultant motor feedback that tells us what things are. The covert process of computing "what is it?"

Informative sequence-A sequence of findings that constitutes the main syndrome of interference manifestation. It has six parts: (1) subjective; (2) case typing; (3) intermediate relationship; (4) dissociated cross-cylinder relationship; (5) equilibrium pattern; (6) amplitude of accommodation.

Inhibition-As applied to the effect of plus lenses on accommodation and the effect of base-in prism upon convergence. There is a change in the postural mechanism as though the stimulus object has been moved further from the eye. Projection is away from the plane of regard and from the organism.

Innate-Patterns of behavior which are present at birth and are therefore present prior to experience.

Input-It is the energy distribution striking the sensory surface.

Integration-The combination and organization of neural excitation within neural centers in such a way as to produce coordinated and adaptive activity.

Interference-The effect, resulting from the disorganization in the central nervous system of the habitual relationships of the neural patterns controlling accommodation and convergence, caused by changes in innervations in the system having the greater susceptibility to fatigue.

Ionic volley-It is the energy propagation along a nerve pathway, due to the initiating reaction at the sensory surface.

Kinesthesis-see Proprioception.

Lag of accommodation-Something that is subtracted from gross near-point accommodative tests; the change that can be effected in the postural-set of the focusing mechanism by the interpositioning of convex lenses, due to the existence of an area of compensation in the convergence pattern (exophoria).

Learning-The process of acquiring the ability to respond adequately to a given situation. The modification of behavior and experience brought about by an organism's response to its environment. It is the modification of response tendencies consequent upon experience.

Lens-A portion of space bounded by a spherical curve. A device or a means of causing the organism to make the maximum change possible in the accommodative pattern without inducing an undesirable change in the convergence pattern. The primary purpose of a lens is to create a space configuration that is in accord with the distortion in the visual behavior pattern occasioned by the unacceptability of the visual task of continued excitation of a sense receptor beyond its refractory phase.

Lens prescription-The lens amounts which are prescribed for the purpose of permanently altering spatial identification and manipulation in order to restore the equilibrium within the visual behavior pattern.

Localization-The placing of a source or stimulation with reference to the organism.

Locus-Meeting place; the center.

Luster-The experience of practically looking through one color at another and obtaining a metallic sheen.

Manipulatory skills-Studies of convergence response. The integrity of the convergence response when the motor impulses must be motivated by the organization in the central nervous system and a moving target is the trigger stimulus.

Maturation-The process of growth whereby the state of complete development is attained.

Mechanistic-Machine-like; automatic; unvarying; precise. Explaining phenomena in terms of mechanics or operating parts.

Minus projection-The minus resulting from the subtraction of a "lag" from the gross cross-cylinder tests; an "active state of inhibition" between the patterns of accommodation and convergence to prevent blurring or doubling. It is present at far when the static retinoscopy test is in minus and the unaided acuity is 20/20 or better. It is found at near when the cross-cylinder nets are in minus and the unaided acuity at near is 20/20 or better.

Molar-Whole or unitary.

Molecular-Atomistic, the opposite of whole, unitary or molar. Emphasis is upon parts.

Monocular Projection-A psychological skill (Renshaw) in which a stereogram (picture) is presented to one eye and a light neutral ground is presented to the other eye. The patient is dissociated by the dissimilar targets. The patient now attempts to touch some portion of the picture using pointers which are held in each hand. The disparate distance between the two pointers indicates the positioning of the postural mechanism. The position of the picture and neutral ground are then reversed and the pointing repeated. The disparate distance should be the same.

Motility-The directed, integrated, rhythmic behavior of the organism.

Motor-Same as Efferent.

Myope, adventitious-A type of environmental adaptation wherein the organism: (a) ablates acuity at far; (b) changes in the behavior pattern of accommodation at far; (c) attains a high level of achievement at near. The stages in this adaptation are: (1) daily recurrent vocational myope; (2) a "fixed" myope with plus available at near; (3) more myopia at far, minus projection at near; (4) equal amounts of myopia at far and at near.

Myopia-The visual condition wherein minus lenses are required to restore standard acuity; a symptom at far point of a condition that stemmed from near point; a type of environmental contraction. An individual who once had standard acuity at far, who has lost it and to whom it can be restored with a concave lens is a myope.

Nearpoint tests-Optometric tests which probe the visual pattern of the patient while the stimulus target is within arm's length.

Nonembedded (see disorganized)-The nonembedded case is one in which the deviation is functional and structure has not yet been altered to conserve energy; there is a less constructed approach possible.

Ocular defects-The end result of visual problems. Stresses imposed upon the visual mechanism from within the organism that produce changes in structure of that mechanism. These structural changes are measured as ocular defects.

Ocular discomfort-The localized projection of discomfort for the purpose of terminating a visual task that has lowered achievement to a degree unsatisfactory to itself.

Optimal-Best.

Optometry-The art and science of visual care.

Organism-A complex cellular structure capable of maintaining its existence as a unitary system. A unified system of energy capable of growth and reproduction.

Organization-The degree of integration of those neural patterns required by the organism to perform the necessary acts of that species.

Organized case-A visual problem in which the organism has made fairly rigid adjustment to the environmental problem encountered and is not in a pliable plastic state of visual habits that will permit easy and quick correction through lens application or visual training. The organism has achieved the best possible equilibrium in space, despite the impairment. There is now a restriction of performance in visual space. The environment that has been constricted is the cultural or symbolic dimension.

Origin-The zero reference point of the measures employed.

Orthophoria-The position of the eyes is not changed when the binocular space lattice is ruptured. It is a condition significant of the absorption of exophoria. It is a signal that a distortion exists in the visual pattern. The loss of potential ability to manipulate space beyond the plane of regard.

Output-The resultant covert or overt movement pattern produced by the organism in response to the initiating input.

Part-Anything that is the result of division, either real or imaginary.

Pattern-A functional integration of discriminable parts, which operates or responds as a unitary whole. The configuration of nervous excitation in the central nervous system which controls conduction to an effector.

Perception-A conscious experience that has a certain degree of organization and meaning. It is the organization of data in the sense that what is given through the receptors is organized into a pattern of response.

Perseveration-The persistent continuation of a line of thought or activity once it is under way.

Phoria-Change in overt action in space. It informs as to how much accommodation may be changed with a lens, without causing an overt change in convergence. They are measurements of the relationships existing to protect the integrity of convergence pattern.

Physical world-The energies that arise from without the organism and excite his sense organs and cause an interaction with his actual surrounds.

Plateau-Learning curves usually exhibit a leveling off, followed by a further rise. This level stretch of little or no measurable improvement in skill is known as a plateau.

Positive relative accommodation-The amount that accommodation may be stimulated (minus lenses) from a given fixation position before blur or diplopia occurs. It is the maximum amount that we can stimulate accommodation with convergence fixed.

Positive relative convergence-The amount that convergence may be stimulated (base-out prism) from a given fixation point before blur or diplopia occurs. It is the maximum amount we can stimulate convergence with accommodation fixed.

Postural movements-The large movements which regulate body position in relation to the forces of gravity and acceleration.

Posture-Position, stance. A pattern of reciprocal innervations resulting in a desired placement of a physical mechanism.

Preparatory set-The bodily attitude or posture which is assumed as the initial stage of a given activity.

Presbyope-An individual who cannot read standard type (20/20) at near with his basic finding (subjective) and to whom standard acuity can be restored by the use of plus lenses.

Prism-A device that causes a change in the convergence pattern.

Probe body-An instrument used to make an exploratory examination or test. Optometrically, these instruments are lenses and prisms.

Processing-The action and speed of the organism in integrating the incoming information into the C.N.S. and this time lag must not exceed 200 m.s. before overt and covert output is effected if maximum meaning is to be gained.

Prodromal-Symptoms preceding and heralding a disease.

Prognosis-Prediction as to the probable course and outcome of a disorder.

Projection-The reference or localization of sensations to the source or place of origin of the stimulus. While the sensory-cerebro-motor processes all take place within the body, we ascribe the position of the object to some locus in space. We see things where we must go in order to touch, feel or manipulate them.

Proprioception-The mass of sensory data received from structures in the muscles, tendons, ligaments, bones, cartilages and membranes of the joints. It forms the basis for the perception of bodily movements, and it provides the necessary afferent impulses which enable the organism to adjust its movements accurately.

Range-The limits within which a thing may vary in degree or magnitude.

Reaction-In biology, the response of the body, or one of its parts, to stimulation.

Reading-The vicarious transfer of one person's visual space world to the visual space world of another person through the use of the visual signs of a language.

Receptor-A sensory structure.

Recovery point-The return to single vision. It is significant of the "degree of organization" between the patterns of accommodation and convergence. If there is poor integration or organization within the visual behavior pattern, it would be necessary to reduce the amount of prism power greatly before single vision would be restored. This would be a low recovery. If a high integration or organization exists, the converse will occur and a high recovery will result.

Redintegration-The process by which the mind again completes a complex mental state.

Reflex-A local movement produced by stimulation of the part in question. A stereotyped contraction of an isolated group of muscles.

Rehabilitation-To restore to former capacity. Reconditioning of the visual pattern by means of lenses, prisms or visual training.

Reorganization (restructuring)-Organism referring activity to lower cortical levels.

Resolution-The ability to continue to see separately and unblurred the details of the visual object as those details are made smaller and closer together.

Retarded reader-A person with excellent acuity, high degree of binocular vision, but whose ability to interpret, to get meaning from the printed page, is below his age, grade or intelligence level.

Retinal rivalry-Monocular alteration. A perceptual response obtained when different targets are presented to each eye which cannot be fused. There is a rhythmic alternation of the targets which is called retinal rivalry and which is usually recorded in cycles of alternation per one minute.

Retinoscopy (static)-The measurement of a relationship between patterns of accommodation and convergence made measurable by the radical sensory interference of the retinoscope (flicker).

The using of projected light beam, whereby the existing relationship of the depth of focus to the retina is observed. When that depth has been moved forward, the observed motion is "against;" when moved backward the observed motion is "with."

Reversal phenomenon-An over action due to continued inhibition of a particular function. Under conditions of maintained inhibition, upon release of that inhibition, an excessive and reversed action occurs. The presence of reversals in the pattern of optometric test measurements indicates an advanced visual problem. In the accommodative interference case (B-type), these reversals are: dissociated cross-cylinder net is less in plus than the subjective finding, negative relative convergence in greater magnitude than the positive relative convergence test; positive relative accommodation in greater magnitude than negative relative, accommodation.

Rotations-The ability of the eye to follow a smoothly moving target in a circular path. It is one of the basic visual skills.

Satiety-Resultant changes produced in the visual pattern by prolonged exposure to stimulation. The disorganization of visual patterns by the process of maintaining fixation under conditions of high contrast and intensity, far beyond the ordinary accepted time limits for effective use of a sense receptor.

Scanning-The neurological process in which the organism "searches" his incoming and previous memory traces for matching information. Internal scanning takes place in the specious present. Memory traces are reviewed as they relate to the input data. From the result, the probable future can be predicted.

Seeing-The identification of reflected light; an activity of the human body and mind. Its end result is human behavior in its fullest sense.

Sensation-It is the specific and constant response produced by the stimulation of a sensory structure. Light, color, contrast and direction seem to be the fundamental visual sensations. An elementary process underlying perception.

Sensory-See Afferent.

Servo-mechanism-A closed loop control system which operates to control the machine of which it is a part.

Set-Orientation of energy mobilization.

Sigma-One thousandth of a second.

Size constancy-Seen objects tend to remain the same size. The physical law that states that the size of an object decreases by the square of the distance from the object to observer does not hold. Objects tend to remain constant in size color and shape.

Skeletal nervous system-Voluntary nervous system. The motor output which controls the posturing mechanism of the systems. One phase of the dual-effector process.

Skew-The distortion of the visual pattern due to the prolonged effect of stress measurable as shifts in the analytical and visual skills test data.

Skew chart-A graphical presentation of optometric test data that indicates the departure of visual tests from their statistical norms.

Skill-A developed or acquired aptitude or ability a motor performance that has become facile and well integrated; ease and precision in performance of motor acts. The ability to bring about some end result with maximum certainty and minimum outlay of energy.

Space-That which surrounds us.

Spastic movements-Tension type movements, uneconomic or ineffective type of movements.

Spatial-Of or pertaining to space.

Standard practice-It is the way "it is done;" the customary procedure in performing a test. It is the standard method which has been validated statistically or by clinical practice.

Stereopsis-Depth perception; tri-dimensionality. The accurate location of objects in space.

Stimulation-It refers to the effect of minus lenses upon the accommodative mechanism and the effect of base-out prism upon the convergence mechanism; it changes the postural set of these mechanisms as if the stimulus object had been moved closer to the eye. An environmental change of sufficient intensity to cause a change in a sensory structure.

Stimuli-The forces that act upon the receptor. A portion of energy presented by the environment.

Strabismus, adventitious-A type of environmental adaptation wherein the organism: (a) ablates binocularity; (b) changes the mechanism of convergence; (c) attains a satisfactory visual adaptation to itself. The complete cycle of adaptation for divergent or exotropia is: (1) intermittent tropia at far, no deviation at near; (2) fixed tropia at far, intermittent at near; (3) increased tropia at far, slight tropia at near; (4) equal degree of deviation at far and near.

Stress-Any conditions impinging on the organism which require adjustive reactions.

Stresses-Forces leading to tension formation are known as stresses.

Stressors-The agents producing stresses.

Structure-A quality of an organized whole, presumably related to the positional interdependence of its parts.

Structured (see "organized") - A visual pattern that is fixed.

Subjective-A measure of the latitude which may be occupied by lenses if there is value to the organism in such a localization. It is the amount of accommodation free of association with convergence. It is the greatest amount of plus or the least minus through which the patient can read 20/20 binocularly.

Subjective, nearpoint-That amount of accommodation free of association with convergence (represented by the basic finding) plus an amount due to the existence of a "learned compensatory relation" with the convergence pattern at near. The cross-cylinder test values at near.

Suppression-A type of cancellation where areas of the total perceptual field have been eliminated by the organism.

Symptoms-The answers given by the modified organism to definite demands. A structural or functional change that indicates the presence of an anomalous condition.

Syndrome-A pattern of factors functionally related in such a manner that if you change one of them, the others will change. It gathers the information contained in the analytical examination into small compass for summation. Denoting the aggregate symptom of a disease or functional disturbance. A characteristic sequence of symptoms.

System-Any totality, the aspect of which are interrelated members of the whole.

Tachistoscope-A variable exposure instrument used for training form and unity of the identification process.

Tension-A state of strain or imbalance in an organism which leads to behavior in the direction of restored equilibrium. A readiness for immediate action.

Texture-The amount of detail or "grain" that the viewer can detect and interpret. The Snellen letters and all objects in the environment have degrees of "texture."

Therapy-Treatment; application of various treatment techniques.

Tonic-Pertaining to muscle tension or contraction; muscle tone.

Tonus-A state of partial contraction of a muscle group.

Toxic typing-A visual problem whose typing syndrome is: (1) static retinoscopy in less plus than the subjective; (2) abduction at far lower in its value than convergence at far; (3) induced phoria at near less than its expected value; (4) negative fusional reserve duction test below its expected value and lower than its mate, positive fusional reserve.

Training-The arranging of conditions that through repeated experience the individual may teach himself.

Transaction-The reaction between the person and an object, his experience and his resultant effector process.

Typing-The process of assembling a significant series of findings indicative of a certain type of problem and needing a certain indicated method of corrective procedure. It refers to: (1) the manner in which lenses will be accepted; and (2) the direction the corrective procedures will be given. We have two basic case types. These are: B-type (accommodative problems) and C-type (convergence problems).

Unorganized case-The visual problem making adjustments or adaptations in visual skills or visual performance to the needs of the individual in the environment in which he lives.

Versions-The ability of the eyes (binocularly) to follow a smoothly moving target.

Visceral nervous system-Involuntary nervous system. The motor out put to control the internal organs of the system. One phase of the dual-effector visual system.

Vision-The means whereby we perceive space as a whole. It is only by vision that spatial relations of objects outside the body and at a distance from it are satisfactorily dealt with in detail. It is all the light related activities of the organism, plus the organism's freedom in its environment to carry through these actions efficiently.

Visual achievement-The ability to interpret the external visual environment by means of the photo (light) receptor.

Visual acuity-The ability to discriminate contours; to tell when there is separation from background and whether there are one, two or three objects and not just a blur. It is the ability to perceive the interspace between two objects when it is very small. It is the reciprocal of the just resolvable visual angle measured in minutes.

Visual behavior pattern-It is made up of the behavior patterns of convergence and accommodation, the other skeletal postural patterns and the other contributory visceral patterns.

Visualize-The ability to remember, know and predict where and what things were, are and will be in space-time.

Visual problem-A visual pattern which has suffered a decrement in performance. It is a distorted response. A distortion in the manipulation of visual space. A stress produced interference with the ability of the organism to mobilize experience for correct or immediate action.

Visual skills-They are performance tests. They are elements in obtaining meaning from the visual environment. They show impairment of visual performance.

Visual space-The external world as perceived through the eyes. The terrain with objects in it which surround the subject.

Visual space world-The learned relationships between objects in space.

Visual training-The alteration of the manipulation of space at a magnitude not tolerable as a consistent performance, but capable of forcing changes that necessitate changes in the visual pattern. The primary objective in visual training is to so disorganize the behavior pattern that lenses can be used at the point of the artificial visual task so that the organism may adequately restructure the visual behavior pattern behind those lenses.

Whole-Anything that has members of phases and yet possesses attributes which distinguish it as a unit from its parts or aspects.

Questions and Answers

1. Where did the expecteds for the various analytical tests come from?

These expected values were determined by averaging the values found in thousands of cases. Other authorities who have checked these values have arrived at the same results. Here is a comparison of the results found by Morgan, Shepard and OEP:

Test No.		Morgan	Shepard	O.E.P.
#9		7-11	9	7-9
#10	break	19	21	19
#10	recovery	10	9	10
#11	break	7	9	9
#11	recovery	4	4	5
#16B	break	21	25	21
#16B	recovery	11	13	15
#17B	break	21	20	22
#17B	recovery	13	11	18

2. Why is the subjective test (#7) taken to 20/20 visual acuity, instead of best visual acuity?

(a) The subjective test values are not necessarily the lenses which are going to be prescribed by the optometrist. They do represent the maximum lens power which may be used at far.

(b) The subjective lens power is a comparison point for all optometric test results. Its stability is, therefore, important. The statistical research of Shepard reveals that test-retest results will have twice the dispersion if taken through the subjective to best visual acuity, as compared with the subjective to 20/20 visual acuity. His exact data is:

#7 (best V.A.) Mean +0.50 std. dv. 1.62 D.
#7 (20/20 V.A.) Mean +0.87 std. dv. 0.87 D.

3. Why is a six-to-one relationship used in computing lags at near, instead of the actual accommodative-convergence relationship?

If the individual reacts to visual space in a physical manner, we would have 2.50 D. of accommodation and 15 diopters of convergence, assuming 60 p.d. and 16-inch fixation distance, or a relationship of 6 p.d. of convergence and 1 of accommodation. We find that the experimentally determined accommodative convergence relationship is so variable that it is difficult to utilize it in determining the lag. In a recent experiment on the effect of prolonged television viewing on certain optometric findings by Stein and Hofstetter, they found the following variations in ACA ratio:

Subject:	G.H.	2:1	Subject:	G.C.	2:1
		1:1			2:1
		3:1			4:1
		4:1			3:1
		3:1			2:1

In using a six-to-one, rather than the experimental value, we usually obtain a net that is too great. This value must then be checked to prevent the prescribing of a near-point lens which is not acceptable to the patient. The acceptance of this lens depends upon its effect upon the equilibrium pattern. If the equilibrium pattern through this lens is similar to the habitual pattern of the individual, the lens is acceptable, if the lens creates an equilibrium pattern that differs from the habitual pattern, it is rejected. The value of this lens must be modified so that the pattern through this lens and the habitual lens are similar. In this case, this new lens amount becomes "the amount of accommodation free of convergence at near-point."

4. What are the factors that influence the acceptance of a single vision lens for constant wear?

These are: (1) nets at near-that portion of the cross-cylinder net which is acceptable in the equilibrium findings; (2) program of lens fitting-formulated from the duction pattern at both far and near; (3) the cross-cylinder net-based upon the gross cross-cylinder tests, less the lag of accommodation, figured from the phoria at near (15A and 15B), the resultant value being modified by the amplitude of accommodation ratio if the amplitude is below 5 diopters.

5. Why do we use a modified lag table for the dynamic retinoscopy finding at 20 inches?

The maximum lag you can have at a 20-inch fixation distance is 2 diopters. The lag is based upon the phoria taken through the dissociated cross-cylinder lenses. This is done because the correlation coefficient between the gross No. 5 and gross No. 14A is 0.8. The phoria taken through the dissociated cross-cylinder lenses is taken at a fixation distance of 16 inches. Therefore, the lag table of the dynamic retinoscopy test is considered as a modified table because of the change in total accommodation possible and the difference in fixation distance.

6. When a reduction in plus is indicated by the duction pattern of the case, what is the minimum and maximum cut?

The minimum cut is 0.25 D. and the maximum cut is 0.75 D.

7. Through what Rx do we take the near-point findings from 16A on down in a case of a myope who has never worn minus glasses?

These near-point test findings are taken through plano.

8. What is minus projection?

It is an active state of inhibition between the patterns of accommodation and convergence to prevent blurring or doubling. It is found at far when the static retinoscopy finding is in minus and the subjective in plano is in plus. It is found at near when the cross-cylinder net is in minus and standard acuity is present at near unaided.

9. If 16B is 15/10 and 17B is 13/6, which duction is low-low?

#16B	15/10	(15/21)
#17B	13/6	(13/22) low-low

13/22 is a lower or smaller fraction than 15/21.

10. What is the difference in significance between "prisms to blur" and "prisms to break?"

Prisms to break (ductions) are used to primarily determine programs of lens fitting (case typing). Prisms to blur (positive and negative relative convergence) are used as the final check on the acceptance of any lens power at near-point.

11. What is visual training?

(a) The alteration of the manipulation of space at a magnitude not tolerable as a consistent performance.

(b) The primary objective in training is to so disorganize the behavior pattern that lenses can be used at the point of the artificial visual task so that the organism may adequately restructure his visual behavior pattern behind these lenses.

(c) The objective of training is to restore achievement in whatever sphere it has been lowered and at the same time to enhance the level of visual achievement in all the visual environment and to bring such attainment to the organism that the intellectual capacity may be raised and the temperamental responses find approval and, therefore, satisfaction.

12. What is the fundamental objective of visual training?

The fundamental objective is to increase achievement. This may require: reducing the degree of amblyopia; increasing the degree of fusion; raising stereopsis; reducing or eliminating the angle of squint; eliminating structured esophoria or exophoria; building plus acceptance at near and far;

stabilizing the refractive error; establishing tolerance to anisometropic correction; improving perceptual skills; increasing spatial manipulation; eliminating suppressions; increasing accommodative amplitude; improving accommodative facility (speed and accuracy).

13. What do we mean by the term "reversal?"

In a "B-type" case, we expect to have plus and base-in tests, but if the visual problem has existed for some time, we find that the relative position of these tests are reversed. Continuous stimulation has finally resulted in a spatial reversal in values. This occurs in other physiological structures. The repeated stimulation of one point may result not only in abatement, but even in reversal of effect, e.g., flexion of the elbow instead of extension. This type of reversal has been reported by Sherrington, Brown, and Goldstein.

14. What are the three basic steps in correcting a visual problem by visual training?

(a) Disorganize the distorted visual behavior pattern; (b) direct visual performance towards desirable reorganization; (c) assist in stabilization at a desirable level.

15. Does every visual problem need visual training?

The answer is yes if we are thinking in terms of prevention and enhancement of visual skills. No individual could help but benefit from visual training. Usually those cases which allow some plus to be prescribed can be handled without visual training. Those visual problems which are recent in time or which are disorganized can be handled by lens application. These cases are B1-1, 2, 3 and B2-1, 2, 3 and 4. But any patient could receive enhancement in visual skills through training. When we realize how competitive modern life has become, the more we realize the importance of visual training for our patients.

16. What information do we obtain from the distant subjective test (#7)?

(a) To determine the maximum spherical dioptric acceptance at far point; (b) to determine the degree of anisometropia; (c) to determine the amount and axis of any existing astigmatism; (d) to determine if the individual is capable of standard acuity.

17. What does a phoria test measure?

A phoria measures the change produced in the convergence pattern and by an associated change in accommodation; determines the lag; determines how long the visual problem has existed.

18. What do we mean by the term "acceptance?"

The term "acceptance" is used to indicate that the amount of the dissociated cross-cylinder test or the binocular cross-cylinder test does not reverse the habitual equilibrium pattern as set by the organism. For example, if our case revealed the following relationships:

habitual pattern	$\frac{16A\text{-}21}{17A\text{-}20}$
14A net	$\frac{16A\text{-}21}{17A\text{-}20}$
14B net	$\frac{16A\text{-}20}{17A\text{-}21}$

we would state that the net plus of the dissociated cross-cylinder test is accepted, while the lens value represented by the binocular cross-cylinder test is rejected.

19. Give the single vision prescription if the corrective framework was as follows:

far:	not over	O.D.	+1.50
		O.S.	+1.00
	not under	O.D.	+1.50
		O.S.	+1.00
near:	not over	O.D.	+1.00
		O.S.	+0.50
	not under	O.D.	+0.50
		O.S.	+plano

The single vision prescription would be: O.D. +1.00; O.S. +0.50.

20. What are the factors which must be considered in prescribing a cylindrical correction?

We must evaluate the following factors: 1. age of patient; 2. previous ocular history; 3. effect of cylinder upon acuity; 4. comparison of amount of cylinder found objectively with that found subjectively; 5. axis of cylinder (oblique vs. with or against R.); 6. the effect of the cylinder upon the visual skills of the patient (fusion and stereopsis); 7. organizational status of the case; 8. amount of cylinder; 9. ocular complaint of the patient; 10. vocational history of the patient.

21. Why do we use a numerical designation for our optometric tests?

It is a short hand method of designating and identifying our optometric tests. It is much easier to say, "15A," than, "The phoria test taken through the plus of the dissociated cross-cylinder test at near."

It is easier to study relationships between tests and to group them into case types, syndromes, and patterns.

Each number designates one test which has been taken by an accepted standard procedure.

22. When does the patient have visual discomfort?

He will have discomfort when his ability to perform visually is not adequate for the demands of his environment. Thus, the visually inefficient child who is forced to perform at nearpoint will have visual discomfort if he cannot develop suppression.

23. What is focus?

It is that particular pattern of light energy distribution upon the retina which at the moment results in standard acuity.

24. Give an example of emmetropia at near.

We have emmetropia at near when the net cross cylinder test is plano. For example:

#14A +1.00
#15A 6 exo (lag is 1.00 D.)
Net 14A is plano

25. Do we have minus projection at near when the subjective finding is in more plus than the M.S.D.A.?

No, we merely have less hyperopia at near than at far. For example:

#7 +1.00, M.S.D.A. +0.50.

26. Does the test distance determine how much accommodation will be in action?

Under special test conditions, it can be shown that as the target approaches the eye of the observer, increased accommodation occurs.

When we check the individual in his normal visual environment we find that the test distance does not correlate too well with the amount of accommodation in play. Emsley (Visual Optics, p. 166) states, "It is not an easy matter to determine precisely the state of accommodation of an eye. The brain is apparently capable of 'seeing' an object distinctly when the eyes optical system is focused for some point nearer or further away than the object." On page 173 he further states, "As already remarked, however, such distinctness cannot be relied upon as indicating unchanged accommodation. It can change within limits because of the depth of focus of the refracted pencils within the eye, and latitude allowed by cortical interpretation."

Pheiffer (Am. J. Optom. 32,543 [1955]) reporting on book retinoscopy states, ". . . The amount of this variation was 0.50 to 0.75 diopter and concurs with the observations made by other workers. Since this change may occur several times during the reading of a line or not at all, it is in all probability not due to the retinoscopist being on or off the visual axis. Seven of the subjects made greater changes in accommodation when reading physics material (0.50 to 1.00) as compared to the digest material (0.25 to 0.75)...." In his conclusion, he estimates that when the subject is reading at 16 inches, accommodation cannot be postured closer than 10 inches or further away than 20 inches. This is, of course, without the subject experiencing blurring or doubling and with the reading material at 16 inches.

27. What is the difference between perceptual skills and manipulatory skills?

Perceptual skills are the measurements of visual abilities which are taken through a stereoscopic device.
Manipulatory skills are those measurements of visual abilities which are taken outside of a stereoscopic device.

28. How does exophoria protect the convergence pattern?

The presence of exophoria prevents doubling by absorbing any excessive stimuli coming to the convergence pattern because of the demands of the environment in which the subject functions. In the morning, this individual may exhibit six exophoria; but by evening it may have decreased to one diopter of exophoria because of the environmental demands. The presence of exophoria, which is an area of inhibition in the central nervous system, absorbs the stimulus coming from other portions of the system, and thereby it protects the convergence mechanism against functioning and resultant diplopia. The exophoria gives the organism a certain latitude or flexibility of functioning of the convergence mechanism.

29. How does hyperopia protect the accommodative pattern?

Changes in the amount of hyperopia make it possible for the subject to maintain standard far point acuity in spite of increased environmental impact.

In early morning he may be a 1.00 diopter hyperope; by late afternoon he may be only a +0.50 diopter hyperope; if he goes bowling that evening we may find a decrease to emmetropia. Hyperopia provides a buffer area in the accommodative pattern which in turn provides the organism with clear vision, even though excessive stimulation may be arising because of the day-to-day stress situations.

30. It has been stated that the relationship between accommodation and convergence is a constant. What is the functional viewpoint?

The functional viewpoint is that the ACA ratio is a variable that fluctuates in amount to about the same degree as the induced phoria at near (#13B). Persons having a well stabilized pattern will also have a less variable fluctuation in the ACA ratio. Persons under intense stress will tend to have a more variable fluctuation in the ACA ratio. For example, Stein and Hofstetter in their investigation of the effect of prolonged viewing of television upon certain optometric tests, measured the ACA ratio after viewing TV for various times (Am. Acad. of Optom. 28,250 [1951]). On subject C.H., they obtained the following values of the ACA ratio: 2:1, 1:1, 3:1, 4:1, 3:1.

The close relationship between ACA ratio and the induced phoria at near (#13B) can be shown by using the data of Fry (Am. Acad. Optom. 17,939 [1940]). In his article, he presents a scatter-diagram which graphically presents this relationship. However, if we use his data and calculate the coefficient of correlation, we obtain a value of 0.92. This shows a very highly significant relationship between the two variables.

Furthermore, Emsley (Visual Optics, p. 204) states that the ACA ratio must change, "When an ametrope is first corrected for distance, the accommodation-convergence relationship to which he has become accustomed is suddenly changed, and a new relationship has to be developed. The corrected myope now requires more accommodation; the hyperope less accommodation than before. Moreover, when a presbyopic addition is first worn, the amount of accommodative effort required for nearwork is suddenly diminished; and again, a new relationship between the two functions in near work has to be met."

31. What do we mean by the term "stimulation?"

Stimulation refers to the change induced in the postural set of the accommodative mechanism by minus lenses or to the change in the convergence mechanism by base-out prism.

Under conditions of stimulation the effect is as if the object of regard had moved closer to the subject.

32. What do we mean by the term "inhibition?"

Inhibition refers to the change induced in the postural set of the accommodative mechanism by plus lenses, or it refers to the change in the postural set of the convergence mechanism by base-in prism.

Under conditions of inhibition the effect is as if the object of regard had moved further away from the subject.

33. What is the role of the case type?

The case typing refers to the modification procedure which follows with the subjective at far and the maximal spherical dioptric acceptance at near. If the case typing is a B1-full plus is acceptable at all points. If the case typing is a B2-5 or less-cut plus at far and prescribe full plus at near. If the case typing is a B2-6 or B2-7 or B1-6 or 7 cut plus at all points. If the case typing is a C-cut plus at both far and near.

34. What is the maximum lag you can deduct from nearpoint accommodative tests?

Dynamic retinoscopy at 20 inches (#5) - Maximum lag is 2.00 D.
Dynamic retinoscopy at 40 inches (#6) - Maximum lag is 0.25 D.
Dissociated cross-cylinder test at near (#14A) - Maximum lag is 2.50 D.
Fused cross-cylinder test at near (#14B) - Maximum lag is 1.75 D.

35. What is the difference between blur, break and recovery tests?

These are portions of a test in which prism is introduced so that the convergence pattern is either stimulated (base-out) or inhibited (base-in) while the patient is fixating at the plane of regard at 16 inches.

The blur portion of the test measures the extent of the learned relationship between accommodation and convergence. It measures the ability of the organism to withstand the probing of the convergence pattern and to inhibit this activity from invading the accommodative pattern and causing a blur. The extent of this magnitude depends upon learning.

When the amount of prism interposed passes the blur point, we are steadily increasing the direct change in the convergence pattern and associated change in the accommodative pattern. How long the patient will tolerate this dilemma depends upon how well integrated these two patterns of accommodation and convergence are. If the integration between accommodation and convergence is poor, the patient will break very shortly past the blur finding; if the integration is good, the patient will show a considerably higher break finding.

After the patient has exceeded his break value and has reported diplopia, we begin to reduce the magnitude of the interposed prism. We approach a situation wherein the photic distribution across retina, in relationship to the macula, is within the organizational ability of the patient, and the patient will regain single vision. If the visual pattern is poorly organized, the amount of prism will have to be reduced considerable before single vision is obtained; if highly organized, the patient will retain single vision very quickly.

36. Why do we obtain a blur in the farpoint base-out duction (no. 9) and why do we not obtain a blur in the farpoint base-in duction (no. 11)?

When the patient is fixating at far and we introduce increased amounts of base-out prism, we are stimulating convergence while accommodation is at the plane of regard. This increased stimulus from convergence will be inhibited until the maximum extent of the learned relationship between accommodation and convergence has been reached. At this point, increased amounts of base-out will result in a blur. This change in convergence is a normal organsmic experience when looking from far to near.

However, when we perform the base-in duction test at far, we are asking the organism to prevent inhibition proceeding towards the accommodative pattern. The patient has never had an opportunity to learn this trick of reflexly inhibiting convergence while fixating at far. Therefore, he will not blur; but he will try to maintain single vision as long as possible. When the extent of Panum's areas have been exceeded, he will experience diplopia.

37. What is the difference in the lag of accommodation?

The lag of accommodation is a correction factor which is subtracted from the gross nearpoint accommodative tests to obtain a nearpoint net accommodative test value. We usually place it in terms of equation: gross - lag = net. Thus, the lag represents the amount of accommodation which is reflexly tied up with convergence.

38. What is the difference between the terms "visual achievement" and "visual acuity?"

Visual acuity refers to the ability of the subject to recognize a standard contour target at a particular distance.

Visual achievement is the sum total of all the visual skills which measure the patient's ability to perform in his environment. Thus, visual acuity is one of the profile skills which aid in determining visual achievement.

39. What is meant by the term "amplitude?"

Amplitude of accommodation is a range of performance in the accommodative pattern for the purpose of preserving clear vision in spite of advancing years.

40. What is the difference between the amplitude of accommodation test (#19) and positive relative accommodation (#20)?
The following outline gives the points of difference:

41. If the duction pattern of a case is 11-17B low: The subjective is +0.75: The maximum plus you could prescribe at far is?
We have a B2 typing. Therefore, plus must be cut at far. The smallest reduction in plus is 0.25 diopter. Hence, the maximum plus you may prescribe as far is +0.50.

42. Check the following duction tests:

#10 17/6 L	#10 20/5 L	#10 10/9 LL
#11 5/4 LL	#11 10/6 H	#11 12/2 L

RULES:
(a) No. 10 Br. must be 19 or higher.
(b) No, 11 Br. must be 9 or higher.
(c) Recovery must be ½ of break or higher.
(d) If both tests are low, the low test is the one with the low break.

43. What statistical evidence do we have that the habitual and induced phoria tests should have the same expected (mean) values?
The following data is based on 500 clinical cases selected at random from the total clinic files at the Illinois College of Optometry.

Habitual Phoria at Far		Induced Phoria at Far	
Mean	0.75 Exo	Mean	0.996 Exo
Median	0.65 Exo	Median	0.84 Exo
Std. Dev.	2.7 d.	Std.Dev.	2.94 d.
Sigma Mean	0.07 d.	Sigma Mean	0.08 d.
Skewness	0.66	Skewness	0.16
Kurtosis	0.25	Kurtosis 0.28	

Habitual Phoria at Near		Induced Phoria at Near	
Mean	4.72 Exo	Mean	4.61 Exo
Median	4.73 Exo	Median	4.74 Exo
Std. Dev.	5.01 d.	Std. Dev.	5.57 d.
Sigma Mean	0.13 d.	Sigma Mean	0.14 d.
Skewness	-0.26	Skewness	-0.21
Kurtosis	0.26	Kurtosis 0.24	

Although this data is based on persons having a visual problem, and we would therefore expect deviations from the magnitude of the expected values on 'Normal' people, still we can compare the habitual and induced values and we see that they have about the same magnitude.

44. How are alterations in visual behavior measured?

The alterations in visual behavior are found by comparing the magnitude of a particular test value with that expected for unimpaired individuals. The greater this difference, the greater the alteration in visual behavior.

Factor	**Amp. of Acc.**	**Pos. Rel. Acct.**
Test distance	13"	16"
Target	0.62 Em. Type	20/20 Reduced Snellen
Control lenses	Subjective	(a) Non-presbyope or hyperope - subjective (b) Myope – Habitual minus (c) Presbyope – fused cross cylinder net
Endpoint of test	Print difficult to read	Complete blur-out
Calculations	a) Non-presbyope – Minus above subjective added to 2.50 b) Presbyope- plus above subjective subtracted from 2.50	Record the amount of minus above the control.
Purpose of test	a) Deterioration of case b) Modification of lag	Comparison between positive and negative relative accommodation indicates acceptance of plus.

45. What are the basic factors which must be considered in evaluating a visual problem?

The following factors must be considered:

1) Case History
   a) Previous ocular difficulty.
   b) Any health difficulty.
   c) Any developmental problem.
   d) Any educational problem.
   e) Any behavior difficulties.
   f) Social-environmental demands.
2) Analytical Examination
   a) Case type and deterioration.
   b) Maximum lens acceptance at far and near.
   c) Are the lens amounts accepted in the equilibrium pattern?
   d) At what stage in time is the visual problem?
   e) Is the erroneous visual behavior embedded or disembedded?
   f) Is there sufficient amplitude for demands?

3) Visual Skills (visual abilities)
   a) In what manner has the patient tried to cope with his problem?
   b) To what extent do we find distortions in the visual pattern?
4) Professional judgment.

46. The patient returning for a progress report reveals a disembedded pattern. Would you expect the patient to have comfort or discomfort?

The presence of disembedding indicates performance at a higher cortical level which is inefficient. Therefore, if the patient is forced to perform a nearpoint task, I would expect him to have discomfort. If he can avoid nearpoint activity, he may have comfort.

47. Classify phoria tests in three different ways?

1. According to test distance
   a) Farpoint tests: #3, #8, #12
   b) Nearpoint tests: #13A, #13B, #18, #15A, #15B
2. According to direction
   a) Lateral tests: #3, #8, # 13A, #13B, #15A, #15B
   b) Vertical tests: #12, #18
3. According to the lenses used
   a) Habitual tests: #3, #8, #13A
   b) Induced tests: #8, #13B, #12, #18, #15A, #15B

48. What is the meaning of the statement: "We can never prescribe more minus for near than for far?"

This statement refers to lens application for the myope, where the distant subjective is in minus. We must never give the patient more minus for near than for far. For example:

#7-1.00
#14A net -2.00
#14B net -1.75

The maximum minus that could be prescribed for near is -.1.00 d.

49.How does the optometrist look at the visual data in order to arrive at a diagnosis?

The skilled visual diagnostician looks at the visual data in somewhat of the following manner:
A. Subjective finding
B. Cross cylinder nets
C. Duction pattern

D. Established case type and deterioration
E. Determine M.S.D.A.
F. Did the plus of the subjective influence the nearpoint phorias significantly (#13A compared to #13B)
G. Corrective framework
H. Organizational status of case
I. Tentative Rx
J. Weigh tentative Rx against information from case history and previous Rx.
K. Philosophy of the visual diagnostician
   a. Prescribing prosthetically
   b. Prescribing for prevention and enhancement
L. Progress examination to verify effect of the visual care.
M. Long-Hop examination to determine visual status of patient so that continuing care may be initiated before serious adaptations have occurred.

50. Why does plus at near when prescribed for the beginning myope tend to block its progression?

The myopic patient is beginning to move accommodation toward himself while maintaining convergence at the plane of regard. Therefore, when we require him to use plus at near we are forcing accommodation to move out to the plane of regard. This is in the opposite direction in which he is set to operate and, therefore, tends to upset his myopic programming. The precaution for this approach to be effective in the stabilization of myopia is that the patient must maintain a maximum reading distance through this plus lens application.

51. What is the significance of the ACA ratio in functional visual analysis?

The ACA ratio gives us an additional clue as to the embeddedness of the existing visual pattern. The embedded visual pattern has a rigid relationship between the accommodative and convergence pattern. Therefore, in the embedded case we would expect to find a normal or high ACA ratio (5:1 or higher). In the disembedded visual pattern we have a loose relationship between the patterns of accommodation and convergence. Thus, for the disembedded pattern we would expect to have a low ACA ratio (4:1 or less).

52. How do we determine the ACA ratio?

Three methods are customarily used for this purpose: (1) the gradient method, (2) the Fry method, and (3) the positive and negative relative accommodative method.

(1) The gradient method. After taking the induced phoria at near (#13B) add an additional plus one diopter of spheres O.U. and repeat the phoria measurement. The change in phoria is equivalent to the ACA ratio.

	#13B	6 Exo
(+1.00)	#13BB	9 Exo

Change in convergence = 9 - 6 - 3 d.
Change in accommodation = 1 d.
Thus, the gradient is 3:1

(2) The Fry method.

$$\text{ACA ratio} = \frac{15 - \#8 + \#13B}{2.50}$$

where, Exo is a minus value
Eso is a plus value.

For example: #8 1 Exo
#13B 6 Exo

$$\text{ACA ratio} = \frac{15 + 1 - 6}{2.50} = \frac{10}{2.50} = 4.0$$

(3) The positive and negative relative accommodative method.
Upon the completion of the positive relative accommodative test (#20) a phoria is taken. Also upon the completion of the negative relative accommodative test (#21) a phoria is taken. Through the minus of the #20 finding an esophoric shift is expected and through the plus of the #21 finding an exophoric shift is expected. The total shift in accommodation is compared to the total shift in convergence to give us a gradient magnitude.

For example:			
	#20	-1.75	2 Eso
	#21	+2.25	4 Exo
		4.00	6

gradient is equal to 6/4 or 1.50.

53. What does the lens directive mean, "Never prescribe a lens greater than the accommodation free of convergence."

This means that the maximum plus you can consider for prescribing at farpoint is the subjective (#7). Also, the maximum plus you can consider for prescribing at nearpoint is the cross-cylinder nets (#14A or #14B nets).

54. Through what control lens do we take the various analytical tests following the cross-cylinder tests (#15B) in the case of a presbyope?

Sufficient plus must be used for near point tests through which the patient will have 20/20 visual acuity at nearpoint. We may use the #14B net or even the #14B gross lenses for this purpose. At times if the patient has shown 20/20 at near through his old Rx, his lens value may be placed in the phoroptor and utilized for nearpoint tests. In any instance, whatever control lenses are used they must be noted on the examination form. In a few instances where the patient has not received visual care for many years it may be desirable to take the nearpoint tests through both the cross-cylinder net and the patient's old nearpoint Rx.

55. What do you mean by the term "embedded?"

The term "embedded" applies to the change that occurs with time to the visual pattern. At first the adaptations to visual stress are completely reversible. A night's sleep and in the morning the visual pattern is back to its optimum operating condition. However, when this cycle has been repeated several times we reach a stage where complete reversal does not occur and the visual pattern has become partially modified. If the visual stress is still maintained, a further restriction in performance occurs which allows the organism maximum performance but within a restricted area. The pattern is now more rigid or set and is less amenable to attack by only lenses. This stage is now considered as embedded and the analytical findings will reveal:

#4 equal to or greater than #7 in plus;
#9 equal to expected or higher;
#10 decrease in break value, recovery above the expected value;
#11 break up, though lower than the mean; recovery in excess of the mean value;
#14B net equal to or in excess of #14A net;
#16B recovery up in excess of the mean (break even lower);
#19 and #20 up (#20 higher for the adult, #19 in child);
CA ratio-ratio is normal or high (5:1 or greater).

56. Since base-out prism and plus lenses allow the patient to converge nearer than he is accommodating, why not prescribe the prism rather than the plus lenses for the B-type case?

It is true that the spatial relationships for both base-out prism and plus lenses are the same. However, there are two additional factors in which they differ.

Spatially: base-out prism—convergence in and accommodation out.
plus lenses—convergence in and accommodation out.
Size change: base-put prism—target gets smaller.
plus lenses—target gets larger.
Plane of regard: base-out prism—toward the patient.
plus lenses—convergence at plane of regard.

Thus, although the spatial qualities of base-out prism and plus lenses are similar, the other effects reveal that these two probe bodies are directly opposite to each other. The increase in size and the movement of accommodation away from the plane of regard that we obtain with our plus lenses are changes that are essential for the success in the treatment of the B-type case.

57. Why is the #9 finding high for the beginning myope?

In the beginning myope we have the movement of accommodation toward the patient with convergence out (spatially). Therefore, as we add base-out prism in the beginning myope we are moving convergence towards accommodation, restoring the initial spatial balance. However, as we continue to add additional amounts of base-out prism we are now moving convergence even closer to the patient measuring how well learned the patterns of accommodation and convergence are at the moment. Since this is a beginning problem there, is a considerable learned ability present. Since the #9 finding in the beginning myope contains both of these components we would expect this finding to be higher than its normal value. In fact the higher it is above nine prism diopters the more certain we can be that the myopia found subjectively is of recent occurrence.

9 (beg. myope) = BO. to restore balance + B.O. learned extent.

58. Why does the duction pattern of abduction at far (#11) and positive fusional reserve (#16B) both low indicate that the case will accept the full plus revealed by the case data?

It is obvious that it was the initial clinical observations that made it possible to determine that when we had #11-#16B low we could prescribe the maximum plus at both far and at near. We can reason that this would be true if we accept the following premises: (a) The visual problem starts at nearpoint and moves from the plane of regard toward the patient. (b) In the initial stages of a visual problem we have no interference at farpoint.

At farpoint fixation distance we have two duction tests which we are comparing: #10 which is a base-out test and #11 which is the base-in test. When we turn base-out prism at this test distance we have no interference at this distance. Since the base-out movement is carrying convergence toward the patient, an experience which he has had many times, we will find this value to be high. However, when we begin to turn base-in prism at the distant fixation distance we are asking the patient to carry convergence out beyond infinity-an experience which he has never experienced before. Therefore, we will have the base-in duction of #11 to be lower.

At the nearpoint fixation distance we are again comparing the base-out duction, #16B with the base-in duction test, #17B. In the beginning visual problem the interference has created spatial disturbances toward the patient. Therefore, when we investigate the spatial manipulative ability of the patient with prism base-out we are forcing the pattern into an area of difficulty and the test magnitude will be low. However, when we turn base-in prism at the near point fixation distance we carry convergence beyond the plane of regard into a spatial area in which the patient has no difficulty and, therefore, #17B will be high.

Whenever we have the pattern of #11-#16B low, we can be certain that the visual problem is of recent origin and maximum plus can be utilized. This is the significance of a B1 typing.

59. Why does the duction pattern of abduction at far (#11) and negative fusional reserve (#17B) both low indicate that we must reduce the plus prescribed at far but we can prescribe full plus at near?

As the explanation given in the answer to question 58 has shown, when #11 is low it indicates a recent visual problem.

However, when we view the nearpoint ductions we find that the visual problem has been in existence long enough so that it has gone beyond the plane of regard at the near point fixation distance. It is for this reason that the base-in prism duction will now become the lower of the two (#17B lower than #16B).

The visual problem is beginning to approach far point. Therefore, it is advisable to reduce the far point plus so that we do not create any additional problems at the spatial position. At nearpoint we need all of the help we can get, therefore, we can utilize the full plus shown in the pattern. We might say that the problem is in transit and can best be stabilized by applying the full plus at near which would block any further visual deterioration at far point. In addition, in order to avoid any possibility of creating any additional difficulties at far point it is advisable to reduce the applied plus spheres at this point.

60. Why does the duction pattern of convergence at far (#10) becoming the lower duction over abduction at far (#11) indicate that we should reduce plus at all points (at both far and at near)?

When the visual problem has lasted for sufficient time and/or has been of such high intensity it will spread in the last stages to the far point fixation distance. When this interference in visual patterning reaches farpoint and we start to turn base-out prism to measure the degree of interference present, as soon as convergence starts moving from the plane of regard we have reached the limit of flexibility possessed by the patient and the target will double. Therefore this finding (#10) becoming the low duction value signals the practitioner that the visual problem is in its latter stage. In this instance it is advisable to reduce the proposed plus lens application below the acceptable in the subjective at far and the M.S.D.A. at near.

The more extensive or intensive the visual problem becomes the more conservative we must be in our lens applications unless aid is also given by means of home or office visual training.

61. Why does OEP use the same expected values for the positive and negative fusional reserves when the control lens through which the test may be performed is the subjective at far (#7), binocular cross-cylinder net (#14B net) or even the habitual minus at near?

The question is concerned with the possible influence that accommodative changes at near would have upon the expected value of the fusional reserve tests at nearpoint. It is common clinical experience that any change in accommodative status is immediately reflected in some change in the magnitude of the blur findings (positive and negative relative convergence). However, the prism tests taken to the limit of single vision is a learned relationship and is relatively independent of accommodative changes. Thus, if a particular patient has a break test value of 30 prism diopters it may consist of 20 diopters of accommodative convergence and diopters of fusional convergence, or it might consist of 15 diopters of accommodative-convergence in combination with 15 diopters of fusional convergence. The total magnitude of the fusional reserve has remained the same.

The lack of effect of accommodation upon the magnitude of total convergence is well illustrated by the lack of effect age has upon the magnitude of the near point of convergence test. In addition, we have the results of the statistical studies of Morgan which found a zero correlation between prism-to-break test at near and dynamic retinoscopy at 20 inches. The same zero correlation was found between these break tests and the cross-cylinder tests at near.

However, an additional statistical study was made by the author upon the effect of additional plus at near upon the magnitude of the fusional reserve tests utilizing the clinical files of the Illinois College of Optometry. One hundred case records were taken at random in the age group of from 25 to 43 in which the nearpoint control lens had been the subjective at far. An additional 100 cases were selected at random in which the ages were from

40 to 72 in which the control lens used averaged 1.74 diopters greater than the subjective at far. The results were as follows:

	Group One	Group Two
Age:	25 -43	40 - 72
Control:	#7	#7 +1.74 D.
Number:	100	100
#16B	M = 20.0	M = 20.4
	Sigma = 7.83	Sigma = 6.78
		C.R. = 0.4 (not a significant difference)
#17B	M = 21.72	M = 22.70
	Sigma = 5.55	Sigma = 5.07
		C.R. = 1.3 (not a significant difference)

Therefore, in spite of the increased plus used in the second group for a control lens it did not have a significant effect upon altering the magnitude of either the positive or negative fusional reserve tests performed at near. Thus, the same expected values for these tests may be used without regard of the magnitude of the control lenses used.

62. Should not the expected values for the various optometric tests be modified for the age of the patient?

Our present clinical knowledge does not seem to indicate the necessity for any modification of expected values for the age of the patient. When you consider that these mean values are the upper range for non-impaired individuals we have sufficient latitude to compensate for the age factor. Haynes (Comparison of Selected Analytical Findings at Various Age Levels, Visual Training Conf., St. Louis, 1959) has published data of this type, and I have selected his duction test values for comparison and have added an additional column to present the expected values used at the present time.

	Expected Values	190 Children 5-6 yrs. age	150 Persons 8-14 yrs. age	150 Persons 25-35 yrs. age
#10 Br.	19	17.7	19.2	19.6
#10 Rec.	10	5.2	6.5	7.0
#11 Br.	9	8 5	8.8	7.8
#11 Rec.	5	2.4	4.2	3.3
#16B Br.	21	22.0	18.1	20.3
#16B Rec.	15	5.7	6.8	6.6
#17B Br.	22	20.7	23.2	22.3
#17B Rec.	18	8.7	13.6	13.1

63. What is the maximum minus projection a case may have?

The least plus that we may have in the cross-cylinder test is emmetropia, and the maximum exophoria we may use for the calculation of the lag is

15 prism diopters. Therefore, the resultant minus projection in such a case would be -2.50 D.

#14A = plano
#15A = 15 exophoria (lag 2.50)
#14A Net = -2.50 D.

64. We may have two similar visual problems with equal magnitudes of minus projection and yet won't they respond differently to lens application?

The following two cases illustrate the situation where we have equal magnitudes of minus projection and yet will respond differently to lens attack.

(A)		(B)	
#14A	+1.50	#14A	Plano
#15A	15 Exo	#15A	6 Exo

Both case (A) and (B) have -1.00 D. nets. If equal plus sphere lens application is utilized, case (A) would respond quicker to the inhibition and develop a plus nearpoint net than case (B).

INDEX

Page numbers followed by f indicate figures; t, tables.